A Clinical Approach to Ultrasound

A Clinical Approach to Ultrasound

Editor: Bradley Hayes

AMERICAN
MEDICAL PUBLISHERS
www.americanmedicalpublishers.com

AMERICAN
MEDICAL PUBLISHERS
www.americanmedicalpublishers.com

Cataloging-in-Publication Data

A clinical approach to ultrasound / edited by Bradley Hayes.
p. cm.
Includes bibliographical references and index.
ISBN 978-1-63927-834-3
1. Ultrasonic imaging. 2. Diagnostic ultrasonic imaging. 3. Ultrasonics in medicine.
4. Diagnostic imaging. I. Hayes, Bradley.
RC78.7.U4 C55 2023
616.075 43--dc23

American Medical Publishers,
41 Flatbush Avenue,
1st Floor, New York,
NY 11217, USA

ISBN 978-1-63927-834-3 (Hardback)

Contents

Preface

Ultrasound is a method of diagnostic imaging that uses high-frequency sound waves to produce images of structures within the body. This method involves the application of a thin layer of gel on the skin, which helps the transducer in transmitting ultrasound waves across the body. This device is placed directly on the skin, vagina or rectum to generate images through wave reflection. In this imaging method, sound travels through fluids and soft tissue which echoes back from denser surfaces for creating an image. Some common techniques used for ultrasound imaging are bone sonometry, abdominal ultrasound, breast ultrasound, echocardiogram, ophthalmic ultrasound, etc. Ultrasound guided biopsies are performed to collect a sample of tissue. Furthermore, it can also be used in the field of anesthesiology for guiding needle placement. This book discusses the clinical approach to ultrasound. It provides comprehensive insights into this area of diagnostic imaging. The book will serve as an invaluable resource for students and professionals.

The researches compiled throughout the book are authentic and of high quality, combining several disciplines and from very diverse regions from around the world. Drawing on the contributions of many researchers from diverse countries, the book's objective is to provide the readers with the latest achievements in the area of research. This book will surely be a source of knowledge to all interested and researching the field.

In the end, I would like to express my deep sense of gratitude to all the authors for meeting the set deadlines in completing and submitting their research chapters. I would also like to thank the publisher for the support offered to us throughout the course of the book. Finally, I extend my sincere thanks to my family for being a constant source of inspiration and encouragement.

Editor

1

Ultrasound findings in critical care patients: the "liver sign" and other abnormal abdominal air patterns

Joseph Dahine[1], Annie Giard[2], David-Olivier Chagnon[3] and André Denault[4,5*]

Abstract

In critical care patients, point of care abdominal ultrasound examination, although it has been practiced for over 30 years, is not as widespread as its cardiac or pulmonary counterparts. We report two cases in which detection of air during abdominal ultrasound allowed the early detection of life-threatening pathologies. In the first case, a patient with severe *Clostridium difficile* was found to have portal venous gas but its significance was confounded by a recent surgery. Serial ultrasonographic exams triggered a surgical intervention. In the second case, we report what we call the "liver sign" a finding in patients with pneumoperitoneum. These findings, all obtained prior to conventional abdominal imaging, had immediate clinical impact and avoided unnecessary delays and radiation. Detection of abdominal air should be part of the routine-focused ultrasonographic exam and for critically ill patients an algorithm is proposed.

Keywords: Ultrasound GI, Critical care/shock, Diagnostic imaging, Echo, Gastroenterology diagnosis

Background

In 2009, the American College of Chest Physicians (ACCP) and La Société de Réanimation de Langue Française (SRLF) proposed guidelines in critical care ultrasound [1]. Those guidelines included not only cardiac but also general critical care ultrasound. The latter included pleural, lung, vascular, and abdominal imaging. Among the technical and cognitive elements required for competence in abdominal ultrasonography, there was no mention of detecting abnormal air in specific areas despite the significant importance of this finding in critically ill patients. Figure 1 illustrates the mechanism of a typical artifact associated with a pneumoperitoneum underlying the liver. Moreover, abdominal ultrasound is a skill that has been practiced for over 30 years in the acute care setting [2, 3]. But over the years, other modalities, such as the focused assessment with sonography in trauma (FAST), have rather gained prevalence in the clinical setting. Given the recent increased availability of point of care ultrasound (POCUS), we submit that perhaps the time has come to include advanced skills as part of the toolbox with which physicians caring for critically ill patients should be familiar. To illustrate this, we report the cases of two patients where such routine use of the focused abdominal ultrasound exam led to the rapid detection of ominous findings of abnormal air patterns as the etiology of the clinical deterioration and expedited care. Written informed consent was obtained from the two patients.

Case presentation 1

A 66-year-old man presented with a 24-h history of severe nausea and abdominal pain. His medical history was remarkable for a rectal adenocarcinoma that was resected 4 months prior to presentation and had left him with a temporary ileostomy. He was otherwise healthy and took no medications. He underwent closure and reanastamosis of his ileostomy 5 days prior to his presentation. Upon arrival to the emergency department, his blood pressure (BP) was 80/40 mmHg and was tachycardic but displayed normal mentation. His examination was remarkable for diffuse abdominal pain and rebound tenderness, but no

*Correspondence: andre.denault@umontreal.ca
[4] Department of Anesthesiology and Division of Critical Care, Montreal Heart Institute, Université de Montréal, 5000 Belanger Street, Montreal, QC H1T 1C8, Canada
Full list of author information is available at the end of the article

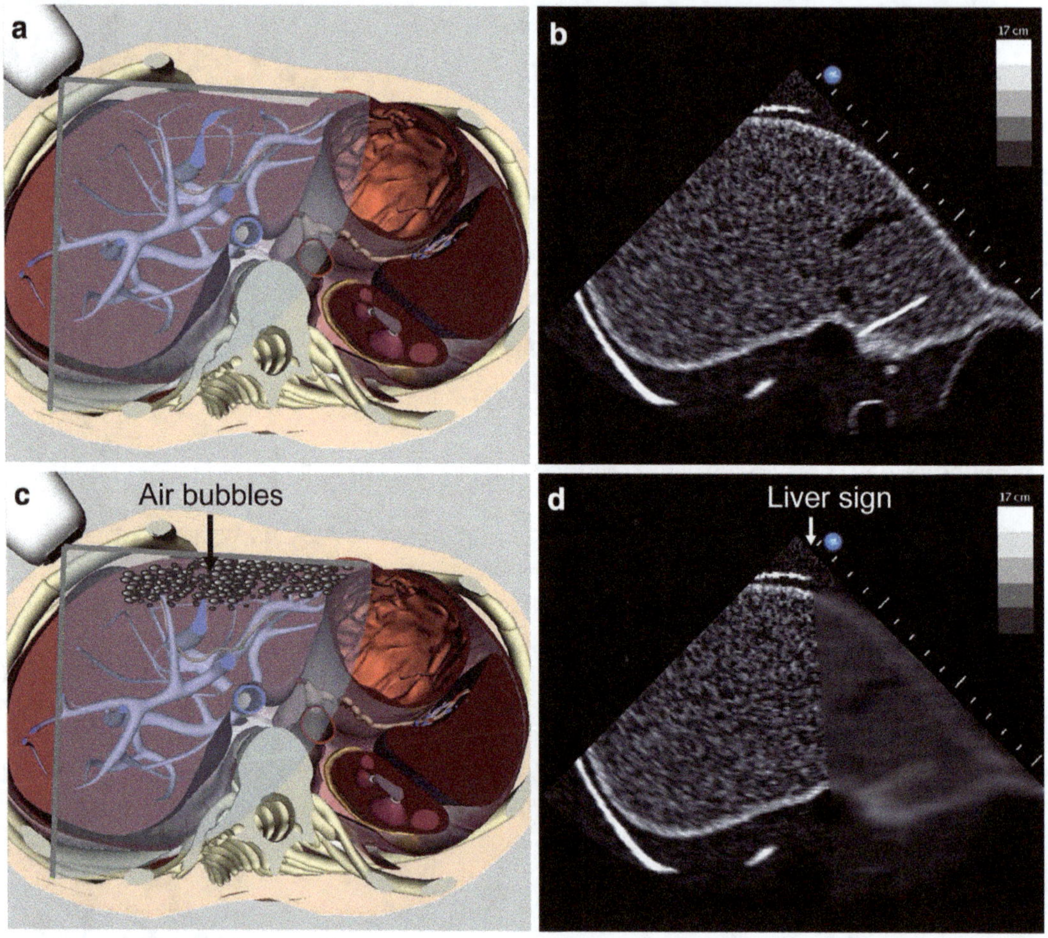

Fig. 1 Pneumoperitoneum. **a**, **b** Normal aspect of the liver using a transverse view at the anterior axillary line. **c** When air is present in the abdomen, it will typically accumulate in the non-dependant region just anterior to a portion of the liver. **d** When the ultrasound beam is positioned over this area, the normal acoustic aspect of the liver will be followed by a sharply demarcated acoustic shadow. The term "liver sign" can be used to describe this abnormal air-liver interface. Anatomical and two-dimensional plane using the Vimedix simulator with permission of CAE Healthcare, Ville St-Laurent, QC, Canada

guarding. Laboratory work revealed acute kidney injury with a creatinine of 180 mmol/L. His pre-operative baseline value was 66 mmol/L. However, his arterial lactate and white blood cell counts (WBC) were normal. The patient received initial fluid resuscitation and underwent a computed tomography scan that showed a dilated cecum (8 cm) and an edematous colon. A *Clostridium difficile* toxin assay returned positive. He was admitted to our intensive care unit (ICU) for monitoring and medical therapy with intravenous metronidazole and oral vancomycin. The patient improved from a hemodynamic, renal as well as abdominal pain point of view, but his WBC and creatinine started to increase 3 days later without new hemodynamic compromise. An abdominal ultrasound (US) was performed and revealed evidence of thumbprinting (Fig. 2a), with the thickened colon wall measured at 17 mm (normal values: <3 mm when measured with high-frequency linear array probes) [4], as well as pneumatosis intestinalis (Fig. 2b) In addition, peripherally located air speckles that follow the portal circulation were present (Fig. 3). These findings were absent on the baseline US exam we performed upon admission. An abdominal X-ray as well as a repeat computed tomography (CT) scan were obtained to confirm the findings (Fig. 2d). The scan was performed with oral but not intravenous contrast in the context of acute kidney injury. A diagnosis of failure of medical therapy was made and a discussion with the surgical team led to a tentative colectomy-saving procedure, namely a redo-ileostomy in order to irrigate vancomycin locally. The patient improved within the next 48 h and was discharged from our ICU.

Case presentation 2

The ICU team was called for immediate assessment of a 61-year-old woman who was hospitalized on the surgical ward with a complaint of desaturation and acute

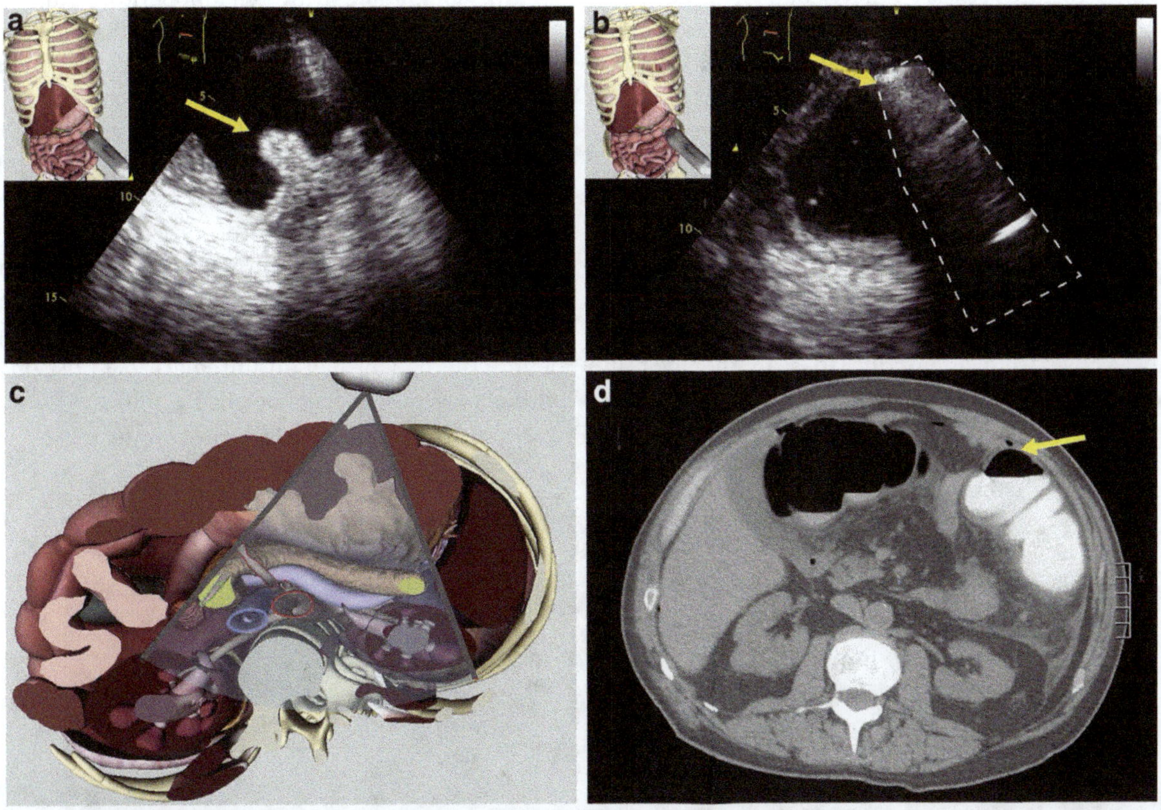

Fig. 2 **a** Left upper abdominal transverse view showing an edematous large bowel typical of a «thumb-printing» aspect. The *yellow arrow* denotes the affected area of edematous bowel wall. **b** Air artifact originating from the bowel wall can be seen. The *yellow arrow* shows an echogenic foci in the bowel wall causing shadowing. **c** Corresponding anatomical plane using the Vimedix simulator (CAE Healthcare, Ville St-Laurent, QC, Canada). **d** Computed tomography showing air within the large bowel wall (*yellow arrows*). (See Additional file 1: Video #S1a and Additional file 2: Video #S1b)

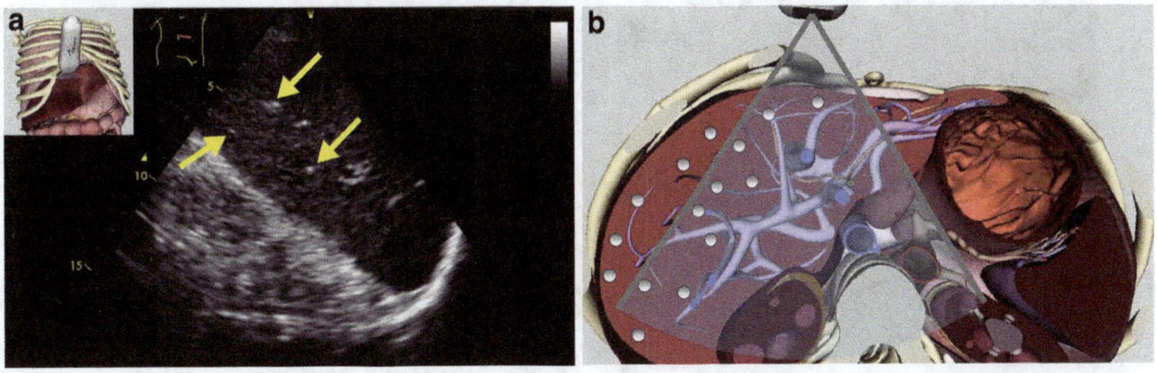

Fig. 3 **a** Right paramedian transverse scan of the liver. Numerous small, round, hyperechoic, punctuate air artifact are seen in the periphery of the liver tissue. **b** Corresponding anatomical plane using the Vimedix simulator (CAE Healthcare, Ville St-Laurent, QC, Canada). (See Additional file 3: Video #S2)

abdominal pain following dilation of a known anal stenosis which occurred 5 days prior. She was otherwise known for multiple abdominal surgeries in the past, ischemic cardiomyopathy with a 45 % ejection fraction, dyslipidemia and history of drug abuse. At the time, she was known to be taking pregabalin, hydromorphone, acetaminophen, aspirin, atorvastatin, and prophylactic subcutaneous heparin. Upon initial assessment, she was afebrile, tachypneic, and normotensive. Her heart rate was 110/min, BP normal but her oxygen saturation was 85 % on 50 % inspired oxygen. Initial examination was aimed at ruling out an acute coronary syndrome with subsequent congestive heart failure, but an electrocardiogram was normal and a focused transthoracic echocardiography (TTE) did not reveal new wall motion abnormalities or a worsening in the cardiac function. As part of our routine ultrasound examination, we looked at the inferior vena cava (IVC) [5, 6] and portal vein in order to determine her fluid status [7–9]. In order to do this, we usually proceed with our probe in the longitudinal axis, starting midline and anteriorly in the abdomen and moving laterally towards the posterior-axillar line. Surprisingly, we discovered an air artifact that obstructed our view as we were attempting to scan the liver in this motion (Fig. 4a). This was unexpected, as this is a finding compatible with pneumoperitoneum, which is not expected as a complication of anal dilation, given that the rectum is a retroperitoneal structure. We hence performed an upright abdominal film that confirmed free air under the diaphragm as well as a CT scan without contrast (Fig. 4b) to document the findings. This information guided our surgeons who took the patient back to the operating room (OR). The findings intraoperatively were that of fecal peritonitis secondary to an anterior faux-conduit that was created iatrogenically by the initial anal dilation attempt and communicated with the peritoneum. The patient had an unremarkable post-op course and was discharged from our ICU.

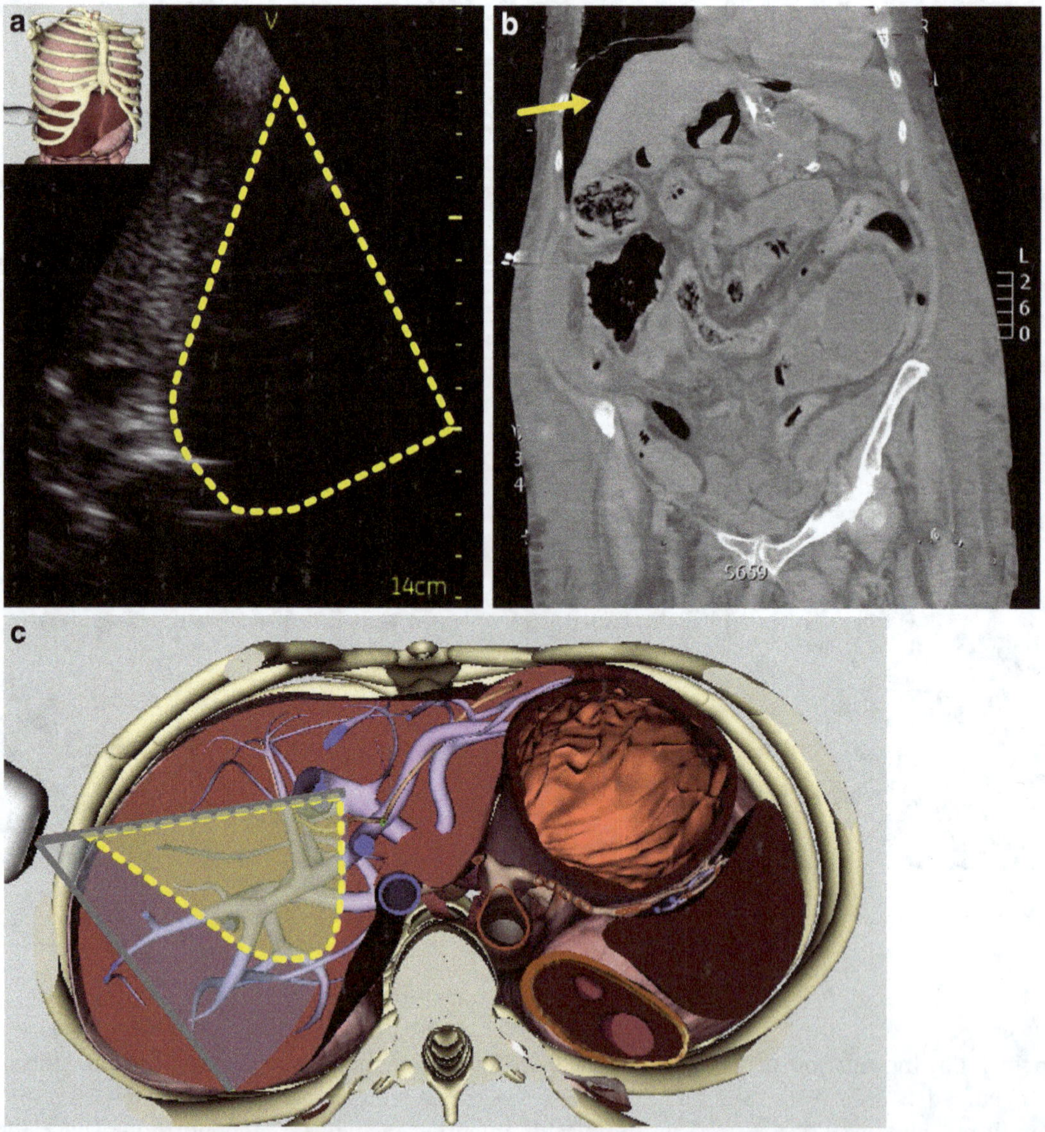

Fig. 4 **a** Mid-axillary transhepatic transverse view of the liver in a patient with acute pneumoperitoneum. Note the acoustic shadowing in the *right-sided portion* of the liver which corresponds to the most anterior part of the liver where air will accumulate. **b** Confirmation was obtained with computed tomography. **c** Corresponding anatomical plane using the Vimedix simulator (CAE Healthcare, Ville St-Laurent, QC, Canada). (See Additional file 4: Video #S3)

Conclusions

In the above cases, we used the ultrasound to observe three abnormal air patterns that should alert the clinician to an intra-abdominal pathology, namely intraperitoneal air (case#2), portal venous gas (case#1), and intramural air (case#1).

Intraperitoneal air can be seen using the liver as an acoustic window. Indeed, the liver offers a unique echogenic window. Although the hepatic flexure of the colon can sometimes be found interposed, there is generally no bowel that creates artifact in the right upper quadrant. Free air will accumulate anteriorly in the supine position and create an air artifact interfering with the normal liver texture (Fig. 1). It is of importance not to press deeply with the ultrasound probe as this can shift small amount of free air away from the US field. This phenomenon of air interposition should be considered abnormal and is similar to the "lung point" shadow that occurs in a pneumothorax where ultrasound reveals loss of normal lung sliding [10]. We propose the term "liver sign" to describe this longitudinal band air artifact that interrupts normal scanning of the liver from the anterior abdominal midline to the posterior axillary in the longitudinal axis.

Traditionally, other studies have described the main ultrasonographic finding of free intraperitoneal air as peritoneal stripe enhancement with associated reverberation artifacts [11, 12] and recommended the use of a linear probe to improve detection [13] similarly to what is recommended in lung ultrasound. Other indirect signs have also been described. Examples include thickened bowel loops (such as in our first case), air bubbles in ascitic fluid and thickening of bowel or gallbladder wall associated with ileus [13]. Another sign is the scissor maneuver, described by Karahan et al. which entails repeatedly applying pressure with the linear ultrasound probe sagitally oriented in the right paramedian epigastric area and looking for a shift in the reverberation (i.e., presence upon releasing probe pressure; disappearance upon increased pressure using the caudal part of the probe) [14].

However, our cases highlight two important points that contrast with the existing literature. First, we did not document a peritoneal stripe enhancement, but the reverberation artifacts were present. Second, the phased array probe was used rather than the typical abdominal convex or linear probe. Several handheld echo devices do not have an abdominal probe. Rather, the phased array probe has become more prominently used as it allows reliable examination of the cardiac structures, which remains at the core of the assessment of the unstable patient. In addition, abdominal, renal, and cranial settings are commonly available when using the cardiac-phased array probe.

Caution has to be exercised in the interpretation of this finding as free air usually resolves rapidly post-laparotomy or laparoscopy but can rarely persist for weeks [15]. In *C. difficile* colitis, such as in our first case, complications such as worsening bowel wall edema, bowel distention and pneumatosis intestinalis can help guide the clinician towards surgical therapy prior to an obvious macrohemodynamic deterioration which would occur after perforation. Furthermore, artifacts that can mimick pneumoperitoneum have been described such as pseudo-pneumatosis intestinalis and pseudo-thickened gut [16]. Interested readers are encouraged to explore this topic further as it is beyond the scope of this article.

Portal air or hepatic portal venous gas can result from mesenteric ischemia or other conditions associated with alteration of the intestinal mucosa [17]. Using sonography, air in the portal vein can be seen as flowing echogenic bubbles mostly in the periphery. In contrast, air in the biliary tree or pneumobilia is commonly seen following biliary instrumentation when the sphincter of Oddi becomes incompetent. It can occur in patients with acute cholecystitis. With ultrasound, reflective linear echoes will be seen. However, they are less mobile, more centrally located, they change with position, are associated with several comet tail artifacts and are not associated with venous flow [18].

Several technical limitations preclude complete visualization of the gastrointestinal tract. Ultrasound itself is operator-dependent. In a small study of 31 patients in the emergency room with abdominal pain in which five patients were found to have pneumoperitoneum by both CT imaging and abdominal X-ray, the sensitivity and specificity of a hand-carried ultrasound were 80 and 81 %, respectively [19]. Hence, clinical suspicion of abdominal pathology without supporting evidence on US should always lead to further imaging by CT scan.

However, a recent study showed that senior physicians with experience in abdominal US can rapidly learn to identify patterns suggestive of pneumoperitoneum with almost 90 % accuracy [20]. The study also indicated that a focused abdominal US exam comprising two views (epigastric and right hypochondrium) was similar

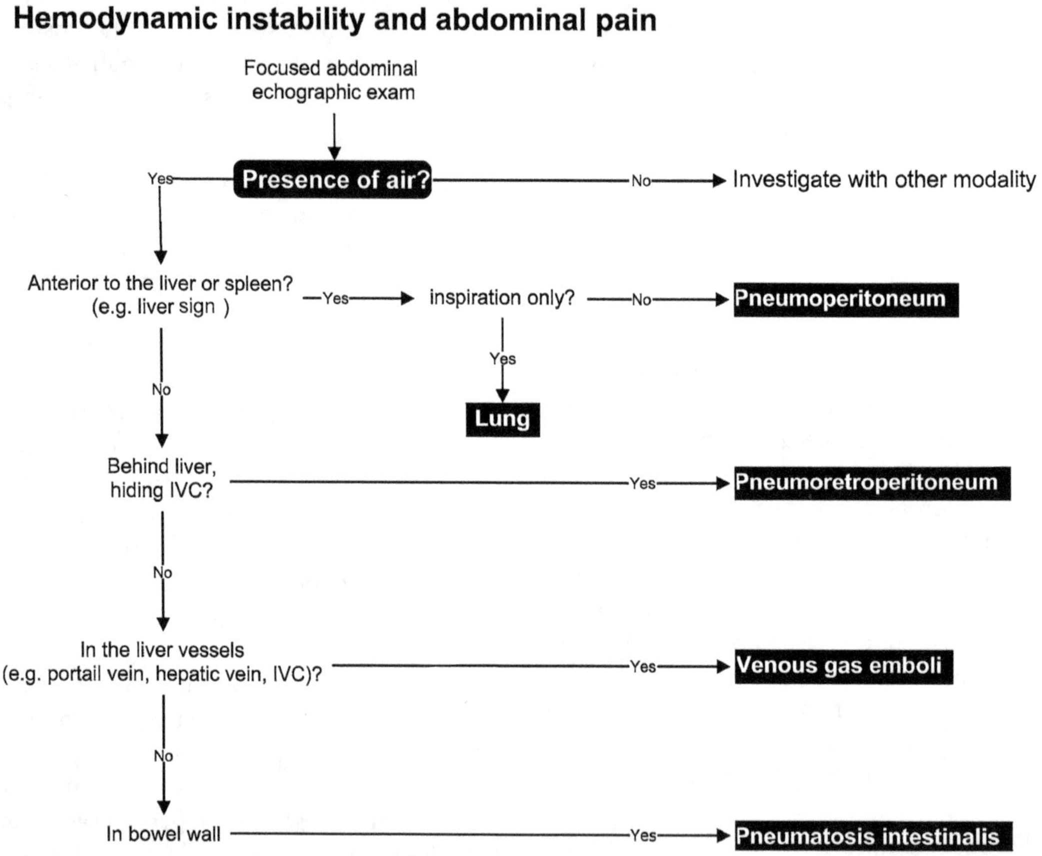

Fig. 5 Proposed approach using bedside ultrasound for patients with abdominal pain and hemodynamic instability. If air is present anterior to the liver or spleen (in the absence of a recent abdominal surgery) during both inspiration and expiration, a pneumoperitoneum should be suspected. A pneumoretroperitoneum will be associated with air behind the liver hiding the inferior vena cava (IVC). Venous gas embolism will be associated with air in the liver typically in the portal vein mostly in the peripheral regions of the liver. Air embolism can also be seen in the hepatic vein and the IVC. Finally pneumatosis intestinalis is characterized by air in the bowel lumen

in sensitivity and specificity to the full abdominal exam. We believe that this further supports the importance of encouraging exposure to abdominal US in the ICU and to ensure clinicians are trained to not only identify abnormal patterns, but first and foremost to acquire images at the bedside autonomously.

The two cases we report offer additional insight into the usefulness of adding a focused abdominal exam to the already well-established focused TTE as proposed by the ACCP, SRLF, and other organizations [1, 21, 22]. Critical impending complications will be suspected when air is present in specific locations such as the peritoneum, the retroperitoneum, the lumen of preformed organs or vessels (such as the bladder or the portal vein), the parenchyma of organs (such as liver or kidney), and the abdominal wall [12]. Figure 5 summarizes an approach for the identification of normal and abnormal abdominal air.

Consent

Written informed consent was obtained from the patient for publication of this case report and any accompanying images.

Additional files

Additional file 1: Video S1a. Pneumatosis–patient view.

Additional file 2: Video S1b. Pneumatosis–simulator view.

Additional file 3: Video S2. Air in the portal circulation.

Additional file 4: Video S3. The liver sign.

Abbreviations

ACCP: American College of Chest Physician; BP: blood pressure; CT: computed tomography; FAST: focused assessment with sonography in trauma; ICU: intensive care unit; IVC: inferior vena cava; OR: operating room; POCUS: point of care ultrasound; SRLF: La Société de Réanimation de Langue Française; TTE: transthoracic echocardiography; US: ultrasound; WBC: white blood cell counts.

Authors' contributions
JD and AD acquired the ultrasound images, drafted the manuscript and drafted the algorithm. AG and DOC made substantial contributions to the manuscript. All authors read and approved the final manuscript.

Author details
[1] Department of Intensive Care, Université de Montréal, Montreal, QC, Canada. [2] Department of Emergency Medicine, Hôpital Sacré-Coeur de Montréal, Montreal, QC, Canada. [3] Department of Radiology, Centre Hospitalier de l'Université de Montréal, Montreal, QC, Canada. [4] Department of Anesthesiology and Division of Critical Care, Montreal Heart Institute, Université de Montréal, 5000 Belanger Street, Montreal, QC H1T 1C8, Canada. [5] Division of Critical Care, Centre Hospitalier de l'Université de Montréal, Montreal, QC, Canada.

References

1. Mayo PH, Beaulieu Y, Doelken P, Feller-Kopman D, Harrod C, Kaplan A, Oropello J, Vieillard-Baron A, Axler O, Lichtenstein D, Maury E, Slama M, Vignon P (2009) American College of Chest Physicians/La Société de Réanimation de Langue Française statement on competence in critical care ultrasonography. Chest 135:1050–1060
2. Seitz K, Reising KD (1982) Ultrasound detection of free air in the abdominal cavity. Ultraschall Med 3:4–6 **German**
3. Moriwaki Y, Sugiyama M, Toyoda H, Kosuge T, Arata S, Iwashita M, Tahara Y, Suzuki N (2009) Ultrasonography for the diagnosis of intraperitoneal free air in chest-abdominal-pelvic blunt trauma and critical acute abdominal pain. Arch Surg 144:137–141
4. Strobel D, Goertz RS, Bernatik T (2011) Diagnostics in inflammatory bowel disease: ultrasound. World J Gastroenterol 17:3192–3197
5. Denault AY, Vegas A, Royse C (2014) A bedside clinical and ultrasound-based approaches to the management of hemodynamic instability. Part I focus on the clinical approach: continuing professional development. Can J Anesth 61:843–864
6. Vegas A, Denault AY, Royse C (2014) A bedside clinical and ultrasound-based approach to hemodynamic instability. Part II bedside ultrasound in hemodynamic shock: continuing professional development. Can J Anesth 61:1008–1027
7. Scheinfeld MH, Bilali A, Koenigsberg M (2009) Understanding the spectral Doppler waveform of the hepatic veins in health and disease. Radiographics 29:2081–2098
8. Toupin F, Denault A, Lamarche Y, Deschamps A (2013) Hemodynamic instability and fluid responsiveness. Can J Anesth 60:1240–1247
9. McNaughton DA, Abu-Yousef MM (2011) Doppler US of the liver made simple. Radiographics 31:161–188
10. Moore CL, Copel JA (2011) Point-of-care ultrasonography. N Engl J Med 364:749–757
11. Chen SC, Wang HP, Chen WJ, Lin FY, Hsu CY, Chang KJ, Chen WJ (2002) Selective use of ultrasonography for the detection of pneumoperitoneum. Acad Emerg Med 9:643–645
12. Hoffmann B, Nurnberg D, Westergaard MC (2012) Focus on abnormal air: diagnostic ultrasonography for the acute abdomen. Eur J Emerg Med 19:284–291
13. Coppolino F, Gatta G, Di Grezia G, Reginelli A, Iacobellis F, Vallone G, Giganti M, Genovese E (2013) Gastrointestinal perforation: ultrasonographic diagnosis. Crit Ultrasound J 5(Suppl 1):S4
14. Karahan OI, Kurt A, Yikilmaz A, Kahriman G (2004) New method for the detection of intraperitoneal free air by sonography: scissors maneuver. J Clin Ultrasound 32:381–385
15. Smith KS, Wilson TC, Luces L, Stevenson AA, Hajhosseini B, Siram SM (2013) Pneumoperitoneum 48 days after laparoscopic hysterectomy. JSLS 17:661–664
16. Wilson SR, Burns PN, Wilkinson LM, Simpson DH, Muradali D (1999) Gas at abdominal US: appearance, relevance, and analysis of artifacts. Radiology 210:113–123
17. Liebman PR, Patten MT, Manny J, Benfield JR, Hechtman HB (1978) Hepatic-portal venous gas in adults: etiology, pathophysiology and clinical significance. Ann Surg 187:281–287
18. Huang J, Stone MB (2010) Ultrasound identification of traumatic pneumobilia. Am J Emerg Med 28(255):e5–e6
19. Schleder S, Jung EM, Heiss P, Stroszczynski C, Schreyer AG (2014) Hand carried and high end ultrasound systems are equally inferior to abdominal radiography and multidetector computed tomography in the diagnosis of pneumoperitoneum. Rofo 186:219–224
20. Nazerian P, Tozzetti C, Vanni S, Bartolucci M, Gualtieri S, Trausi F, Vittorini M, Catini E, Cibinel GA, Grifoni S (2015) Accuracy of abdominal ultrasound for the diagnosis of pneumoperitoneum in patients with acute abdominal pain: a pilot study. Crit Ultrasound J 7:15
21. Via G, Hussain A, Wells M, Reardon R, ElBarbary M, Noble VE, Tsung JW, Neskovic AN, Price S, Oren-Grinberg A, Liteplo A, Cordioli R, Naqvi N, Rola P, Poelaert J, Gulic TG, Sloth E, Labovitz A, Kimura B, Breitkreutz R, Masani N, Bowra J, Talmor D, Guarracino F, Goudie A, Xiaoting W, Chawla R, Galderisi M, Blaivas M, Petrovic T et al (2014) International evidence-based recommendations for focused cardiac ultrasound. J Am Soc Echocardiogr 27:683.e1–683.e33
22. Arntfield R, Millington S, Ainsworth C, Arora R, Boyd J, Finlayson G, Gallagher W, Gebhardt C, Goffi A, Hockman E, Kirkpatrick A, McDermid R, Waechter J, Wong N, Zavalkoff S, Beaulieu Y (2014) Canadian recommendations for critical care ultrasound training and competency. Can Respir J 21:341–345

2

Pediatric emergency medicine point-of-care ultrasound: summary of the evidence

Jennifer R. Marin[1*], Alyssa M. Abo[2], Alexander C. Arroyo[3], Stephanie J. Doniger[4], Jason W. Fischer[5], Rachel Rempell[6], Brandi Gary[7], James F. Holmes[8], David O. Kessler[9], Samuel H. F. Lam[10], Marla C. Levine[11], Jason A. Levy[6], Alice Murray[12], Lorraine Ng[9], Vicki E. Noble[13], Daniela Ramirez-Schrempp[14], David C. Riley[15], Turandot Saul[16], Vaishali Shah[17], Adam B. Sivitz[18], Ee Tein Tay[19], David Teng[20], Lindsey Chaudoin[9], James W. Tsung[19], Rebecca L. Vieira[6], Yaffa M. Vitberg[21] and Resa E. Lewiss[22]

Abstract

The utility of point-of-care ultrasound is well supported by the medical literature. Consequently, pediatric emergency medicine providers have embraced this technology in everyday practice. Recently, the American Academy of Pediatrics published a policy statement endorsing the use of point-of-care ultrasound by pediatric emergency medicine providers. To date, there is no standard guideline for the practice of point-of-care ultrasound for this specialty. This document serves as an initial step in the detailed "how to" and description of individual point-of-care ultrasound examinations. Pediatric emergency medicine providers should refer to this paper as reference for published research, objectives for learners, and standardized reporting guidelines.

Keywords: Pediatric emergency medicine, Point-of-care ultrasound, Diagnostic, Procedures

In the last 20 years "clinician-performed" or "point-of-care" ultrasound has expanded from a screening test in trauma to being used by almost every medical specialty for diagnosis, monitoring or procedural guidance [1]. Much of this revolution was initiated in tertiary care centers; but with increasing pressure for expedited diagnosis and efficient use of manpower resources throughout healthcare, point-of-care ultrasonography (POCUS) has been adopted across the entire spectrum of clinical settings from outpatient clinics to critical care units. With its affordability, limited infrastructural, maintenance, and resource requirements, ultrasonography has an especially important role in environments where diagnostic imaging resources are limited. In such settings, ultrasound provides information that has a significant impact on patient outcomes and can change the way medicine is practiced [2, 3].

Pediatric emergency POCUS has been part of this movement, with published scanning protocols describing its use in the evaluation of trauma, abdominal pain [4, 5], dyspnea [6], and musculoskeletal complaints [7, 8], among others. This is much the same range of complaints that are the focus of adult emergency and critical care ultrasound. Indeed, it could be argued that the rationale for the use of clinician-performed ultrasonography is even more compelling in the care of children since the goal of minimal exposure to ionizing radiation is most important in this age group [9]. However, in contrast to adult emergency [10] and critical care medicine [11], there is currently no standard for the practice of pediatric emergency POCUS.

The following document is an initiation of this process. It is our hope that it will serve to define the field, establish standards of practice, delineate training requirements, and point to needed areas of scientific investigation. If

*Correspondence: jrmmarin@yahoo.com
[1] Children's Hospital of Pittsburgh, 4401 Penn Ave, AOB Suite 2400, Pittsburgh, PA 15224, USA
Full list of author information is available at the end of the article

adult emergency and critical care ultrasound are any guide, it is likely that an effect of this process will be the recognition of clinician-performed ultrasonography as a core competency of pediatric emergency care that requires a place in training programs at both post-graduate and undergraduate levels [12].

To develop this document, we assembled a group of thought leaders and content experts to review the scientific literature and use it to formulate evidence-based statements about emergency POCUS. For this initial effort, we assembled members of a pediatric emergency POCUS work group, which wrote the recently published POCUS guidelines for pediatric emergency physicians [13, 14]. With collaboration from additional content experts in the field, who had either completed an ultrasound fellowship or specialty training in pediatric emergency POCUS, we sought to create a comprehensive document summarizing the current evidence. For each application, the evidence is reviewed with respect to indications, current knowledge (or lack of it), curriculum objectives for learners, and identified pitfalls. We also developed standardized reporting guidelines for each ultrasound indication. The reporting guidelines are intended as templates that sonologists may choose to use as a method of extracting and documenting appropriate information about ultrasound exams for reporting, quality assurance, and if desired, research. They are not intended as stepwise instructions on how to complete exams. Each section was written by members of the core group of content experts and then edited by the lead authors (JRM, REL), and by Anthony J. Dean, MD, *Critical Ultrasound Journal* supervising editor for this piece.

Given the exponential growth of POCUS and descriptions of new exams, techniques, and indications, this document should not be viewed as a comprehensive summary of POCUS. Further, while we realize there is overlap between emergency medicine and other disciplines, such as critical care medicine, the purviews are different and the focus of this document is the pediatric emergency medicine provider. We recognize that a methodological limitation of this document is the absence of global representation among its authors, as well as a validated consensus process. Moreover, we acknowledge that many leaders in the field of POCUS, and particularly pediatric emergency POCUS are not included in our author group. Since this is the first step in an iterative process, we strongly hope that future versions of this document will draw more extensively on the expertise of pediatric emergency physicians worldwide. We hope that this document will provide a framework for both ongoing practice and serve as a springboard for continuing efforts in training and research.

Diagnostic applications of ultrasound

Ultrasound evaluation of the appendix

Evidence

1. Summary/brief explanation of indication
   - POCUS has proven to be a valuable imaging examination in the evaluation of right lower quadrant abdominal pain to assess for findings of appendicitis.

2. Relevant adult-specific literature
   - In a meta-analysis on the use of radiology ultrasound versus computed tomography (CT) for acute appendicitis, it was determined that CT had superior sensitivity (94 vs. 83 %) with similar specificity (93 vs. 94 %) [15].
   - The American college of radiology (ACR) recommends CT over ultrasound in the routine evaluation of adults with suspected appendicitis [16].
   - There have been several studies where emergency medicine physicians used POCUS to evaluate acute appendicitis. In 2000, Chen et al. examined 147 patients and reported a sensitivity of 96 % and specificity of 68 % with an accuracy of 89 %. This was significantly more favorable than the surgeon's clinical accuracy of 71 % ($p < 0.005$) [17]. Fox et al., in 2008, using primarily emergency medicine residents for the POCUS evaluation, enrolled 132 patients and found a sensitivity of 65 % and a specificity of 90 % [18]. While the sensitivity was too low to recommend POCUS as a screening test for appendicitis, the specificity, similar to that reported in the radiology literature, suggested that a positive study could preclude further CT imaging. Similar results were reported by Mallin [19].
3. Relevant pediatric-specific literature
   - In the radiology literature, sensitivity of ultrasound examination in pediatric patients ranges between 50–100 %, and specificity between 88–99 % [15, 20]. In a large multicentered study, ultrasound sensitivity matched that of CT when the patient had symptoms for greater than 48 h [21].
   - In 2010, the ACR reaffirmed that ultrasonography should be the first-line imaging study in children under 14 years and in pregnant women [16].
   - In a subanalysis of the study by Fox et al., the authors reported the sensitivity and specificity for the 2–17 year population ($n = 42$) to be 74 and 85 %, respectively [18].
   - Out of concern for the radiation risks associated with (CT) [22, 23] several authors have proposed staged imaging strategies with ultrasound as the

initial imaging study, followed by CT in equivocal or non-visualized studies [24–26]. This "sono-first" approach was found to be cost effective [27].

- Two recent studies have evaluated PEM physician conducting POCUS for appendicitis. Sivitz et al. [28], with 264 POCUS studies by PEM fellows and attendings, found a sensitivity of 85 % (95 % CI 75–95), specificity of 93 % (85–100), positive likelihood ratio of 11.7 (6.9–20), and negative likelihood ratio of 0.17 (0.1–0.28). Elikashvili et al. [29], looking at 150 patients also demonstrated the specificity of PEM-performed POCUS to be 94 % (95 % CI 88–97), indicating that a positive POCUS exam can be acceptable as a rule-in study. They also demonstrated a significantly decreased length of stay for patients with disposition by POCUS compared to radiology (154–288 min) without any cases of missed appendicitis.
- To address the limited availability of radiologic ultrasonography at one institution, one study evaluated use of teleultrasonography to diagnose appendicitis in children. Accuracy of emergency medicine resident-performed POCUS interpreted in real time by a remote expert was high and similar (sensitivity 100 %, specificity 98 %, positive predictive value 95 %, negative predictive value 100 %) to that of onsite expert-performed ultrasonography [30].

4. Outstanding questions to be answered/voids in the literature to date
   - While the minimum appendiceal measurement for acute appendicitis is generally stated at 6 mm, in a study of healthy patients without any abdominal complaints, 23 % of subjects had an appendiceal diameter greater than 6 mm, and 9 % were greater than 7 mm [31]. Therefore, a measurement greater than 6 mm does not necessarily indicate acute appendicitis. Some have suggested using a diameter cutoff at 7 mm to avoid false-positive diagnosis [32].
   - As can be seen from the previous discussion, published data on accuracy of POCUS for appendicitis are somewhat limited and inconsistent in their findings. There are no studies to our knowledge regarding the training that is needed to achieve competence in this application of POCUS.

Curriculum objectives

1. Describe the *indications* for POCUS evaluation of the appendix
   - The indication for performing a right lower quadrant ultrasound is in a patient who presents with a history or examination concerning for acute appendicitis.
2. Describe the *limitations* of the POCUS evaluation of the appendix
   - The primary limitation of sonography for appendicitis is the lack of consistent visualization of the normal appendix. Published visualization rates have ranged from 22 to 98 % [20].
   - While increased body habitus has often been cited as a limitation for ultrasound, Sulowski et al. demonstrated that compared to normal weight children, there were no statistically significant differences in outcomes or CT utilization for obese children undergoing evaluation for acute appendicitis [33].
   - Measurement of the appendiceal diameter alone may not be sufficient to diagnose appendicitis. The presence or absence of other variables such as appendiceal wall thickness, the presence of an appendicolith, free fluid, or periappendiceal inflammatory changes may also help to identify positive or negative cases [32, 34].
   - It can be difficult to visualize a perforated appendix due to the inability to perform a graded compression exam on a patient with peritonitis. The presence and constellation of secondary findings such as complex fluid collections, dilated bowel and RLQ echogenic fat may help distinguish perforated appendicitis from uncomplicated appendicitis [35, 36].
3. Describe the *relevant anatomy* to be identified in the POCUS evaluation of the appendix
   - Structures in the right lower quadrant that aid in identification of the appendix include the psoas muscle, iliac artery and vein, terminal ileum, cecum and ascending colon. The relationship between the psoas muscle and iliac vessels remains constant, as does the ascending colon being the most lateral right-sided intra-abdominal structure. However, the cecum's position is not consistent in every patient, and may reside in the (normal) cecal fossa, or in a more cephalad, medial, or pelvic location. This can make finding the appendix difficult, as its origin off the medial portion of the cecum 1–2 cm from the ileocecal valve may be equally hard to find. In addition, finding the appendix with a normally positioned cecum may be compromised by a retro-cecal position.
   - Performing the examination requires a graded compression technique, where gentle downward pressure is applied with the ultrasound transducer. This helps to visualize the non-compressible appendix by localizing the source of pain, as well as compressing away small bowel and displacing artifacts caused by bowel gas [37].

- The normal appendix is a blind ending, aperistaltic, tubular structure arising from the medial cecum, and measuring less than 6 mm in diameter. In the transverse orientation, it takes on a target-shaped appearance. A normal appendix appears round to ovoid and compressible [38]. When ovoid, the diameter should be measured along the narrow part of the oval in order not to overestimate the diameter. Measurements are taken from outer wall to outer wall.
- In acute appendicitis, the appendix will assume a rounded shape, and the diameter should be greater than 6 mm. Increasing wall thickness makes acute appendicitis increasingly likely and 1.7 mm (measured from hyperechoic mucosa to hyperechoic serosa) is used by some authors as a cutoff value [32].
- There may also be secondary signs of inflammation such as periappendiceal inflammation, free fluid, appendicolith, or hyperemia of the appendiceal wall [17].
- The sonographic appearance of the submucosal layer, ranging from sharply delineated to hazy to absent in advanced disease, has been suggested as a tool to grade acute appendicitis [39].
- In perforated appendicitis, a phlegmon or abscess may be seen, while the appendix may appear decompressed or may not be visualized [35, 36].

4. Recognize specific *pitfalls* involved with POCUS evaluation of the appendix
   - Misidentifying normal small bowel or folds of the bowel wall for an appendix.
   - Visualization of only the normal portion of a diseased appendix, where inflammation is isolated to the tip (false negative).
   - Misdiagnosing a normal appendix as inflamed secondary to other intra-abdominal processes, such as Crohn's disease or pelvic inflammatory disease (false positive).
   - Misdiagnosing acute appendicitis based on a diameter greater than 6 mm in an ovoid appearing compressible appendix and/or without any secondary signs of inflammation.

Reporting Guideline for Ultrasound Evaluation of the Appendix

Patient Demographics:

Patient Name:
Patient Gender: ☐Male ☐Female

DOB: _/_/__
MR#:
Date & Time: _/_/__ _:_

Examination Demographics:

☐Initial Exam
☐Repeat Exam

Operator Name(s): ________

Operator Training: ☐Attending ☐Fellow ☐Resident ☐Medical Student ☐Other: ________

☐Patient consents to these images being used for educational purposes
☐Patient consents to these images being used for research purposes

Indication(s) for exam:

☐Abdominal pain/tenderness ☐ Focal right lower quadrant tenderness ☐Peritonitis
☐Educational ☐ Other: ____________

Views:

Appendix-				
	Short axis:	☐Adequate	☐Limited	☐Not obtained
	Long axis:	☐Adequate	☐Limited	☐Not obtained
	Blind end:	☐Adequate	☐Limited	☐Not obtained

Findings:

Appendix	☐Visualized	☐ Not Visualized	
AP Diameter > 6mm	☐Absent	☐Present	☐Indeterminate
Appendix Compressibility	☐Absent	☐Present	☐Indeterminate
Peristalsis	☐Absent	☐Present	☐Indeterminate
Sonographic McBurney's	☐Absent	☐Present	☐Indeterminate
Appendicolith	☐Absent	☐Present	☐Indeterminate
Periappendiceal inflammation	☐Absent	☐Present	☐Indeterminate
Free fluid	☐Absent	☐Present	☐Indeterminate
Peritoneal Abscess	☐Absent	☐Present	☐Indeterminate

Interpretation:

☐Normal exam ☐Appendicitis ☐Perforated Appendicitis ☐Indeterminate

Quality assurance:

Image Quality: ☐Adequate ☐Inadequate

Accuracy of interpretation: ☐Agree ☐Disagree ☐Unable to assess

Accuracy of interpretation as compared to a gold standard: ☐Not performed ☐TP ☐TN ☐FP ☐FN

Comments:

Ultrasound evaluation of the biliary tract

Evidence

1. Summary/brief explanation of *indications*
   - The use of POCUS for hepatobiliary disease centers on identifying the presence of gallstones. A secondary goal is identification of evidence of biliary inflammation and/or biliary obstruction. Although still considered a rare disease in the pediatric population, rates have been on the rise over several decades [40]. This is thought to be due to increasing rates of obesity and better availability of diagnostic imaging [41, 42].
   - Pediatric patients may present with atypical or intermittent symptoms, making misdiagnosis or delay in diagnosis common.
2. Relevant adult-specific literature
   - Research in adult populations has shown that emergency medicine physicians can accurately perform and interpret gallbladder POCUS [43, 44].
   - POCUS evaluation of the gall bladder can decrease emergency department length of stay, especially during times when department of radiology studies is not available (e.g., evening and nighttime hours) [45–47].
   - Clinician sonologists who had performed over 25 biliary POCUS exams showed excellent agreement in image interpretation as compared with experienced sonologists [48].
   - Patients are overwhelmingly satisfied with POCUS performed in the emergency department. A high percentage of patients would rather stay in the ED to have a POCUS performed than being transported to the radiology suite for the exam [49].
3. Relevant pediatric-specific literature
   - In a recent case series of 13 pediatric patients with cholecystitis or biliary tract disease, no patient had the classic presentation of fever, elevated leukocyte count and an acute abdomen. POCUS may help avoid missing this important disease entity [50].
4. Outstanding questions to be answered/voids in the literature to date
   - There are limited published data on the use of POCUS in the assessment of the biliary system of the pediatric patient.
   - It is unclear how much training is required to develop competence in performing ultrasonography for acute cholecystitis in the pediatric population. In one study of adult patients, EM residents' accuracy was similar to that of an experienced member of faculty [44]. In another study involving adult patients, performance of up to 50 emergency ultrasound examinations appeared to have little effect on the accuracy of right upper quadrant ultrasound [51]. In a third study as noted previously, sonologists who had performed over 25 ultrasounds showed excellent agreement in image interpretation as compared with experienced sonographers, with increasing accuracy correlating with increasing experience in those with less than 25 examinations [48]. Rather than simply requiring an arbitrary number of examinations, another method of competency assessment may be necessary [51].

Curriculum objectives

1. Describe the *indications* for biliary tract POCUS
   - The primary indications for biliary tract POCUS are the identification of cholelithiasis and acute cholecystitis.
   - Clinical indications for performing gallbladder ultrasound are symptoms, signs, or laboratory abnormalities that prompt concern for biliary tract disease. These include but are not limited to the following: patients presenting with upper abdominal pain or tenderness, nausea, vomiting fever, jaundice.
2. Describe the *limitations* of biliary tract POCUS
   - Since it is a focused exam, POCUS is not intended to identify all abnormalities and pathologies of the right upper quadrant. POCUS should be interpreted in the context of the clinical picture and if the findings are non-diagnostic, further imaging studies may be warranted.
   - Pathology of structures surrounding the gall bladder, such as the liver, pancreas or portal system, may not be identified by a focused exam.
   - Biliary POCUS may be technically limited by overlying bowel gas, adipose tissue and patient discomfort.
3. Describe the *relevant anatomy* to be identified with biliary tract POCUS
   - The gallbladder usually lies posterior to the inferior margin of the liver in the mid-clavicular line. In some patients, the fundus may extend several centimeters below the costal margin; in others, the gallbladder may be high in the porta hepatis surrounded by liver parenchyma.
   - The gallbladder should be evaluated with the highest frequency range that provides adequate depth and penetration using an abdominal transducer. Images may be obtained subcostally or by looking through the rib spaces more superiorly.

- If these maneuvers do not provide adequate images, it may be helpful to place the patient in a left lateral decubitus position.
- When imaging the gallbladder with the transducer placed below the costal margin, a deep inspiration by the patient lowers the diaphragm and liver and may allow better visualization of the hepatobiliary structures.
- When imaging the gallbladder with the transducer placed between rib spaces, sonographic shadowing may be decreased by orienting the transducer parallel to the ribs directing the ultrasound beam through the intercostal spaces.
- A sonographic Murphy's sign if present should be noted. It is obtained by eliciting tenderness reproducing the patient's symptoms when probe pressure is applied directly over the gallbladder, with the absence of symptoms when probe pressure is applied either medially or laterally to the gallbladder.
- The gallbladder wall should be measured along the anterior wall between the lumen and the liver parenchyma. Measurement of the posterior wall may be inaccurate due to difficulty in delineating the outer wall of the gallbladder which usually abuts gas-filled intestinal structures. Posterior acoustic enhancement or the presence of gallstones may further degrade the precision of measurement of the posterior wall.
- Pericholecystic fluid may appear as an anechoic stripe seen along the anterior surface of the gallbladder or as a heterogeneously echogenic fluid collection adjacent to the fundus or posterior wall of the gallbladder. It may also appear as a hypoechoic region within the hepatic parenchyma adjacent to the wall of the gallbladder.
- Evaluation of the common bile duct may also be performed for abnormalities including dilatation and choledocholithiasis. The common bile duct usually lies anterolateral to the portal vein with the common hepatic artery lying anteromedial. Color Doppler may be used to help differentiate between the two. The common bile duct should be measured and evaluated for dilation.
- To determine whether gallstones are mobile or impacted in the gallbladder neck, the patient can be turned into the left lateral decubitus position or asked to sit up or stand from the supine position.

4. Recognize specific *pitfalls* involved with biliary tract POCUS
   - Missing findings by not scanning through the entire organ in two orthogonal planes.
   - Mistaking other fluid-filled right upper quadrant structures for the gallbladder. These structures may include the portal vein, the inferior vena cava, and hepatic or renal cysts. Scanning in two planes and being mindful of surrounding anatomy will reduce this possibility. In addition, looking for the "exclamation point" sign with the gallbladder as the exclamation and the right portal vein as the point will help to verify the anatomy.
   - Mistaking loops of small bowel for a gallbladder containing gallstones. The wall of the bowel is anatomically very similar to the wall of the gallbladder, and bowel gas can cause intense shadowing. This misreading can be avoided by systematically scanning through the entire organ, demonstrating that it is cystic and not tubular, and searching for peristalsis.
   - Mistaking the common hepatic artery for the common bile duct. The common bile duct usually lays anterolateral to the portal vein with the common hepatic artery lying anteromedial. The common bile duct has thin walls, and the hepatic artery has thicker and more echogenic walls. Color Doppler may help make the distinction, as there should be no detectable flow in the common bile duct. If the common bile duct is of normal diameter, the distinction is usually moot, since both vessels have similar diameter, which is significantly smaller than that of the portal vein.
   - Failure to measure the gallbladder wall on the surface that abuts the liver.
   - Failure to measure the gallbladder wall exactly at right angles to its surface. Such measurements will exaggerate the thickness of the gallbladder wall.
   - Gallbladder wall thickening also occurs when the gallbladder is contracted. This is normal in the postprandial state.
   - Many nonsurgical diseases also cause gallbladder wall thickening including malnutrition, renal failure, liver failure, congestive heart failure, hypoproteinemia, hypoalbuminemia, and in patients receiving total parenteral nutrition.
   - The gallbladder may be difficult to identify in chronic cholecystitis, especially when filled with stones. A gallbladder filled with one large stone or with a collection of stones may create the "wall echo shadow" (WES) sign, a finding that may result in failure to identify the gallbladder or mistakenly identifying it as the duodenum or transverse colon.
   - Small gallstones may be overlooked or confused with artifact from adjacent bowel gas. The entire

gallbladder should be scanned in multiple planes and if not well visualized the patient repositioned to evaluate for mobility of gallstones. Common bile duct stones are often not be visualized and may be suspected only by the shadowing they cause.

- Cholesterol stones are smaller and less echogenic than calcium containing stones, and frequently float to the anterior wall of the gallbladder.
- Stones in the gallbladder neck may be overlooked due to edge shadowing artifact. Small gallstones, which are intrinsically the most difficult to identify, are the most likely to cause obstruction by becoming impacted in the gallbladder neck. This area should be imaged in several planes to avoid missing a stone.
- Pneumobilia and emphysematous cholecystitis may be identified by increased echogenicity due to air artifact in the gallbladder wall and biliary tree.
- For most of their natural history, most gallstones are asymptomatic. The presence of gallstones does not rule out other life-threatening emergencies of the thorax and abdomen.
- Bowel gas may prevent adequate examination. Slow, graded compression can be used, or the patient may be repositioned. If the study is still inadequate, the limitation should be documented and other methods of evaluation should be used.

Reporting Guideline for Ultrasound Evaluation of the Biliary Tract

Patient Demographics:

Patient Name:
Patient Gender: ☐Male ☐Female

DOB: _/_/___
MR#:
Date & Time: _/_/___ _:_

Examination Demographics:

☐Initial Exam
☐Repeat Exam

Operator Name(s): _______

Operator Training: ☐Attending ☐Fellow ☐Resident ☐Medical Student
☐Other: _______

☐Patient consents to these images being used for educational purposes
☐Patient consents to these images being used for research purposes

Indication(s) for exam:

☐ Abnormal labs ☐ Abdominal pain ☐ Fever ☐ Jaundice
☐ Nausea/Vomiting ☐ Pancreatitis ☐Educational ☐ Other: __________

Views:

Gallbladder long axis:	☐ Adequate	☐ Limited	☐ Not obtained
Gallbladder short axis:	☐ Adequate	☐ Limited	☐ Not obtained
Common bile duct:	☐ Adequate	☐ Limited	☐ Not obtained
Portal vein:	☐ Adequate	☐ Limited	☐ Not obtained

Findings:

Gallstone(s):	☐Absent	☐Present	☐Indeterminate
Gallbladder wall >3mm:	☐Absent	☐Present	☐Indeterminate
Pericholecystic fluid:	☐Absent	☐Present	☐Indeterminate
Sonographic Murphy's sign:	☐Absent	☐Present	☐Indeterminate
Common bile duct wall >6mm:	☐Absent	☐Present	☐Indeterminate
Other: _____			

Interpretation:

☐Normal exam ☐Cholelithiasis ☐Cholecystitis ☐Choledocholithiasis
☐Acalculous cholecystitis ☐Indeterminate ☐Other:____

Quality assurance:

Image Quality: ☐Adequate ☐Inadequate

Accuracy of interpretation: ☐Agree ☐Disagree ☐Unable to assess

Accuracy of interpretation as compared to a gold standard: ☐Not performed ☐TP ☐TN ☐FP ☐FN

Comments:

Ultrasound evaluation of bladder volume

Evidence

1. Summary/brief explanation of indications
   - POCUS can be used to determine the presence of urine in the bladder before attempting urethral catheterization in infants and children.
   - If the bladder appears empty by ultrasound, the clinician may defer the procedure until the child's bladder contains urine, therefore, avoiding failed procedure attempts [52].
   - POCUS assessment of bladder volume may confirm urine production or urinary retention.

2. Relevant adult-specific literature
   - Ultrasound of the bladder can evaluate suspected urinary retention, measure post-void residual volume and evaluate for bladder stones [53].
   - In adult patients, the following equation has been utilized as an estimation of bladder volume: depth (cm) × width (cm) × height (cm) × correction factor 0.75 = bladder volume (cc) [54].

3. Relevant pediatric-specific literature
   - A successful urethral catheterization is considered a urine volume sufficient for urinalysis and culture, usually considered about 2–2.5 ml [55–57].
   - Milling et al. defined the urinary bladder index in infants (<2 years) as the product of anterior–posterior and transverse bladder diameters expressed in centimeters squared. A value of 2.4 cm^2 was found to correlate with a bladder volume of 2 ml. In this study, all infants with a bladder index greater than 2.4 cm^2 had a successful catheterization attempt and all children who had a urinary bladder index less than 2.4 cm^2 had a failed catheterization attempt [54].
   - Two other studies demonstrated that the use of a POCUS estimation of bladder volume in infants led to increased success rates of emergency department urethral catheterization [56, 57]. These studies advocated repeating the ultrasound every 30 min until adequate urine volume was achieved before catheterization attempt.
   - Bladder POCUS can also be used in older children to determine if they are making urine. Bladder ultrasound may provide additional information in patients who otherwise appear euvolemic, but have reports of a prolonged interval since their last void.
   - Qualitative assessment of bladder volume by health care providers can be learned with a brief, 10 min training session [58]. Specialized bedside bladder scanners may also be used if a bedside ultrasound system is not available [52].
   - Bladder volume in children >3 years of age can be estimated by (depth × height × width) × 0.68 + 4 [59].

4. Outstanding questions to be answered/voids in the literature to date
   - Further study on this topic may include determining how performing POCUS for pediatric bladder volume assessment affects emergency department length of stay, time to antibiotic administration, and parental satisfaction.

Curriculum objectives

1. Describe the *indications* for POCUS for bladder volume assessment

   Indications for pediatric bladder volume assessment include:
   - Evaluation for urine in the bladder prior to urethral catheterization attempts in infants or those children who are unable to provide a sterile clean-catch specimen.
   - Assessment for urine production in children with a history of a prolonged time period since their last void.

2. Describe the *limitations* of POCUS for bladder volume assessment
   - Determination of bladder volume becomes less accurate with small bladder volumes.

3. Describe the *relevant anatomy* to be identified when performing bladder volume assessment
   - The bladder can be recognized as an anechoic, fluid-filled, structure residing in the anterior inferior pelvis. When empty, it is located immediately behind the pubic symphysis. With increasing distention, the dome of the bladder extends in a cephalad direction above the pubic symphysis.
   - Measurements should be taken in three dimensions if possible, allowing for calculation of bladder volume. In infants, the urinary bladder index can be calculated based solely on a transverse and anteroposterior measurement in the transverse plane.

4. Recognize specific *pitfalls* with POCUS of the urinary tract
   - Failure to place the transducer caudal enough on the lower abdomen to visualize the bladder and the pubic symphysis.
   - Mistaking other fluid-filled pelvic structures (e.g., ovarian cyst) for the bladder.
   - Failure to measure the maximal diameter of the bladder in any one view and, consequently, underestimating bladder volume.

*Discussion of ultrasound-guided suprapubic bladder aspiration can be found in the procedures section.

Reporting Guideline for Ultrasound Evaluation of Bladder Volume

Patient Demographics:

Patient Name:
Patient Gender: ☐Male ☐Female

DOB: _/_/___
MR#:
Date & Time: _/_/___ _:_

Examination Demographics:

☐Initial Exam
☐Repeat Exam

Operator Name(s): ________

Operator Training: ☐Attending ☐Fellow ☐Resident ☐Medical Student ☐Other: ________

☐Patient consents to these images being used for educational purposes
☐Patient consents to these images being used for research purposes

Indication(s):

☐ Urine Catheter ☐ Suprapubic Aspiration ☐ Decreased urine output
☐ Other:_____

Views:

Bladder sagittal: ☐ Adequate ☐ Inadequate ☐ Indeterminate
Bladder transverse: ☐ Adequate ☐ Inadequate ☐ Indeterminate

Findings:

Bladder size: x:_____cm y:_____cm z:_____cm
Bladder volume: _______cm^3

Interpretation / Outcome:

Bladder volume for urine collection: ☐ Adequate ☐ Inadequate
Other:_____

Quality assurance:

Image Quality: ☐Adequate ☐Inadequate

Accuracy of interpretation: ☐Agree ☐Disagree ☐Unable to assess

Accuracy of interpretation as compared to a gold standard: ☐Not performed ☐TP ☐TN ☐FP ☐FN

Comments:

Ultrasound evaluation of deep venous thrombosis

Evidence

1. Summary/brief explanation of indications
   - Deep vein thrombosis (DVT) should be suspected in patients who present with limb pain and/or swelling and with risk factors such as trauma, prolonged immobilization, malignancy, congenital heart disease, hypercoagulable disorders (including neoplastic disease and nephrotic syndrome), pregnancy, or patients with indwelling catheters.
   - DVT in can be detected using compression ultrasonography. The presence of clot is demonstrated by the inability to compress the vein with the ultrasound probe, while it is being sonographically visualized.
   - POCUS is most commonly used to assess the deep venous systems, since these can give rise to pulmonary emboli. Deep venous systems include those of the lower extremity (femoral and popliteal veins), those of the upper extremity (subclavian, axillary, brachial veins), and the internal jugular veins.
   - POCUS can also easily identify thrombosed superficial veins.
2. Relevant adult-specific literature
   - A meta-analysis from 2008 estimated an overall sensitivity of POCUS of 95 % (95 % CI 87–99 %) and a specificity of 96 % (95 % CI 87–99 %) when radiology ultrasound was used as the reference standard [60].
   - One study of 156 patients with a suspected lower extremity DVT demonstrated that POCUS had excellent agreement with that performed in the radiology department (kappa = 0.9), and patients were evaluated more than 2 h faster with POCUS [61].
   - POCUS may yield high negative predictive value for DVT evaluation, avoid unnecessary anticoagulant treatment, and may be performed when radiology studies are not available with good accuracy [62, 63].
   - In adults, proximal lower extremity DVT can be excluded by a limited compression study of just the common femoral and the popliteal veins. If these veins can be compressed and the patient has a negative d-dimer study, DVT is excluded. If the veins can be compressed and the d-dimer study is positive, the patient requires another ultrasound test in 3–5 days to assess for distal venous thrombosis [64].
3. Relevant pediatric-specific literature
   - To date, there is only a case series of POCUS utilized in the pediatric ED to evaluate for DVTs [65].
4. Outstanding questions to be answered/voids in literature to date
   - There is limited description of POCUS for the diagnosis of DVT in children. All comparative studies between POCUS and radiology studies have been performed in adult patients. Assessing accuracy of POCUS for pediatric DVT will be difficult given that it is a rare entity in emergency departments. However, the technique has been shown to be simple and rapid to perform in adults and can be easily applied to children.

Curriculum objectives

1. Describe the *indications* for the POCUS evaluation for DVT
   - Indications: DVT POCUS should be considered in patients with risk factors for DVT, who present with extremity pain, swelling, and/or shortness of breath.
   - Risk factors for DVT include indwelling central venous catheters, congenital heart disease, inherited or acquired hypercoagulable disorders, history of pregnancy or malignancy, or history of trauma or medical illness requiring immobilization or hospitalization.
2. Describe the *limitations* of the POCUS evaluation for DVT
   - Upper extremity and thoracic DVTs may be difficult to visualize on ultrasound in patients with indwelling catheters due to rib shadowing and air in the thorax.
   - Clavicles and ribs prevent compression assessment of the proximal internal jugular, subclavian, and thoracic veins.
   - Abdominal contents prevent compression assessment of the Iliac veins and the IVC.
   - Imaging and compression of veins in patients with a high body mass index may be more challenging.
3. Describe the *relevant anatomy* to be identified with POCUS evaluation for DVT
   - Compression ultrasonography verifies venous patency using an ultrasound transducer to compress and obliterate the vein lumen under direct visualization [66]. Comparison of contralateral sides may assist in diagnosis, as can the use of color and spectral Doppler.
   - Pressure is applied through the transducer until the adjacent artery is seen to start to compress. If the vein does not compress with this amount of force, it is deemed noncompressible.

- Femoral vein: Evaluation starts at the inguinal ligament with compression every centimeter until 1–2 cm beyond its bifurcation into superficial and deep branches [66].
- Popliteal vein: Evaluation starts with vein compression superior to the popliteal crease and continues until the trifurcating terminal branches of the popliteal veins are identified [66]. The bony landmarks of the femoral condyles and the tibial plateau should be identified to confirm that the popliteal vessels are indeed being examined. When examined from the popliteal fossa, the popliteal artery lies immediately superficial/posterior to these bony landmarks, and the popliteal vein is immediately superficial/posterior to the artery.
- Internal jugular vein: compression starts at the level of the clavicle and continues superiorly until the base of the skull [66].
- The veins of the upper extremity to be assessed by compression include the axillary, brachial, and the antecubital.

4. Recognize specific *pitfalls* involved with POCUS evaluation for DVT

- Misidentifying lymph nodes or arteries as noncompressible veins.
- Mistaking a noncompressible vein for an artery.
- Mistaking large compressible collateral superficial veins for deep veins, when the deep veins are actually occluded by thrombus.
- Assuming that the presence of color flow or spectral Doppler signal rules out DVT. Many DVTs do not completely occlude the vein, hence the need for compression evaluation.
- Assuming that acute thrombus will be echogenic and, therefore, directly visualized on ultrasound. Acute thrombus is anechoic, hence the need for compression evaluation. With the passage of time, some thrombus becomes calcified and thus identifiable on B-mode with appropriate gain adjustments.
- Possible clot dislodgement during evaluation.
- Evaluation of chronic DVTs is an advanced skill that should be done by a vascular lab or radiology department with access to previous imaging or with scanning protocols that evaluate chronic DVTs.

Reporting Guideline for Ultrasound Evaluation of Deep Venous Thrombosis

Patient Demographics:

Patient Name:
Patient Gender: ☐Male ☐Female

DOB: _/_/__
MR#:
Date & Time: _/_/__ _:_

Examination Demographics:

☐Initial Exam
☐Repeat Exam

Operator Name(s): _______

Operator Training: ☐Attending ☐Fellow ☐Resident ☐Medical Student
☐Other: _______

☐Patient consents to these images being used for educational purposes
☐Patient consents to these images being used for research purposes

Indication(s) for exam:

☐ Leg pain	☐ Leg swelling	☐ Leg erythema	☐ Dyspnea
☐ Tachypnea	☐ Pleurisy	☐Educational	☐ Other: ________

Views:

Right saphenofemoral junction:	☐Adequate	☐Limited	☐Not obtained
Right femoral vein:	☐Adequate	☐Limited	☐Not obtained
Right popliteal vein:	☐Adequate	☐Limited	☐Not obtained
Right internal jugular vein:	☐Adequate	☐Limited	☐Not obtained
Other: ____________	☐Adequate	☐Limited	☐Not obtained
Left saphenofemoral junction:	☐Adequate	☐Limited	☐Not obtained
Left femoral vein:	☐Adequate	☐Limited	☐Not obtained
Left popliteal vein:	☐Adequate	☐Limited	☐Not obtained
Left internal jugular vein:	☐Adequate	☐Limited	☐Not obtained
Other: ____________	☐Adequate	☐Limited	☐Not obtained

Findings:

Right

Saphenofemoral junction:	☐Compressible	☐NOT compressible	☐Indeterminate
Femoral vein:	☐Compressible	☐NOT compressible	☐Indeterminate
Popliteal vein:	☐Compressible	☐NOT compressible	☐Indeterminate
Internal jugular vein:	☐Compressible	☐NOT compressible	☐Indeterminate
Other: ____________	☐Compressible	☐NOT compressible	☐Indeterminate

Left

Saphenofemoral junction:	☐Compressible	☐NOT compressible	☐Indeterminate
Femoral vein:	☐Compressible	☐NOT compressible	☐Indeterminate
Popliteal vein:	☐Compressible	☐NOT compressible	☐Indeterminate
Internal jugular vein:	☐Compressible	☐NOT compressible	☐Indeterminate
Other: ____________	☐Compressible	☐NOT compressible	☐Indeterminate

Interpretation:

☐ Normal exam ☐ Deep Vein Thrombosis ☐ Indeterminate

Quality assurance:

Image Quality: ☐ Adequate ☐ Inadequate

Accuracy of interpretation: ☐ Agree ☐ Disagree ☐Unable to assess

Accuracy of interpretation as compared to a gold standard: ☐Not performed ☐TP ☐TN ☐FP ☐FN

Comments:

Ultrasound evaluation of the eye

Evidence

1. Summary/brief explanation of indication
   - POCUS evaluation of the eye (ocular POCUS) allows visualization of the components of the globe and the optic nerve. Many pathologies can be diagnosed using ultrasound including foreign body, retinal detachment, vitreous hemorrhage, and lens dislocation [67]. Ocular POCUS can also be used in the evaluation of patients with signs and symptoms of increased intracranial pressure (ICP).

2. Relevant adult-specific literature
   - *Intra-ocular pathology* Ocular ultrasound is widely utilized in the ophthalmologist's diagnostic evaluation of eye pathology. Several case reports describe an array of conditions diagnosed with emergency physician-performed POCUS. Blaivas et al. found that POCUS by emergency physicians had a sensitivity of 100 % and specificity of 97.2 % in the detection of ocular pathology when compared with computed tomography (CT) and evaluation by the ophthalmology service [68]. A meta-analysis found ocular POCUS to have excellent sensitivity of 97–100 % and specificity of 83–100 % in the diagnosis of retinal detachment [69].
   - *Optic nerve sheath diameter measurement* In addition to assessment of intra-ocular pathology, changes in the optic nerve sheath diameter (ONSD) correlate with increased ICP. Small adult studies have shown excellent sensitivity and specificity of ONSD measurements in the detection of increased ICP in both the emergency department and intensive care unit [70–73].

3. Relevant pediatric-specific literature
   - *Intra-ocular pathology* There are limited data regarding the use of emergency physician-performed POCUS to evaluate for intra-ocular pathology in children. An isolated case report describes the diagnosis of retinal detachment in a pediatric patient with POCUS in the emergency department [74]. Additionally, POCUS identification of optic drusen, retinoblastoma, and retinal hemorrhage in the setting of abusive head trauma has been reported [75–77].
   - *Optic nerve sheath diameter measurement* Pediatric normal values for the measurement of optic nerve sheath size have been established and several publications have described the use of these measurements in the evaluation of children at risk of increased intracranial pressure (ICP) in neurosurgical clinics [78–81]. A case–control study noted a significant difference between the ONSD of patients with signs of increased ICP diagnosed by CT when compared to controls [82]. Studies of ED physician-performed ONSD measurements are limited to small prospective case series regarding the use of POCUS in pediatric patients undergoing evaluation for increased ICP [83, 84]. Using CT or invasive measurement techniques as the reference standard, one study found a sensitivity of 83 % and specificity of 38 % of ONSD measurements performed by emergency medicine physicians and interpreted by ophthalmologic ultrasonographers. In this study, when ONSD measurements were performed and interpreted by emergency physicians, they found a sensitivity and specificity of 96 and 38 %, respectively. Further study focused on ONSD measurements in patients with suspected pediatric ventriculoperitoneal shunt failure and found ONSD measurements to have sensitivity of 61.1 % and specificity of 22 % for detecting shunt malfunction [85]. A study of children with hydrocephalus found utility in using a patient's own baseline

ONSD measurements as a comparison for when they are symptomatic, particularly when there are no changes noted with neuroimaging [86].

4. Outstanding questions to be answered/voids in the literature to date:
   - Further studies are needed to evaluate the role of ocular POCUS in the assessment of ocular pathology and increased ICP in the pediatric population as current literature has demonstrated variable results.

Curriculum objectives

1. Describe the *indications* for ocular POCUS
   - Indications for ocular POCUS include, but are not limited to: change in visual acuity, ocular pain, foreign body, eye trauma, and concern for increased intracranial pressure.
2. Describe the *limitations* of ocular POCUS
   - Post-surgical changes or congenital anomalies of the eye may create scarring that prevents the expected changes in size in the optic nerve sheath with increase in intracranial pressure.
   - To date, there are limited data regarding the accuracy of POCUS for measuring ONSD as a proxy for intracranial pressure. One study suggests a high sensitivity but suboptimal specificity.
   - Differentiation of vitreous detachment from retinal detachment has been shown to be difficult for novice ultrasonographers leading to inaccurate diagnosis of retinal detachment [87].
3. Describe the *relevant anatomy* to be identified with ocular POCUS
   - The anterior and posterior segments of the eye and the optic nerve should be examined. The cornea, the most anterior structure of the anterior segment, is identified as a thin, hypoechoic tissue superficial to the anechoic fluid of the anterior segment. The lens, located posteriorly within the anterior segment, is an anechoic thin structure flanked by the iris and the ciliary body, which are seen as echogenic structures extending centrally from the lateral walls of the globe. Deep to the lens, the posterior segment is filled with anechoic vitreous. The posterior wall of the globe contains the retina and choroidal layers that are not well visualized in the normal eye. Behind the globe, the optic nerve is a hypoechoic, elongated structure extending posteriorly and, in the evaluation of ONSD, is measured 3 mm from the interior surface of the optic cup.
4. Recognize specific *pitfalls* with ocular POCUS
   - The measurement of the optic nerve sheath requires a scanning plane in the middle of the nerve (to avoid underestimation of diameter). Images that are low in quality or resolution can lead to inaccurate measurements.
   - Ocular POCUS after traumatic injury to the eye or face should be performed without applying any transducer pressure to the eyeball. If there is a possibility of globe rupture, a thick layer of gel should be used to prevent contact between the eyelid and transducer. A study of 40 patients demonstrated small, transient elevation in intraocular pressure during ocular POCUS, but pressure change was similar to that caused by physical exam [88].
   - POCUS may be limited in its ability to diagnose retinal detachment; therefore, sonologists should be cautious in ruling out the diagnosis.

Reporting Guideline for Ultrasound Evaluation of the Eye

Patient Demographics:

Patient Name:
Patient Gender: ☐Male ☐Female

DOB: _/_/___
MR#:
Date & Time: _/_/___ _:_

Examination Demographics:

☐Initial Exam
☐Repeat Exam

Operator Name(s): _______

Operator Training: ☐Attending ☐Fellow ☐Resident ☐Medical Student ☐Other: _______

☐Patient consents to these images being used for educational purposes
☐Patient consents to these images being used for research purposes

Indication(s) for exam:

☐Eye traumas	☐Vision change	☐Suspect foreign body
☐Visual loss	☐Head injury	☐Headache
☐Altered Mental Status	☐Vomiting	☐Suspect VP shunt failure
☐Eye pain	☐Educational	☐ Other_______

Views:

Right eye transverse:	☐Adequate	☐Limited	☐Not obtained
Right eye longitudinal:	☐Adequate	☐Limited	☐Not obtained
Left eye transverse:	☐Adequate	☐Limited	☐Not obtained
Left eye longitudinal:	☐Adequate	☐Limited	☐Not obtained

Findings:

Retinal contour R:	☐Normal	☐Abnormal	☐Indeterminate	☐Not obtained
Retinal contour L:	☐Normal	☐Abnormal	☐Indeterminate	☐Not obtained
Lens R:	☐Normal	☐Dislodged	☐Indeterminate	☐Not obtained
Lens L:	☐Normal	☐Dislodged	☐Indeterminate	☐Not obtained
Vitreous body R:	☐Normal	☐Abnormal	☐Indeterminate	☐Not obtained
Vitreous body L:	☐Normal	☐Abnormal	☐Indeterminate	☐Not obtained
ONSD R:	☐Normal	☐Enlarged	☐Indeterminate	☐Not obtained
ONSD L:	☐Normal	☐Enlarged	☐Indeterminate	☐Not obtained

Other:_______

Interpretation:

☐Normal exam ☐Intraocular foreign body ☐Lens dislocation
☐Retinal detachment ☐Vitreous detachment ☐Vitreous hemorrhage
☐Increased ONSD ☐Papilledema ☐Indeterminate
☐Other: _________

Quality assurance:

Image Quality: ☐Adequate ☐Inadequate

Accuracy of interpretation: ☐Agree ☐Disagree ☐Unable to assess

Accuracy of interpretation as compared to a gold standard: ☐Not performed ☐TP ☐TN ☐FP ☐FN

Comments:

Ultrasound evaluation of abdominal trauma-focused assessment with sonography for trauma (FAST)

Evidence

1. Summary/brief explanation of indications
   - The focused assessment with sonography for trauma (FAST) examination seeks to detect intraperitoneal fluid (hemoperitoneum), pericardial fluid (hemopericardium), and intrathoracic fluid (hemothorax) in patients after blunt or penetrating truncal trauma. The "extended" FAST (e-FAST) examination also assesses the chest for pneumothorax.

2. Relevant adult-specific literature
   - In adults when CT scan is readily available a large meta-analysis determined that there was no demonstrable benefit in mortality with the use of ultrasound in blunt abdominal trauma [89].
   - In two randomized controlled trials, the FAST examination safely decreased abdominal CT use in injured adults [90, 91] as well as decreased the time to the operating room, hospital length of stay, and complications [90].
   - Evidence indicates that both emergency medicine physicians and surgeons can accurately perform the FAST examination [92–94].
   - Competency in performing and interpreting the FAST examination may be accomplished after performing 10–30 examinations in adult patients [95–97] with error rates as low as 5 % [96].
   - Lung ultrasound is more accurate than supine anterior chest radiograph for diagnosing pneumothorax [98].

3. Relevant pediatric-specific literature
   - The sensitivity of the FAST examination for hemoperitoneum in pediatric trauma patients is variable, ranging from 31–100 % [99–101]. The sensitivity improves in the most severely injured patients [102]. This suggests that an ED evaluation protocol using abdominal ultrasound in children may have clinical utility. Patient sampling, selection bias, ultrasound protocols, and outcome definitions were highly variable in prior pediatric studies and account for the reported variation in test characteristics [101].
   - The results of a meta-analysis of 25 observational studies of 3838 children demonstrate that FAST has a sensitivity of 80 % when used to identify those with hemoperitoneum [101]. The sensitivity of FAST, however, drops to 66 % when those patients with intra-abdominal injuries, but without hemoperitoneum, are included in the outcome of interest. Failure to identify patients with intra-abdominal injury without hemoperitoneum is a known limitation of the FAST examination. Furthermore, imaging the solid organs in addition to evaluating for intraperitoneal fluid resulted in only a modest increase in ultrasound sensitivity.
   - The sensitivity of the FAST examination for children undergoing operative intervention or blood transfusion for their abdominal injury is 88 % [103].
   - FAST examination may be incorporated into other aspects of the trauma evaluation to improve the accuracy of the test. One small study found that when combined with an AST or ALT > 100 IU/L the specificity of the FAST examination was 98 %, suggesting a negative FAST and transaminases <100 IU/L should result in patient observation instead of abdominal CT scanning [104].
   - Observational data demonstrate that the FAST examination has limited impact on abdominal CT use in injured children at very low (<1 %) and very high risk (>10 %) of intra-abdominal injury. However, use of the FAST examination in children considered to have 1–10 % risk of intra-abdominal injury safely decreased abdominal CT use [105]. In addition, surgeons desire for abdominal CT scanning decreases once a FAST examination has been obtained [103].
   - The only evidence in children for pneumothorax detection with ultrasound is a case series describing needle placement for treatment of the pneumothorax [106].

4. Outstanding questions to be answered/voids in the literature to date
   - Limited published data exist on pediatric FAST examinations as a screening tool. Currently, no published randomized control trials of the FAST examination in pediatric patients exist.
   - The role of contrast-enhanced FAST to improve detection of solid organ injury in children requires exploration.
   - There are limited data on test characteristics of POCUS for diagnosing pneumothorax in pediatrics.

Curriculum objectives

1. Describe the *indications* for the FAST examination.
   Indications for the FAST examination include:
   - For hypotensive pediatric trauma patients, the FAST examination can rapidly identify hemoperitoneum, hemothorax, or cardiac tamponade and expedite operative intervention and/or transfusion of blood products.
   - In hemodynamically stable patients, a positive FAST examination will typically require further evaluation with abdominal CT scan. If one cannot be obtained in a timely manner or the patient

becomes unstable, serial FAST examinations can be performed to determine active bleeding by assessing for increasing amounts of intraperitoneal fluid.

- In hemodynamically stable patients with negative FAST examinations, abdominal CT scans may be obtained depending on risk factors for intra-abdominal injury [107], or patients may be followed by serial FAST examinations.

2. Describe the *limitations* of the FAST examination
   - The FAST examination does not effectively evaluate solid organs for injuries. In addition, approximately, 25 % of intra-abdominal injuries in children do not have hemoperitoneum [107], thus the FAST examination may be normal despite the presence of an intra-abdominal injury.
   - False-positive FAST examinations (up to 4 % of FAST examinations [101]) may lead to abdominal CT scans that would otherwise not have been obtained.
3. Describe the *relevant anatomy* to be identified with the FAST examination
   - The FAST examination utilizes four specific locations to evaluate for intraperitoneal, intrathoracic, and pericardial fluid. The protocol includes views of the right and left upper quadrant (RUQ, LUQ), pelvis and heart.

1. In the RUQ, a thorough examination visualizes from the diaphragm superiorly to the inferior portion of the liver. Visualization above the diaphragm evaluates for right-sided hemothorax. Morison's pouch (interface of the liver and kidney) is the dependent space of the upper abdomen in the supine position and the most common location to identify hemoperitoneum in adults [108]. Imaging the inferior pole of the right kidney evaluates for fluid in the paracolic gutter.
2. The LUQ is evaluated similar to the RUQ. A thorough examination should visualize from the diaphragm to the inferior portion of the spleen. Visualization above the diaphragm evaluates for left-sided hemothorax. The splenorenal space differs from Morison's pouch due to the configuration of the splenorenal ligament as well as the relatively small size of the spleen compared to the liver. Depending on whether hemorrhage in the left upper quadrant is occurring inside or outside of the lesser sac, free fluid may accumulate circumferentially around the spleen, below the diaphragm (subphrenic), at the inferior pole of the spleen, or in the splenorenal fossa. Visualization of the inferior pole of the left kidney evaluates for hemorrhage in the left paracolic gutter.
3. The pelvis is visualized for intraperitoneal fluid with both transverse and sagittal views. The urinary bladder is used as a landmark to evaluate for hemoperitoneum. Intraperitoneal fluid may accumulate superiorly and/or posteriorly to the bladder. The pelvis is the most common location for free fluid in pediatric patients [109].
4. The FAST examination of the heart is primarily directed to the detection of intra-pericardial fluid. The most common FAST views make use of the subxiphoid window. The image displayed includes the liver and the heart. If the subxiphoid view is inadequate or difficult to obtain, the parasternal long axis view may be used.
   - The e-FAST examination includes imaging the chest to evaluate for pneumothoraces
     - The transducer (a linear is usually used) is placed anteriorly in the mid-clavicular line in a longitudinal plane. The lungs should be visualized from the diaphragm to the clavicles.
     - If lung sliding or B lines or lung pulse are seen, pneumothorax is excluded; underneath the transducer at this point of the chest. If all 3 of these are absent, pneumothorax may be present. In addition, the presence of a lung point (also referred to as the "leading-edge") is pathognomonic for the presence of pneumothorax.
     - Color Doppler and motion mode (M-mode) can be used as adjuncts for evaluating lung sliding.

4. Recognize specific *pitfalls* involved with the FAST examination.

   Pitfalls to avoid when performing the FAST examination include the following:
   - Mistaking the IVC, aorta, gallbladder or intraluminal intestinal fluid as intraperitoneal fluid (false positive).
   - Interpretation of ascites, pleural effusion, or pericardial effusion as being due to traumatic hemorrhage. In most cases, there are clinical or historical clues to the correct diagnosis.
   - Failure to identify all spaces within a given region as described above and concluding that the examination is negative (false negative).
   - Failure to reduce the gain when evaluating the pelvis, and, therefore, being unable to identify intraperitoneal fluid behind the bladder due to posterior acoustic enhancement (false negative).
   - Failure to utilize parasternal views, when unable to visualize the heart via the subxiphoid window.
   - Pitfalls to avoid when performing the e-FAST examination include the following:

- Incomplete evaluation of the lungs concluding the exam is negative for pneumothorax (false negative).
- Interpreting lack of lung sliding due to pleural adhesions or right mainstem intubation as pneumothorax (false positive). Frequently, in such situations the presence of lung pulse and/or B-lines points to the absence of pneumothorax.
- Failing to identify free fluid in the pelvis due to the posterior acoustic enhancement overlying the area behind the bladder

Reporting Guideline for the Focused Assessment with Sonography for Trauma (FAST) examination

<u>Patient Demographics:</u>

Patient Name:
Patient Gender: ☐Male ☐Female

DOB: _/_/___
MR#:
Date & Time: _/_/___ _:_

<u>Examination Demographics:</u>

☐Initial Exam
☐Repeat Exam

Operator Name(s): ________

Operator Training: ☐Attending ☐Fellow ☐Resident ☐Medical Student ☐Other: ________

☐ Patient consents to these images being used for educational purposes
☐ Patient consents to these images being used for research purposes

<u>Indication(s) for exam:</u>

☐ Blunt trauma ☐ Penetrating trauma ☐ Other: ___________

<u>Views:</u>

Right Upper Quadrant	☐Adequate	☐Limited	☐Not obtained
Left Upper Quadrant	☐Adequate	☐Limited	☐Not obtained
Suprapubic	☐Adequate	☐Limited	☐Not obtained
Pericardial	☐Adequate	☐Limited	☐Not obtained
R thorax: lung sliding	☐Adequate	☐Limited	☐Not obtained
R thorax: free fluid	☐Adequate	☐Limited	☐Not obtained
L thorax: lung sliding	☐Adequate	☐Limited	☐Not obtained
L thorax: free fluid	☐Adequate	☐Limited	☐Not obtained

Findings:

RUQ Free Fluid	☐Absent	☐Present	☐Indeterminate
Qualitative Amount:	☐Small	☐Moderate	☐Large
LUQ Free Fluid	☐Absent	☐Present	☐Indeterminate
Qualitative Amount:	☐Small	☐Moderate	☐Large
Suprapubic	☐Absent	☐Present	☐Indeterminate
Qualitative Amount:	☐Small	☐Moderate	☐Large
Pericardial effusion	☐Absent	☐Present	☐Indeterminate
Qualitative Amount:	☐Small	☐Moderate	☐Large
R thorax: lung sliding	☐Absent	☐Present	☐Indeterminate
R thorax: lung point	☐No	☐Yes	☐Indeterminate
R thorax: free fluid	☐Absent	☐Present	☐Indeterminate
Qualitative Amount:	☐Small	☐Moderate	☐Large
L thorax: lung sliding	☐Absent	☐Present	☐Indeterminate
L thorax: lung point	☐No	☐Yes	☐Indeterminate
L thorax: free fluid	☐Absent	☐Present	☐Indeterminate
Qualitative Amount:	☐Small	☐Moderate	☐Large

Interpretation:

☐Normal exam	☐Intraabdominal free fluid	☐Pericardial free fluid
☐R thoracic free fluid	☐R pneumothorax	
☐L thoracic free fluid	☐L pneumothorax	☐Other:____

Quality assurance:

Image Quality: ☐Adequate ☐Inadequate

Accuracy of interpretation: ☐Agree ☐Disagree ☐Unable to assess

Accuracy of interpretation as compared to a gold standard: ☐Not performed ☐TP ☐TN ☐FP ☐FN

Comments:

Ultrasound evaluation of the heart and inferior vena cava

Evidence

1. Summary/brief explanation of indications
   - Focused cardiac ultrasound (FOCUS) [110, 111], which may include the evaluation of the heart as well as the inferior vena cava (IVC), is a limited focused clinician-performed cardiac evaluation directed to identifying specific cardiac disease states in addition to assessing the functional condition of the heart. FOCUS is used in a wide range of clinical conditions and not limited to diagnosing cardiac pathology. Specifically, FOCUS is used to evaluate the functional assessment of the heart in the setting of various shock states to guide appropriate management. FOCUS may fail to identify pathological findings revealed by comprehensive pediatric echocardiography [112] or targeted neonatal echocardiography [113]. FOCUS is not intended to supplant these extended comprehensive examinations.
   - FOCUS can be utilized to rapidly assess global cardiac systolic function in critically ill patients with tachycardia, hypotension or dysrhythmias. Evaluating global cardiac systolic function may help to differentiate cardiac from other causes of hypoxia or shock [110, 111, 114, 115].
   - Assessing pericardial effusion by FOCUS is critical for the evaluation of suspected cardiac tamponade in both the nontraumatic and trauma setting [115–120].
   - The international pediatric basic and advanced life support recommendations state that "FOCUS may be considered to identify potentially treatable causes of a cardiac arrest, but the benefits must be carefully weighed against the known deleterious consequences of interrupting chest compressions" [121] and was reaffirmed by an international consensus panel of experts [110].
   - Evaluation of the inferior vena cava can estimate intravascular volume status [110, 111].
   - Serial FOCUS exams can help to gauge the patient's response to resuscitative interventions, such as fluid boluses, inotropic support and pericardiocentesis [110, 111].

2. Relevant adult-specific literature
   - One of the first uses of FOCUS was to evaluate the heart for pericardial effusion as part of the Focused Assessment with Sonography for Trauma (FAST) examination [115].
   - Several case series have suggested that emergency department echocardiography in penetrating trauma patients is sensitive for identification of cardiac injuries and leads to rapid diagnosis and improved survival [115, 116].
   - Emergency physicians have also demonstrated the ability to accurately detect pericardial effusions not secondary to penetrating trauma [117–119].
   - With limited training, emergency physicians have been shown to accurately characterize left ventricular systolic function in hypotensive patients [122].
   - Several studies have shown that emergency physicians can determine hemodynamic parameters, like ejection fraction and other hemodynamic information comparable to data obtained with comprehensive echocardiography [122, 123].
   - FOCUS may be helpful in cardiac arrest scenarios to help predict outcomes of resuscitative efforts, with a lack of sonographic cardiac activity indicating poor survival [124, 125].
   - Unlike more comprehensive sonographic cardiac assessments, FOCUS can be rapidly deployed and incorporated into advanced life support algorithms without prolonging interruptions in chest compressions, delaying medications or other cardiopulmonary resuscitation measures [125–128].
   - In the adult with hypotension, ultrasound measurements of the inferior vena cava (IVC) have been used to estimate central venous pressure [127]. Dynamic assessments of the IVC have shown that with inspiration complete collapse of the IVC may indicate hypovolemia, while decreases in diameter of less than 50 % may represent fluid overload or increased right atrial pressures [129–131]. Other data from studies in trauma patients suggest that the aorta to IVC ratios may be a more reliable measure of hypovolemia [132]. Dynamic evaluation of the IVC in conjunction with thoracic ultrasound can help with assessing fluid responsiveness for patients in shock [133].
   - There are various arithmetic formulas used for the assessment of IVC collapse, the most common being the collapsibility index [(IVC max diameter-IVC min diameter)/IVC max diameter]. Some have advocated for using clinical gestalt of IVC collapse to estimate volume status [134] (Fields JM, AEM).

3. Relevant pediatric-specific literature
   - In a survey from 2008, 61 % of pediatric emergency departments reported using ultrasound clinically, with 59 % specifying evaluation for cardiac activity, 59 % for pericardial effusion and 7 % using POCUS for advanced cardiac applications [135].
   - Literature describing the use of POCUS in detecting significant cardiac pathology in children such as cardiac tamponade, dilated cardiomyopathy from myocarditis, congenital heart disease and infective endocarditis has been described in a number of case reports [128, 136–141].

- Pediatric critical care and pediatric emergency medicine physicians with focused training were able to diagnose pericardial effusions, cardiac contractility abnormalities, and left ventricular enlargement with an accuracy of 91 % [142, 143].
- Studies have shown that pediatric emergency medicine physicians with POCUS training are both reliable and accurate in assessing left ventricular function and preload by estimating IVC collapsibility when compared to cardiologists/echocardiographers [144, 145].
- The literature on FOCUS evaluation during cardiac arrest in pediatrics is limited to case reports or series. One series of fourteen patients showed good correlation between the presence or absence of a pulse on physical examination and the presence or absence of cardiac activity on ultrasound. [128].
- Both the ratio of aorta to IVC and the dynamic assessment of IVC collapsibility with inspiration have been investigated in the pediatric population as assessments of hydration status and both metrics may correlate with fluid status [146–148].

4. Outstanding questions to be answered/voids in the literature to date
   - More research is needed to create an evidence-based sonographic assessment for pediatric shock and undifferentiated tachycardia similar to guidelines developed for adult patients [149].
   - More evidence is needed on the use of POCUS during pediatric resuscitation [110, 128].
   - Normal values for different ages, disease states and populations are still needed for sonographic identification of fluid status in children, as well as investigations into the utility and impact of incorporating ultrasound into clinical pathways for dehydration [146–148].
   - Investigation is needed into the potential use of communications technology to facilitate real-time tele-echocardiography/POCUS image transfer for consultation with pediatric intensivists or resuscitation experts in critical care or emergency scenarios [110, 150–152].

Curriculum objectives

1. Describe the *indications* for FOCUS
   - FOCUS should be considered for patients with signs of potential cardiac pathology such as shortness of breath, chest pain, syncope, hypotension/shock, a new murmur, and cardiac arrest.
   - The use of FOCUS in infants and children by physicians is still in its investigatory phase. As more outcome-driven evidence is attained, indications are likely to evolve. At the current time, FOCUS may assess for the following:.
   - Assessment of cardiac contractility, pericardial effusion, and hypovolemia, in the setting of undifferentiated shock or tachycardia.
   - Diagnosis of pericardial effusion and tamponade as part of the FAST exam, and in non-traumatized patients.
   - Intravascular volume assessment of patients with hypovolemia secondary to vomiting and diarrhea.
   - Assessment of cardiac motion and/or reversible causes of PEA in cardiac arrest.

2. Describe the *limitations* of FOCUS
   - FOCUS is not primarily directed to the diagnosis or exclusion of congenital heart disease or its complications.
   - Cardiovascular assessment/windows may be limited by injuries, dressings, or body habitus (including cachexia, obesity, scoliosis, and contractures).
   - Standard measurements of the IVC/aorta are not well established for all age groups. Serial exams may be more useful to guide resuscitation than an exam at a single point in time.
   - Inotropic medications and positive pressure ventilation may affect the size and elasticity of the IVC.
   - Foreshortening may distort the normal circular appearance of the left ventricle in short-axis views leading to incorrect estimation of LV function.

3. Describe the *relevant anatomy* to be identified with FOCUS
   - Relevant anatomy is dependent on the indication for FOCUS and the question to be answered.
   - Standard cardiac assessment includes views in the sub-xiphoid, parasternal long-axis, parasternal short axis and apical four-chamber windows with additional views as necessary, such as suprasternal views and extended apical views [110].
   - The IVC is usually assessed in a sub-xiphoid longitudinal plane as it travels through the liver parenchyma, crosses the diaphragm and enters the right atrium. Dynamic assessment may include measurements of vessel diameter during inspiration and expiration using m-mode. The descending aorta is typically viewed in its sub-xiphoid location and measurements of maximum size during systole are compared to the IVC in the transverse plane, usually at the level of the renal arteries.

4. Recognize specific *pitfalls* involved with FOCUS. Pitfalls to avoid when performing cardiac FOCUS include the following:

- Prolonged pauses in chest compressions for more than 10 s while performing FOCUS during pediatric cardiac arrest [110, 114, 128].
- Misinterpreting pericardial fat as a pericardial effusion or pleural effusions as pericardial effusions.
- Positive pressure ventilation and vasopressors may have variable impact on the size and respiratory variation of the IVC [153, 154].
- Mistaking the IVC for the Aorta during the assessment of volume status. The aorta can be identified based on the knowledge of anatomical branching, different flow pattern on pulsed wave Doppler, and a thicker pulsatile wall.
- In the presence of a pericardial effusion, severe tachycardia can impede the identification of diastolic collapse of the right ventricle and/or collapse of the right atrium, resulting in failure to diagnose tamponade. Although not routinely a part of the FOCUS exam, other methods for assessment of cardiac tamponade may be used, including M-mode assessment of respiratory variations in left ventricular diameter, Doppler assessment of mitral inflow velocity variation and visualization of a plethoric IVC [155].
- Confusion of right and left heart chambers and major aortic arch vascular branches may occur due to improper transducer orientation, especially in the setting of congenital heart disease [110, 156].

*Discussion of ultrasound-guided pericardiocentesis can be found in the procedures section.

Reporting Guideline for Ultrasound Evaluation of the Heart and Inferior Vena Cava

Patient Demographics:

Patient Name:
Patient Gender: ☐Male ☐Female

DOB: _/_/___
MR#:
Date & Time: _/_/___ _:_

Examination Demographics:

☐Initial Exam
☐Repeat Exam

Operator Name(s): ________

Operator Training: ☐Attending ☐Fellow ☐Resident ☐Medical Student ☐Other: ________

☐Patient consents to these images being used for educational purposes
☐Patient consents to these images being used for research purposes

Indication(s) for exam:

☐Cardiac arrest ☐Shortness of breath ☐Chest pain ☐Syncope
☐Cyanosis ☐Shock ☐Hypotension ☐Dyspnea
☐Murmur ☐Tachycardia ☐Fever ☐Palpitations
☐Educational ☐Other: ________

Views:

Cardiac-

Subxiphoid:	☐Adequate	☐Limited	☐Not obtained
Parasternal long axis:	☐Adequate	☐Limited	☐Not obtained
Apical four-chamber:	☐Adequate	☐Limited	☐Not obtained
Parasternal short axis:	☐Adequate	☐Limited	☐Not obtained

IVC-

Longitudinal:	☐Adequate	☐Limited	☐Not obtained
Transverse:	☐Adequate	☐Limited	☐Not obtained

Findings:

Global Ventricular Function: ☐Normal ☐Reduced ☐Severely Reduced ☐Standstill ☐Hyperdynamic ☐Indeterminate

Pericardial effusion: ☐Absent/trace ☐Small ☐Moderate (circumferential) ☐Large (concern for tamponade) ☐Indeterminate

Right Ventricular Size: ☐Normal ☐Dilated ☐Hypertrophied ☐Indeterminate
Left Ventricular Size: ☐Normal ☐Dilated ☐Hypertrophied ☐Indeterminate

☐ IVC diameter (maximum):_______ ☐IVC diameter (minimum):_______

☐ IVC collapse index [(IVCmax-IVCmin)/IVCmax]: _________%

Interpretation:

☐Normal exam ☐Cardiac standstill ☐Impaired global ventricular function

☐Pericardial effusion without tamponade ☐Pericardial effusion with tamponade

☐ IVC collapsed ☐ IVC dilated ☐ IVC normal

☐Other:_________

☐ Indeterminate

Quality assurance:

Image Quality: ☐Adequate ☐Inadequate

Accuracy of interpretation: ☐Agree ☐Disagree ☐Unable to assess

Accuracy of interpretation as
compared to a gold standard: ☐Not performed ☐TP ☐TN ☐FP ☐FN

Comments:

Ultrasound evaluation of intussusception

Evidence

1. Summary/brief explanation of indication
   - Ultrasound has become the diagnostic test of choice in the evaluation of patients with suspected *ileocolic* intussusception.
   - In addition to making the diagnosis of intussusception, ultrasound can be utilized to determine if blood flow is still present to the affected bowel, or to identify free fluid, which may prognosticate the success of enema reduction.
2. Relevant adult-specific literature
   - While there are stark differences between the pathophysiology, presentation, and treatment of intussusception in adults and children, the sonographic findings remain the same. In one illustrative case report, an EM physician recognized classic signs of intussusception in a patient with chronic abdominal pain [157].
3. Relevant pediatric-specific literature
   - The use of ultrasound in the diagnosis of intussusception was initially described in 1977 [158]. Since then, the safety, ease, and accuracy of sonography have largely replaced plain radiographs as the initial screening modality [159, 160]. Sonography has since reported sensitivities of 98–100 % and specificities of 88–100 % when performed by imaging specialists [161–164].
   - Radiologists have noted that even junior residents can interpret the typical sonographic findings, often as well as their supervising attendings [161, 164].
   - There has been a single prospective, observational study involving POCUS for the evaluation of intussusception. Eighty-two patients underwent POCUS as well as ultrasound in the department of radiology. POCUS demonstrated a sensitivity of 85 % (95 % CI 54, 97 %) and a specificity of 97 % (95: 89, 99 %), suggesting that POCUS could be used to rule in a diagnosis of intussusception [165].
4. Outstanding questions to be answered/voids in the literature
   - Prospective studies from pediatric emergency centers are needed to determine what level of training is adequate to become competent in the use of bedside sonography as a screening tool for intussusception.
   - Evaluation is needed into outcome measures such as time to fluoroscopic reduction and emergency department length of stay when POCUS is used for the evaluation of intussusception.
   - With only a single observational study to date, further investigation is needed to characterize the performance characteristics of POCUS assessment of intussusception in different emergency settings.

Curriculum objectives

1. Describe the *indications* for POCUS for the evaluation of intussusception
   - POCUS is indicated for the evaluation of children presenting with clinical findings concerning for the presence of an *ileocolic* intussusception. These may include all or some combination of the following: vomiting, bloody or guaiac-positive stool, "currant jelly stool," colicky abdominal pain, or a sausage-shaped palpable mass on the *right side* of the abdomen.
2. Describe the *limitations* of POCUS for intussusception
   - *Ileocolic* intussusceptions may spontaneously reduce before or after the POCUS examination. In the former case, this will result in a missed diagnosis. In the latter case, a positive ultrasound examination will be followed by a negative barium or air enema study [166].
   - Positive identification of an intussusception may not address the presence of a pathologic lead point. These should be considered in patients who present outside the typical age range, or with a suggestive history or physical examination findings.
3. Describe the *relevant anatomy* to be identified in the POCUS examination for intussusception
   - The primary area of concern for an ileocolic intussusception is the ascending colon found in the right lateral abdomen. This is imaged in transverse and sagittal planes from the hepatic flexure down to the area of the ileocecal valve in the right lower quadrant. A normal appearing ileocecal valve rules out an ileocecal intussusception. When normal appearing colonic anatomy is not found, a further search along the path of the transverse and descending colon may be undertaken.
   - Sonographically, the intussusception has been described as a "target" or "doughnut" in transverse view, and as a "pseudokidney," or "hayfork" in an oblique or longitudinal view.
   - Small bowel intussusceptions may be encountered and should be distinguished from ileocolic intussusceptions. Beyond recognizing a normal appearing cecum, small bowel intussusceptions are also smaller and shorter in length.
   - Further evaluation of the intussusception is directed at the identification of signs suggesting advanced disease and, consequently, the unlikelihood of successful enema reduction. These include loculated free

fluid surrounding the intussusception, or "interloop" fluid within the intussusception. These findings are suggestive of bowel wall injury [167, 168]. Free intraperitoneal fluid has been noted with intussusception and is not associated with poor outcomes [169].

- Another sign of bowel wall ischemia is the absence of blood flow on color Doppler imaging. Several authors compared groups of patients with intact and absent flow, and found a decrease in the success of enema reduction in those patients without color flow [170, 171]. This is, however, not necessarily an absolute contraindication for attempted enema reduction [172].
- The presence of echogenic foci has been described in large bowel intussusceptions as well as in necrotizing enterocolitis [173, 174]. These foci, which are representative of air within the bowel wall, are suggestive of reduction failure and perforation.

4. Recognize specific *pitfalls* involved in the POCUS examination for intussusception.
   Pitfalls to avoid when performing a sonographic examination for intussusception include the following:

- Mistaking thickened bowel loops, stool or other abdominal masses for an intussusception.
- Imaging the bowel in only one plane or incompletely visualizing the posterior wall increases the chances of misinterpreting other abdominal masses as an intussusception. Always look for the "target sign" in cross section and the "pseudokidney" in long axis.
- Not recognizing the presence of poor prognostic findings prior to attempted enema reduction.
- Color Doppler assessment should only be performed by sonologists with experience in its use

Reporting Guideline for Ultrasound Evaluation of Intussusception

Patient Demographics:

Patient Name:
Patient Gender: ☐Male ☐Female

DOB: _/_/__
MR#:

Date & Time: _/_/___ _:_

Examination Demographics:

☐Initial Exam
☐Repeat Exam

Operator Name(s): ________

Operator Training: ☐Attending ☐Fellow ☐Resident ☐Medical Student ☐Other: ________

☐Patient consents to these images being used for educational purposes
☐Patient consents to these images being used for research purposes

Indication(s) for exam:

☐ Abdominal pain ☐ Abdominal mass ☐ Vomiting
☐ Bloody stool ☐ Altered mental status ☐ Educational
☐ Other: ____________

Views:

Short axis:	☐Adequate	☐Limited	☐Not obtained
Long axis:	☐Adequate	☐Limited	☐Not obtained

Findings:

Target sign (short axis)	☐Absent	☐Present	☐Indeterminate
Pseudokidney/Sandwich sign (long axis)	☐Absent	☐Present	☐Indeterminate
Trapped free fluid	☐Absent	☐Present	☐Indeterminate
Normal ileocecal valve/cecum	☐Absent	☐Present	☐Indeterminate

Interpretation:

☐Normal exam ☐ Intussusception ☐ Indeterminate

Quality assurance:

Image Quality: ☐Adequate ☐Inadequate ☐Indeterminate

Accuracy of interpretation: ☐Agree ☐Disagree ☐Unable to assess

Accuracy of interpretation as compared to a gold standard: ☐Not performed ☐TP ☐TN ☐FP ☐FN

Comments:

Ultrasound evaluation of the lung

Evidence

1. Summary/brief explanation of indications
   - POCUS can be incorporated into the evaluation of pediatric patients presenting with respiratory distress and/or hypoxemia to assess for the presence of pneumothorax, hemothorax, or pleural effusion [175–177].
   - The lungs can be evaluated sonographically in pediatric patients presenting with any respiratory symptoms or complaints to differentiate between pneumonia and bronchiolitis/viral pneumonia, as well as parapneumonic pleural effusion vs. empyema [175, 177].

2. Relevant adult-specific literature
   - POCUS detection of a pneumothorax in emergency department and intensive care unit patients has become highly prevalent, due to its high sensitivity and specificity [175, 178–182].
   - Pleural effusions: The sensitivity of POCUS for identifying pleural fluid has been shown to be 92 % with a specificity of 93–97 % [182]. POCUS can be used for thoracentesis-guidance/assistance of pleural effusions accurately [182].
   - Pneumonia: Several studies have looked at the ability of POCUS to detect pneumonia in the setting of critically ill patients. Results show a sensitivity of 88–90 % and a specificity of 95–98.5 % using CT as the reference standard [183, 184]. A study done by ED physicians demonstrated that POCUS had a sensitivity of 96.9 % (31/32) for diagnosing pneumonia, compared with that of only 75 % (24/32) for chest radiograph (CXR), with CT confirming pneumonia in 8 US-positive CXR-negative patients [185].

3. Relevant pediatric-specific literature
   - Pneumonia: There have been studies and a meta-analysis that examined the diagnosis of pneumonia by POCUS with high sensitivity and specificity [185–193]. An Italian study demonstrated that of 79 children with suspected pneumonia, 60 had pneumonia detected by ultrasound and 53 had CXR diagnosis of pneumonia; 4/7 which were US-positive and CXR-negative had CT confirmation of pneumonia and 3/7 had a clinical course consistent with bacterial pneumonia [186]. Another study of POCUS demonstrated 86 % sensitivity and 97 % specificity for detection of pneumonia confirmed by CXR [189]. A meta-analysis demonstrated a pooled sensitivity of 96 % (95 % CI 94–97 %) and specificity of 93 % (95 % CI 90–96 %); positive likelihood ratio of 15.3 (95 % CI 6.6–35.3) and negative likelihood ratio of 0.06 (95 % CI 0.03–0.11) [191]. Similar test performance characteristics (sensitivity 87 % [95 % CI 62–96 %] and specificity 94 % [95 % CI 88–97 %) for POCUS have been reported for Acute Chest Syndrome in children with Sickle Cell Disease [192]. Randomized controlled trial evidence suggests that lung ultrasound may be a feasible and safe substitute to chest radiography when evaluating children for pneumonia [193], which may benefit limited resource settings [194].
   - Bronchiolitis/viral pneumonia: Lung ultrasound findings for bronchiolitis/viral pneumonia have been described and characterized in children. In studies performed in children with a diagnosis of bronchiolitis or viral pneumonia, ultrasound findings consisted of small sub-pleural consolidations (typically 0.25 cm in depth) with associated pleural line abnormalities, single or confluent B lines [6, 195, 196]. In general, the presence of more sonographic findings in the lungs correlated with more severe bronchiolitis/viral pneumonia [195], and the need for supplemental oxygen [6]. These ultrasound findings were helpful in distinguishing bacterial versus viral pneumonia during the H1N1 influenza A epidemic in 2009 with high inter-observer agreement [196].
   - Pleural effusions: chest CT may be replaced by a POCUS with or without chest radiography in evaluating complex effusions/empyema [197].
   - Pneumothorax: ultrasound has been shown to be highly accurate to diagnose pneumothoraces in the neonatal ICU in 2 prospective observational studies [198, 199]. Ultrasound has also been reported to assist with needle aspiration of a spontaneous pneumothorax in a preterm infant [200] and in a series of pediatric ED patients by tracking the sonographic "lung point" [106, 201].
   - Other pulmonary pathologies: There are reports on the use of ultrasound in children to diagnose or distinguish among different pulmonary pathologies. These range from conditions such as respiratory distress syndrome (RDS) and transient tachypnea of the newborn (TTN) seen in the neonatal ICU [202], to others such as pulmonary contusions from trauma and chemical pneumonitis [203, 204], as well as different causes of wheezing in children [205].

4. Outstanding questions to be answered/voids in the literature to date
   - To date, no studies have evaluated if POCUS can be used to improve antibiotic stewardship when evaluating for pneumonia.
   - Serial lung POCUS evaluation may have a role in the management of ventilator-supported critically ill children and neonates.
   - Additional studies are needed to investigate the role of ultrasound in administration of surfactant and respiratory support in pre-term neonates, differentiating between lower respiratory tract infections, as well as causes of wheezing in infants and children.

Curriculum objectives

1. Describe the *indications* for lung POCUS
   - Pediatric trauma patients to assess for the presence of pneumothorax and hemothorax.
   - Patients presenting with respiratory symptoms to evaluate for pneumonia versus bronchiolitis/viral pneumonia and the presence of pleural effusion versus empyema.
   - Premature or full-term infants presenting with respiratory distress to assess for RDS and/or TTN [202].

2. Describe the *limitations* of lung POCUS
   - Lung ultrasound may not recognize centrally located pneumonias that do not abut the chest wall (1.5 % of cases) [184, 189].

3. Describe the *relevant anatomy* to be identified with lung POCUS
   - For a complete lung examination, each lung should be scanned in the longitudinal and transverse orientation in the mid-clavicular line anteriorly and posteriorly, and the mid-axillary line for a total of six scanning zones. One should scan superiorly and inferiorly from apices/clavicles to the diaphragm with liver on right, and the diaphragm and stomach or spleen on left are visualized [186, 189].
   - Different relevant lung ultrasound characteristics should be identified such as A lines, B lines, confluent B lines, lung sliding, and lung consolidations with air bronchograms and small subpleural consolidations (0.25 cm with no air bronchograms).
   - M-Mode may be used to confirm the presence or absence of lung sliding and a diagnosis of pneumothorax [175, 176].

4. Recognize specific *pitfalls* involved in lung POCUS
   Pitfalls to avoid when evaluating the lung include the following:
   - Care must be taken to identify the left diaphragm, as the combination of spleen and air in stomach may be mistaken for pneumonia (lung consolidation with air bronchograms) [189].
   - Mistaking pneumonia for thymus—thymus may appear as a lung consolidation on ultrasound but the absence of air bronchograms should differentiate tissue from pneumonia [189].
   - Turn image processing features off (e.g., tissue harmonic imaging, multi-beam imaging) when assessing for lung sliding or B lines.

*Discussion of ultrasound-guided thoracentesis can be found in the procedures section.

Reporting Guideline for Ultrasound Evaluation of the Lung

Patient Demographics:

Patient Name:
Patient Gender: ☐Male ☐Female

DOB: _/_/__
MR#:
Date & Time: _/_/__ _:_

Examination Demographics:

☐Initial Exam
☐Repeat Exam

Operator Name(s): ________

Operator Training: ☐Attending ☐Fellow ☐Resident ☐Medical Student ☐Other: ________

☐Patient consents to these images being used for educational purposes
☐Patient consents to these images being used for research purposes

Indication(s) for exam:

☐ Tachypnea ☐ Respiratory distress ☐ Chest pain
☐ Blunt trauma ☐ Penetrating trauma ☐ Hypoxia
☐ Educational ☐ Other: ____________

Views:

Right anterior thorax:	☐Adequate	☐Limited	☐Not obtained
Right lateral thorax:	☐Adequate	☐Limited	☐Not obtained
Right posterior thorax:	☐Adequate	☐Limited	☐Not obtained
Left anterior thorax:	☐Adequate	☐Limited	☐Not obtained
Left lateral thorax:	☐Adequate	☐Limited	☐Not obtained
Left posterior thorax:	☐Adequate	☐Limited	☐Not obtained

Findings:

Right Thorax:

Lung Sliding:	☐ Present	☐ Absent	☐ Indeterminate
Lung Point:	☐ Present	☐ Absent	☐ Indeterminate
Interstitium:			
A-lines:	☐ Present	☐ Absent	☐ Unable to assess
B-lines:	☐ Present	☐ Absent	☐ Unable to assess
Confluent B-line:	☐ Present	☐ Absent	☐ Unable to assess
Small Sub-pleural Consolidations (0.25 cm):	☐ Present	☐ Absent	☐ Indeterminate
Pleural effusion:	☐ Present	☐ Absent	☐ Unable to assess
Lung consolidation:	☐ Present	☐ Absent	☐ Unable to assess
Air bronchograms:	☐ Present	☐ Absent	☐ Unable to assess

Left Thorax:

Lung Sliding:	☐ Present	☐ Absent	☐ Indeterminate
Lung point sign:	☐ Present	☐ Absent	☐ Indeterminate
Interstitium:			
A-lines:	☐ Present	☐ Absent	☐ Unable to assess
B-lines:	☐ Present	☐ Absent	☐ Unable to assess
Confluent B-lines:	☐ Present	☐ Absent	☐ Unable to assess
Small Sub-pleural consolidations (0.25 cm):	☐ Present	☐ Absent	☐ Indeterminate
Pleural effusion:	☐ Present	☐ Absent	☐ Unable to assess
Lung consolidation:	☐ Present	☐ Absent	☐ Unable to assess
Air bronchograms:	☐ Present	☐ Absent	☐ Unable to assess

Interpretation:

☐Normal exam	☐Thoracic free fluid	☐Pneumothorax
☐Pneumonia	☐Bronchiolitis/Viral Pneumonia	☐Pleural Effusion
☐Atelectasis	☐ Other______	☐ Indeterminate

Quality assurance:

Image Quality:	☐Adequate	☐Inadequate			
Accuracy of interpretation:	☐Agree	☐Disagree	☐Unable to assess		
Accuracy of interpretation as compared to a gold standard:	☐Not performed	☐TP	☐TN	☐FP	☐FN

Comments:

Ultrasound evaluation of musculoskeletal pathology

Evidence

1. Summary/brief explanation of indication
   - In the setting of trauma, POCUS can be used to evaluate for fractures or soft tissue injuries. It also may be used to assess proper bone alignment after fracture reduction.
   - Joints can be visualized to assess for effusion, as well as to determine the best approach for and to guide arthrocentesis.
   - Tendons can be visualized after trauma to evaluate for rupture or tears.
2. Relevant adult-specific literature
   - Fractures:
     - A study done by Marshburn et al. showed that emergency physicians with minimal training were able to identify long bone fractures in adult trauma patients with better sensitivity than clinical impression (92.9 vs. 78.6 %) [206].
     - Detection of rib fractures is described in the radiology literature. Several of these studies show an increased sensitivity in detection of rib fractures by ultrasound as compared to X-ray [207, 208]. However, increased time and pain involved may outweigh the benefits of ultrasound in these settings.
     - Platon et al. compared ultrasound by a radiologist to CT for identifying scaphoid fractures in patients with normal initial radiographs. Their study showed that ultrasound detected 12 out of 13 (92 %) scaphoid fractures that were missed on X-ray, but identified on CT [209].
   - Joints:
     - There are several cases reported in the literature regarding emergency physician use of POCUS to identify hip and ankle joint effusions and to guide arthrocentesis [210–213].
     - There are also several descriptions of using ultrasound in the emergency setting to guide intra-articular blocks [214, 215].
   - Tendons:
     - A few case reports have been published describing the diagnosis of various tendon ruptures or tears using POCUS in the emergency department. Tendon injuries described include quadriceps rupture [216, 217], patellar tendon rupture [218, 219], triceps tear [220], hand injury with tendon laceration [221] and Achilles tendon rupture [222].
3. Relevant pediatric-specific literature
   - Fractures:
     - The best described applications in the pediatric literature include identification of long bone fractures [223–227] and using ultrasound as a tool in fracture reduction [228–231].
     - Hubner et al. [223] prospectively evaluated 163 children who underwent POCUS to evaluate for a suspected fracture. Ultrasound was most successful at identifying diaphyseal fractures of the humerus, femur, and forearm. Ultrasound was less accurate at identifying compound fractures, small-bone hand and foot fractures, and fractures close to joints.
     - In a prospective study of 130 pediatric patients, emergency providers used POCUS to evaluate the elbow, when there was concern for elbow injury. POCUS was used to identify abnormally positioned posterior fat pads and lipohemarthrosis. The study found 98 % sensitivity (95 % confidence interval [CI] 88–100 %) of POCUS to identify the presence of a fracture [232].
     - Weinberg et al. further reported on the accuracy of POCUS for identifying an elevated posterior fat pad as an indication of an elbow fracture. The study demonstrated a sensitivity of 80 % (95 % CI 51–95 %) and a specificity of 87 % (95 % CI 58–98 %) among emergency physicians with minimal training. In addition, none of the 212 pediatric patients reported any pain with the POCUS [226].
     - Studies looking at pain in ultrasound versus radiographs have found similar if not lower pain scores associated with POCUS [233–235].
     - POCUS has demonstrated accuracy when compared to radiography in identifying suspected forearm fractures [224, 235].
     - Effective ultrasound-guided fracture reduction of the forearm has been described [228–231]. Ultrasound for this purpose has the potential to reduce the number of X-rays, associated patient transport times, and limit the use of fluoroscopy. One limitation found by Dubrosvsky et al. was that although POCUS identified patients whose reduction was successful using fluoroscopy as criterion standard, it overestimated the number needing further reduction [231].
     - Additional fractures identified by POCUS in the pediatric literature include scaphoid [236], skull [237–239] and clavicle fractures [226, 233, 234].

- Joints:
    - Two case series describe the use of POCUS to evaluate children presenting with acute onset of limp or hip pain [211, 240]. In one study, POCUS and the history and physical examination were able to appropriately differentiate toxic synovitis from septic arthritis and osteomyelitis in all five children [240].
    - Vieira et al. [241] prospectively evaluated 28 patients who required hip ultrasonography as part of the emergency department evaluation. They determined the test characteristics of POCUS using ultrasounds performed in the Department of Radiology as the reference standard and found a sensitivity of 80 % (95 % CI 51, 95 %), and a specificity of 98 % (95 % CI 85, 99 %).
    - Rabiner et al. [242] prospectively evaluated the use of POCUS in patients suspected of having radial head subluxation. They determined that although some patients with radial head subluxation had abnormal posterior fat pads (14 %), if the POCUS showed no evidence of effusion or lipohemarthrosis, reduction maneuvers could be safely attempted even if there was an unclear history of injury. The "J-sign" is a technique for verifying radial head subluxation and demonstrating successful reduction that was derived prospectively [243]. More research is needed to compare diagnostic performance of these two techniques.
    - There is one case report describing the use of ultrasound-guided intra-articular lidocaine block to aid in shoulder reduction [244].

- Tendons:
    - To date, there are no published studies of POCUS for the evaluation of tendon injuries in pediatric patients. There are publications in orthopedic and rheumatologic journals regarding radiology-performed ultrasound to evaluate the patellar [245], Achilles [246], and wrist [247] tendons.

4. Outstanding questions to be answered/voids in the literature to date
    - Further prospective data collection is needed to clarify the utility of POCUS for the many potential musculoskeletal applications discussed above.
    - It remains unclear if POCUS should be utilized in lieu of other testing, or whether it is best used as a tool for the clinician to decide which subsequent imaging study to obtain or how urgently to obtain other imaging modalities.
    - More research is needed into the feasibility of teaching musculoskeletal POCUS to pediatric emergency physicians and exploring what is needed to achieve competence.

Curriculum objectives

Fractures

1. Describe the *indications* for POCUS for fracture evaluation
    - POCUS is indicated in the setting of trauma to evaluate for fracture, or post-reduction of a fracture to confirm satisfactory alignment prior to splinting/casting.

2. Describe the *limitations* of POCUS for fracture evaluation
    - Ultrasound has not been shown to be as effective as radiographs at identifying compound or small extremity bone fractures or fractures near joints.
    - Although frequently described as less painful than the positioning that is required for plain radiographs, pain during exam or lack of cooperation may limit the quality or feasibility of the POCUS study.

3. Describe the *relevant anatomy* to be identified with POCUS for fracture evaluation
    - Bones should be evaluated along their full length to evaluate the integrity of the cortex. A fracture will appear as a discontinuity in the cortex. In the case of a buckle fracture, this may be a small irregular bump in the cortical line.
    - Cartilage and growth plates are hypoechoic and may be confused for a cortical irregularity (or fracture) on POCUS.
    - Comparative ultrasound of the unaffected contralateral side is often helpful to differentiate fracture from normal anatomy.
    - Each bone should be evaluated separately and in at least two planes.

4. Recognize specific *pitfalls* involved in POCUS for fracture evaluation
    - Misdiagnosing a growth plate or cartilage as a fracture site. Evaluation of the unaffected contralateral side may prevent this error.
    - Mistaking a skull suture line as a fracture line. Sutures will lead to fontanelles if open, or will be in predictable anatomic locations.
    - Failure to perform a complete examination after identifying a single fracture. There may be an additional fracture present.
    - In the transverse plane, failure to scan the entire circumference of the bone along its entire length may lead to missing small non-displaced fractures.

- For longitudinal scanning, bones should be scanned through their entire length in two orthogonal planes.

Joints

1. Describe the *indications* for POCUS evaluation of joints
   - POCUS may be performed when a patient presents with joint pain or when there is suspicion for a joint effusion. This is especially useful in the evaluation of the pediatric hip joint in a child who presents with a limp.
   - POCUS should be used to guide arthrocentesis of the hip, and may be useful for arthrocentesis of other joints.
2. Describe the *limitations* of POCUS evaluation of joints
   - Pressure on the inflamed joint or movement of the joint during POCUS may cause discomfort or pain, and possibly limit images obtained in young children.
3. Describe the *relevant anatomy* to be identified with POCUS evaluation of joints
   - Affected joints should be compared to contralateral asymptomatic joints. In the evaluation of the hip joint, the anterior synovial recess (between the iliofemoral ligament anteriorly and the femoral neck posteriorly) is measured [248]. An effusion will usually appear hypoechoic, and a measurement of greater than 5 mm or a greater than a 2-mm difference from the contralateral hip indicates a positive examination [241].
4. Recognize specific *pitfalls* involved in POCUS evaluation of joints
   - Bilateral effusions will not allow for valid contralateral comparisons and may make the diagnosis of a joint effusion challenging.
   - Anterior synovial recess measurements vary with hip position. Therefore, it is important to ensure the same positioning in both the affected and contralateral normal leg so that measurements are consistent and accurate.
   - Patients may have symptomatic effusions that are smaller than the established parameters for pathology, and could lead to a false-negative exam [249].
   - Transducer pressure may obliterate effusions, especially if small or superficial.

Tendons

1. Describe the *indications* for POCUS evaluation of tendons
   - Tendon evaluation by POCUS is indicated when a patient presents with loss of function normally attributed to a given tendon (flex/extend), penetrating trauma in the region of tendon path, or other signs concerning for a tendon injury.
2. Describe the *limitations* of POCUS evaluation of tendons
   - Location, particularly the depth of various tendons may limit the ability to use POCUS as a diagnostic tool.
3. Describe the *relevant anatomy* to be identified with POCUS evaluation of tendons
   - The tendon should be evaluated along its length to look for discontinuity, retraction, thickening, thinning, changes in the architecture or effusions around the tendon.
   - Tendons should be evaluated in longitudinal and transverse views. The contralateral side should be evaluated for comparison.
   - It is important to be aware of the sonographic difference between tendons with and without sheaths. Normal tendons with sheaths (wrist and ankle tendons) will appear hyperechoic with a 1–2 mm hypoechoic rim of sheath. Tendons without sheaths (Achilles, patellar) are hyperechoic without the hypoechoic encasing [249].
4. Recognize specific *pitfalls* involved in POCUS evaluation of tendons
   - A hematoma or edema may distort the sonographic view of a tendon.
   - Knowledge of whether the tendon being imaged is covered by a synovial sheath or dense connective tissue is important to evaluate for tendonitis, tear or rupture. (i.e., in tendonitis, those surrounded by a synovial sheath will have fluid within the sheath, causing a hypoechoic rim around the tendon greater than 2 mm. Those without sheaths will manifest tendonitis with tendon thickening. With a partial tear of sheathed tendons, ultrasound may have anechoic clefts in the tendon and effusion in the sheath in contrast to tendons without sheaths, which will appear as a hypoechoic defect within the tendon [248].
   - Healthy tendons display anisotropy: tendon fibers appear anechoic if the incident ultrasound beam is not perpendicular to the long axis of the fibers. At sites of injury, tendons lose their characteristic anisotropy.

*Discussion of ultrasound-guided arthrocentesis can be found in the procedures section.

Reporting Guidelines for Ultrasound Evaluation of Musculoskeletal Pathology

Patient Demographics:

Patient Name:
Patient Gender: ☐Male ☐Female

DOB: __/__/____
MR#:
Date & Time: __/__/____ __:__

Examination Demographics:

☐Initial Exam
☐Repeat Exam

Operator Name(s): ________

Operator Training: ☐Attending ☐Fellow ☐Resident ☐Medical Student
☐Other: ________

☐Patient consents to these images being used for educational purposes
☐Patient consents to these images being used for research purposes

Indication(s) for exam:

☐ Swelling ☐ Mass ☐ Decreased range of motion
☐ Redness ☐ Deformity ☐ Pain
☐ Fever ☐ Educational ☐ Procedural
☐ Other: ___________

Views:

Anatomy scanned: ☐Clavicle ☐Forearm ☐Hip ☐Knee
☐Other Extremity:____
☐Other Joint:____
☐Other:____

Affected side:
Muscle: ☐Adequate ☐Limited ☐Not obtained
Tendon: ☐Adequate ☐Limited ☐Not obtained
Joint: ☐Adequate ☐Limited ☐Not obtained
Bone: ☐Adequate ☐Limited ☐Not obtained

Contralateral side:
Muscle: ☐Adequate ☐Limited ☐Not obtained
Tendon: ☐Adequate ☐Limited ☐Not obtained
Joint: ☐Adequate ☐Limited ☐Not obtained
Bone: ☐Adequate ☐Limited ☐Not obtained

Findings:

Affected side:
Muscle Appearance: ☐Normal ☐Irregular ☐Indeterminate
Muscle Disruption: ☐None ☐Partial ☐Complete

Tendon Appearance: ☐Normal ☐Irregular ☐Indeterminate
Tendon Disruption: ☐None ☐Partial ☐Complete ☐Indeterminate

Joint: ☐Fluid ☐No fluid ☐Indeterminate
Maximal joint space: _____ mm
Contralateral joint space: ______ mm
Difference in joint space: _____ mm

Bone Appearance ☐Normal ☐Irregular ☐Indeterminate
Bone Disruption ☐None ☐Aligned ☐Angulated ☐Indeterminate
Bone post-reduction: ☐Aligned ☐Angulated ☐Other: _______ ☐Indeterminate

Interpretation:

☐Normal exam ☐ Joint effusion ☐Tendon injury ☐Muscle injury
☐Fracture ☐ Other:______ ☐Indeterminate

Quality assurance:

Image Quality: ☐Adequate ☐Inadequate

Accuracy of interpretation: ☐Agree ☐Disagree ☐Unable to assess
Accuracy of interpretation as compared to a gold standard: ☐Not performed ☐TP ☐TN ☐FP ☐FN

Comments:

Ultrasound evaluation of the female pelvis

Evidence

1. Summary/brief explanation of indications
   - The female reproductive organs can be visualized sonographically in non-pregnant pediatric females who present with abdominal pain for the evaluation of ovarian cysts, pelvic inflammatory disorder (PID)/tubo-ovarian abscess (TOA), and ovarian torsion.
2. Relevant adult-specific literature
   - Pelvic inflammatory disorder (PID)/tubo-ovarian abscess (TOA):
     - A prospective study demonstrated that a POCUS bimanual examination performed with an endovaginal transducer in place of the internal examining hand (i.e., the sonographic bimanual examination,) was able to provide higher confidence in clinical assessment of uterine and adnexal tenderness than traditional digital bimanual examination in patients, regardless of body mass index (BMI) [250].
     - Adhikari et al. demonstrated that POCUS was able to diagnose TOA in non-pregnant patients who presented with pelvic pain [251]. Of the 20 study patients, ranging from 14 to 45 years old, 14 (70 %) patients had a complex adnexal mass, 5 (25 %) patients had echogenic fluid in the cul-de-sac, and 3 (15 %) patients had pyosalpinx identified on POCUS.
     - TOAs have been traditionally diagnosed on pelvic ultrasounds performed in the department of radiology, with a sensitivity of 93 % and specificity of 98 % [252]. POCUS has been shown to be less sensitive (56–93 %) and specific (83–98 %) in the diagnosis, suggesting that POCUS evaluation of TOA should be used judiciously [253].
   - Ovarian torsion:
     - There are case reports of emergency physicians diagnosing ovarian torsion using POCUS [254, 255].
3. Relevant pediatric-specific literature
   - There is currently no literature specifically evaluating the utility of POCUS in the evaluation of ovarian cysts, pelvic inflammatory disorder or ovarian torsion in the pediatric population. However, data may be extrapolated from the studies conducted in adult patients, as many of them included adolescents in the study population, which represents the majority of the population affected by these conditions [251, 253].
4. Outstanding questions to be answered/voids in the literature to date
   - As noted, there are no published data on the use of POCUS for assessing ovarian cysts, PID, TOA, and ovarian torsion among children. The majority of the data are drawn from the adult population. There are also limited data on how pelvic POCUS might be incorporated into medical decision making. Currently, there are no guidelines or protocols.

Curriculum objectives

1. Describe the *indications* for the gynecologic POCUS examination
   - When ovarian or other gynecologic pathology is suspected such as in a female with lower abdominal pain, vaginal bleeding, or discharge.
   - A ruptured ectopic pregnancy should be strongly suspected in a post-menarchal females with hypotension, syncope, and a positive pregnancy test.
2. Describe the *limitations* of the gynecologic POCUS examination
   - Operator ability in consistently identifying normal ovaries, and in identifying and diagnosing other pelvic masses within the pelvis, particularly in patients with a retroverted uterus.
   - Limited ability to rule out the diagnosis of ovarian torsion by POCUS, due to the fact that blood flow in the involved ovary does not exclude the diagnosis of ovarian torsion. It is difficult to demonstrate both venous and arterial waveforms in all cases and torsion may be intermittent, demonstrating variability in detectable blood flow on color Doppler.
3. Describe the *relevant anatomy* to be identified with the gynecologic POCUS examination
   - Pediatric gynecology can be evaluated either in a trans-abdominal, transperineal/translabial, or trans-vaginal approach. However, the trans-vaginal approach should be avoided in pre-coital, prepubescent females.
   - The bladder appears as a well-circumscribed, rectangular, fluid-filled, anechoic structure in the transverse plane. The cervix can be visualized just posterior to the bladder with the body of the uterus and uterine stripe cephalad and the vaginal stripe caudal to the cervix. The uterus appears as an isoechoic structure with thick walls and a well-defined border. Retained mucous secretions prior to ovulation may make the endometrium appear heterogeneously echogenic and should not be confused with intrauterine tumors. If an intrauterine

device (IUD) is in place, this will typically appear as a hyperechoic linear structure with reverberation artifact. An appropriate location within the body of the uterus, not perforating the myometrium, should be confirmed. The posterior cul-de-sac, or Pouch of Douglas, is posterior to the uterus and may be the site of free fluid collection. A small amount of physiologic free fluid is acceptable, but clinical correlation is advised. Ovaries appear as isoechoic to hypoechoic structures containing multiple anechoic follicles, giving an appearance similar to that of a 'chocolate chip cookie.'

- Ovarian cysts: Simple cysts of less than a centimeter in diameter are defined as ovarian follicles. Simple cysts should be anechoic, smooth walled structures with posterior acoustic enhancement. More complex appearances may be due to hemorrhagic cysts, which may have varying appearances depending on the stage of the clot. Complex, multiloculated cysts require further evaluation with follow-up US or MRI.
- Pelvic inflammatory disorder (PID)/tubo-ovarian abscess (TOA): The normal fallopian tube is not always visible on ultrasound. PID can present with a thickened tubular adnexal structure that is representative of an inflamed fallopian tube. Edematous walls and endosalpingeal folds have been described as the 'cogwheel sign.' A blocked fallopian tube may become dilated and fill with fluid, showing a hydrosalpinx or pyosalpinx. A TOA may cause loss of the architectural definition of the adnexa, with multiple thick-walled, dilated fluid-filled structures that contain fluid-debris and air-fluid levels.
- Ovarian torsion: A torsed ovary will often appear enlarged, amorphous and hypoechoic due to edema from obstruction of lymphatic and venous drainage. Free fluid may be present in the pelvis. Doppler evaluation of the ovary and any adjacent masses should be performed. The whirlpool sign is a dynamic sign demonstrated by placing the ultrasound transducer at right angles to the axis of the ovarian pedicle and fanning it to and fro. The whirlpool sign appears as "a clockwise or counterclockwise wrapping of the hypoechoic ovarian vessels around the central axis" of the pedicle [256]. The ovaries have a dual blood supply and many articles have described normal Doppler flow with torsion [257, 258]. However, studies consistently reveal that venous flow is lost before arterial flow; therefore, optimizing power Doppler settings to detect venous flow significantly enhances the ability to identify partial or early torsion.

4. Recognize specific *pitfalls* with the gynecologic POCUS evaluation
    - Failure to ensure a full bladder for use as an acoustic window in the transabdominal view and an empty bladder for the endovaginal examination.
    - Failure to recognize an enlarged ovary as ovarian torsion, until proven otherwise, despite the presence of blood flow.
    - Misidentifying uterine vasculature as a thin-walled hydrosalpinx on cross-sectional image planes. Doppler evaluation can usually resolve this issue.
    - Misidentifying bowel loops for ovarian or other adnexal structures.
    - Failure to identify abnormal adnexal masses and/or significant pathologic ovarian abnormalities

Reporting Guideline for Ultrasound Evaluation of the Female Pelvis

Patient Demographics:

Patient Name:
Patient Gender: ☐Female

DOB: _/_/___
MR#:
Date & Time: _/_/___ _:_

Examination Demographics:

☐Initial Exam
☐Repeat Exam

Operator Name(s): ________

Operator Training: ☐Attending ☐Fellow ☐Resident ☐Medical Student ☐Other: ________

☐Patient consents to these images being used for educational purposes
☐Patient consents to these images being used for research purposes

Indication(s) for exam:

☐ Vaginal bleeding ☐ Vaginal discharge ☐ Pelvic pain
☐ Abdominal pain ☐ Back pain ☐ Syncope
☐ Hypotension ☐ Educational ☐ Other: ____________

Views obtained:

Trans-abdominal sagittal	☐Adequate	☐Limited	☐Not obtained
Trans-abdominal transverse	☐Adequate	☐Limited	☐Not obtained
Endo-vaginal sagittal	☐Adequate	☐Limited	☐Not obtained
Endo-vaginal coronal	☐Adequate	☐Limited	☐Not obtained
Cul-de-sac	☐Adequate	☐Limited	☐Not obtained
Left adnexa	☐Adequate	☐Limited	☐Not obtained
Right adnexa	☐Adequate	☐Limited	☐Not obtained
Hepatorenal space	☐Adequate	☐Limited	☐Not obtained

Findings:

Uterus: ☐Anteroverted ☐Retroverted ☐Indeterminate

Endometrium :
☐Endometrial stripe thickness: ____mm
☐Heterogeneous material present
☐Fibroid present
☐Indeterminate

Cul-de-sac fluid:	☐Absent	☐Present	☐Indeterminate
Qualitative amount:	☐Small	☐Moderate	☐Large
Hepato-renal space fluid	☐Absent	☐Present	☐Indeterminatc
Qualitative amount:	☐Small	☐Moderate	☐Large

<u>R adnexa</u>

Ovarian Cyst	☐Absent	☐Present	☐Indeterminate
Ovarian measurement: ____mm			
Ovarian mass	☐Absent	☐Present	☐Indeterminate
Color Doppler color flow	☐Absent	☐Present	☐Indeterminate
Power Doppler color flow	☐Absent	☐Present	☐Indeterminate

<u>L adnexa</u>

Ovarian Cyst	☐Absent	☐Present	☐Indeterminate
Ovarian measurement: ____mm			
Ovarian mass	☐Absent	☐Present	☐Indeterminate
Color Doppler color flow	☐Absent	☐Present	☐Indeterminate
Power Doppler color flow	☐Absent	☐Present	☐Indeterminate

<u>Interpretation:</u>

☐Normal exam ☐Simple Ovarian cyst ☐Complex Ovarian cyst ☐Adnexal mass
☐Fibroid ☐Pelvic free fluid ☐Peritoneal free fluid
☐Pelvic inflammatory disease ☐Tubo-ovarian abscess
☐Ovarian torsion ☐Other: ____ ☐Indeterminate

<u>Quality assurance:</u>

Image Quality: ☐Adequate ☐Inadequate

Accuracy of interpretation: ☐Agree ☐Disagree ☐Unable to assess

Accuracy of interpretation as compared to a gold standard: ☐Not performed ☐TP ☐TN ☐FP ☐FN

Comments:

Ultrasound evaluation of the pelvis in the first trimester of pregnancy

Evidence

1. Summary/brief explanation of indications
   - The female reproductive organs can be sonographically visualized in adolescent females who present with abdominal pain or vaginal bleeding in their first trimester of pregnancy. The primary indication for clinician-performed sonographic evaluation of the female pelvis in the first-trimester pregnancy is in the identification of an intrauterine pregnancy; thereby, effectively excluding ectopic pregnancy in the vast majority of patients. There are some defined groups of patients at high risk for ectopic pregnancy in whom this approach is not adequate to exclude ectopic/heterotopic pregnancy. POCUS in the evaluation of first-trimester pregnancy can also be used to determine fetal heart rate, gestational age, and identification of abdominal free fluid. With higher levels of training and experience, point-of-care ultrasound may also assist in the diagnosis of intrauterine demise, anembryonic gestation, gestational trophoblastic disease, various abortion states (inevitable, incomplete, complete, etc.) and adnexal pathology.

2. Relevant adult-specific literature
- IUP:
    - Jang et al. assessed the learning curve of emergency physicians for first-trimester pregnancy POCUS and found that the sensitivity and specificity for identifying an IUP were 80 and 86 %, respectively, for their first 10 examinations, and increased to 100 % sensitivity and specificity after performing 40 examinations [259].
    - McRae et al. conducted a systematic review which demonstrated that POCUS was able to identify a definitive intrauterine pregnancy with a sensitivity of 90 % and a specificity of 98 % in women presenting with pelvic pain and/or bleeding during their first trimester of pregnancy [260].
    - In patients in whom an IUP was determined by bedside ultrasound, the ED length of stay was 21–28 % shorter than when ultrasound was performed by the department of radiology [261]. In a more recent study, patients who received bedside ultrasonography for complications of first-trimester pregnancy had more than 2 h of time savings in average length of stay whether they received transabdominal ultrasound (2.8 h lower length of stay) or transvaginal ultrasound (2.2 h no length of stay). In both cases, this represented a greater than 35 % decrease in length of stay for patients receiving POCUS [262].
- Ectopic pregnancy:
    - A meta-analysis by Stein et al. demonstrated that emergency physicians were able to screen for an ectopic pregnancy with POCUS with a sensitivity of 99.3 %, negative predictive value of 99.96 % and a negative likelihood ratio of 0.08 across a wide variety of practice environments [263].
    - Moore et al. found that in patients with suspected ectopic pregnancies on pelvic POCUS, free intraperitoneal fluid found in Morison's pouch could be rapidly identified by POCUS and was predictive of the need for operative management, with a positive likelihood ratio of 112 [264].
    - Tayal et al. found that earlier identification of an indeterminate POCUS pelvic ultrasound with the eventual diagnosis of an ectopic pregnancy had a higher rate of medical methotrexate treatment and a reduced rate of invasive surgical treatment (36 vs. 83 %) compared with ectopic pregnancy patients diagnosed at initial ED visit [265]. The generally accepted "discriminatory zone", or minimal level of β-HCG at which the first sign of an intrauterine pregnancy (a double decidual sac) can be sonographically visualized, is 1500 mIU/ml. However, many ectopic pregnancies present with β-HCG levels less than 1500 mIU/ml, and many of these have sonographic evidence of ectopic pregnancy [266–269]. Furthermore, many point-of-care sonologists consider the double decidual sac insufficiently specific to rule in intrauterine pregnancy definitively, and the discriminatory zone *cannot* be extrapolated to expected levels at which any of the more definitive sonographic signs of IUP such as yolk sac, fetal pole, or cardiac motion should be seen. These considerations argue that POCUS pelvic ultrasounds should be performed regardless of β-HCG levels in any pregnant patient with a suspicion for ectopic pregnancy.
- Heterotopic pregnancy is much more prevalent in women who have received ovarian induction therapy, and may be diagnosed by POCUS [270]. Although the primary focus of clinician-performed ultrasonography in first-trimester pregnancy is the identification of intrauterine gestation, it is prudent to evaluate the adnexa for signs of heterotopic pregnancy even after an IUP has been identified. Women who have received assistive reproductive therapies should always be evaluated for the presence of ectopic or heterotopic pregnancy even when an IUP is identified. Since identification of extrauterine pregnancy is not a primary indication of the POCUS evaluation, this examination should usually be performed by imaging specialists.
- When POCUS does not identify a definitive IUP (absence of gestational sac with a yolk sac or fetal pole), timely follow-up by gynecologists and/or further ultrasonography by imaging specialists will be required. If the POCUS is suggestive of an ectopic pregnancy (tubal ring, adnexal mass, pseudogestational sac, free fluid in the abdomen, endometrial mantle measuring less than 5–8 mm concerning for an interstitial pregnancy), patients should undergo urgent ultrasonography by imaging specialists and gynecology consultation [271, 272].
- The use of POCUS has demonstrated decreased time to surgery for ectopic pregnancies, shortened lengths of ED stay for patients with normal pregnancies, and decreased number of return ED visits with a subsequent ruptured ectopic [260, 273].

3. Relevant pediatric-specific literature
   - The use of POCUS in pregnant pediatric patients between the ages of 13–21 years old reduced ED length of stay from 149 min (range 7–506 min) to 82 min (range 1–901 min) ($p < 0.001$) when an intrauterine pregnancy was identified on POCUS as compared to when ultrasound was performed by the department of radiology [274].
   - There have been limited studies to date specifically evaluating the application of POCUS in adolescents who present to a pediatric ED with first-trimester pregnancy complaints to differentiate between an IUP and an ectopic pregnancy as well as to diagnose a threatened abortion. However, with further training and credentialing, it is likely that pediatric point-of-care sonologists will attain similar accuracy in identifying and managing first-trimester pregnancy as their colleagues in the adult ED.
4. Outstanding questions to be answered/voids in the literature to date
   - Published data on the use of POCUS in the pediatric ED in assessing adolescents with first-trimester pregnancy are limited.
   - There are no data in children, and limited data in adults regarding the use of POCUS as an adjunct in the evaluation of other common emergency gynecological conditions, such as pelvic inflammatory disease and ovarian torsion.

Curriculum objectives

1. Describe the *indications* for POCUS in first-trimester pregnancy
   - Indications for first-trimester POCUS include evaluation for IUP, identification of yolk sac, fetal pole, detection of fetal heart rate, determination of gestational age, and identification of abdominal free fluid. Understand the principle of exclusion of ectopic pregnancy by identification of IUP.
2. Describe the *limitations* for POCUS in first-trimester pregnancy
   - Limitations include the ability to rule out ectopic pregnancy when ultrasound does not show definitive evidence of an IUP. In this case, an 'indeterminate' exam revealing an empty uterus or a nonspecific intrauterine sac or endometrial fluid collection/echogenic material requires correlation with the patient's quantitative beta hCG and other clinical findings.
   - Patients who have undergone assisted reproductive technology are at high risk for heterotopic pregnancies, and, therefore, require an ultrasound examination by the imaging specialists to rule out the presence of an ectopic pregnancy.
   - POCUS is not sufficient for identifying or ruling out fetal anomalies or for evaluating pelvic anatomy after vaginal-rectal surgery.
3. Describe the *relevant anatomy*/findings to be identified with POCUS in first-trimester pregnancy
   - First-trimester pregnancy should be evaluated in a transabdominal and/or transvaginal approach, depending on clinician training, the availability of equipment, and the gestational age of the fetus
     - Transvaginal ultrasound can identify an intrauterine pregnancy at approximately 5 weeks gestation, and transabdominal ultrasound can identify an intrauterine pregnancy at approximately 6–7 weeks gestation.
   - The first sonographic confirmation of an IUP is the yolk sac at 5–6 weeks, followed by an embryo with cardiac activity at 6 weeks, and finally a fetal pole at approximately 7 weeks. An intradecidual sac can be seen at 4–5 weeks, followed by a double decidual sac at 5 weeks; however, neither of these definitively confirms the diagnosis of an IUP.
   - If the pregnancy is intrauterine, the endomyometrial mantle should be measured. An endomyometrial mantle thickness of at least 5–8 mm is considered normal and minimizes the risk of an interstitial or cornual ectopic pregnancy.
   - In most cases, transabdominal sonography is facilitated by the presence of a full bladder. Conversely, transvaginal ultrasonography is generally easier with empty bladder. The bladder should be identified as a well-circumscribed, fluid-filled, anechoic structure. The uterus appears as a hypoechoic structure with thick walls and a well-defined border. In a typical anteroverted and anteroflexed uterus, the cervix appears just posterior to the bladder angle with the uterine body superior to the bladder and the vaginal stripe immediately posterior to the bladder in the sagittal view. The rectouterine cul-de-sac, or Pouch of Douglas, is posterior to the cervix and may be the site of free fluid collection. The ovaries may be visualized lateral to the uterus on either side and appear as isoechoic to hypoechoic structures containing multiple anechoic follicles. The ovaries should be identified in two orthogonal planes, where possible. This may be limited by the patient's habitus, bowel gas, pelvic anatomy, sonologist skill, or the quality of the ultrasound machine.
   - Depending on the sonographic size, certain presets on the ultrasound machine may allow for gestational dating based on crown-rump length.

- If cardiac activity is noted, M-Mode can be used to measure the fetal heart rate. Doppler should not be used in the first trimester to determine fetal heart rate, as this carries a theoretical risk of exposing the fetus to excessive levels of ultrasound energy with the potential for fetal damage and birth defects.
- In addition to evaluating for an intrauterine pregnancy, the pelvis should be interrogated for evidence of free fluid.
- In unstable patients, the right upper quadrant (Morison's pouch) should also be evaluated as free fluid in this area in a pregnant female should be considered as a ruptured ectopic pregnancy with significant hemorrhage until proven otherwise.

4. Recognize specific *pitfalls* involved in performing POCUS in first-trimester pregnancy

- Attributing an empty uterus to a very early IUP, an ectopic pregnancy, or a completed spontaneous abortion (all of these entities are possible in the "indeterminate exam").
- Mistaking a nonspecific intrauterine sac or a pseudogestational sac for a gestational sac.
- Incorrectly identifying a pregnancy as within the uterus, when in fact it is outside the uterus or interstitial.
- Failure to consider or to identify heterotopic pregnancy.
- Misidentifying an adnexal mass for an ectopic pregnancy.
- Failure to identify an embryonic demise, or diagnosing embryonic demise in a live IUP.
- Failure to perform a POCUS study when the βHCG is below 1500 mIU/L

Reporting Guideline for Ultrasound Evaluation of the Pelvis in the First Trimester of Pregnancy

Patient Demographics:

Patient Name:
Patient Gender: ☐Female

DOB: _/_/___
MR#:
Date & Time: _/_/___ _:_

Examination Demographics:

☐Initial Exam
☐Repeat Exam

Operator Name(s): ________

Operator Training: ☐Attending ☐Fellow ☐Resident ☐Medical Student
☐Other: ________

☐Patient consents to these images being used for educational purposes
☐Patient consents to these images being used for research purposes

Indication(s) for exam:

☐b-HCG Positive	☐Pregnant by history	☐Abdominal pain
☐Vaginal bleeding	☐Pelvic pain	☐Hypotension
☐Syncope	☐Educational	☐Other:_____________

Views:

Trans-abdominal sagittal	☐Adequate	☐Limited	☐Not obtained
Trans-abdominal transverse	☐Adequate	☐Limited	☐Not obtained
Endo-vaginal sagittal	☐Adequate	☐Limited	☐Not obtained
Endo-vaginal coronal	☐Adequate	☐Limited	☐Not obtained
Cul-de-sac	☐Adequate	☐Limited	☐Not obtained
Left adnexa	☐Adequate	☐Limited	☐Not obtained
Right adnexa	☐Adequate	☐Limited	☐Not obtained
Hepatorenal space	☐Adequate	☐Limited	☐Not obtained

Findings:

Intrauterine pregnancy:	☐Absent	☐Present	☐Indeterminate
Appearance:	☐Double decidual sign		
	☐Gestational sac		
	☐Yolk sac		
	☐Fetal pole		
	☐Fetal pole with heart rate		

Fetal heart rate:____bpm
Gestational Age:____

Cul-de-sac fluid:	☐Absent	☐Present	☐Indeterminate
Qualitative amount:	☐Small	☐Moderate	☐Large
Hepato-renal space fluid	☐Absent	☐Present	☐Indeterminate
Qualitative amount:	☐Small	☐Moderate	☐Large
Molar pregnancy:	☐Absent	☐Present	☐Indeterminate
Simple ovarian cyst:	☐Absent	☐Present	☐Indeterminate
	☐Right	☐Left	
Adenexal mass:	☐Absent	☐Present	☐Indeterminate
	☐Right	☐Left	

Interpretation:

☐IUP	☐No IUP	☐Fetal Demise
☐Molar pregnancy	☐Ectopic pregnancy	☐Simple Ovarian cyst
☐Adnexal mass	☐Pelvic free fluid	☐Peritoneal free fluid
☐Other: ____	☐Indeterminate	

Quality assurance:

Image Quality: ☐Adequate ☐Inadequate

Accuracy of interpretation: ☐Agree ☐Disagree ☐Unable to assess

Accuracy of interpretation as compared to a gold standard: ☐Not performed ☐TP ☐TN ☐FP ☐FN

Comments:

Ultrasound evaluation of pyloric stenosis

Evidence

1. Summary/brief explanation of indication
   - The pylorus can be evaluated sonographically in infants in whom there is clinical concern for idiopathic hypertrophic pyloric stenosis (HPS).
   - The typical history includes non-bilious, projectile vomiting in a one-month old infant shortly after feeding. The classic physical exam finding of a palpable "olive" and the laboratory findings of hypochloremic hypokalemic metabolic alkalosis are not commonly seen [275–279].
2. Relevant pediatric-specific literature
   - Ultrasound has been utilized by radiologists to diagnose HPS since 1977 and is now the primary modality used to diagnose HPS [280].
   - Recent literature describes the ability of both emergency physicians [281] and resident surgeons [282, 283] to accurately diagnose HPS by bedside ultrasonography.

- A prospective study of PEM fellows and a PEM attending physician found 100 % (95 % CI 62–100 %) sensitivity and 100 % (95 % CI 92–100 %) specificity when evaluating patients with suspected HPS, with measurements of pyloric muscle wall width and length that were not statistically different ($p = 0.50$ and $p = 0.79$, respectively) from those of Radiology specialists [284].

3. Outstanding questions to be answered/voids in the literature
   - Literature from the emergency medicine and surgery publications describes either small case series, or high probability patients. The test characteristics of POCUS in the evaluation of the pylorus for HPS require continued evaluation.
   - Variable measurements have been used in radiology texts to establish the diagnosis for HPS [285–289]. There is currently no definitive consensus regarding absolute measurements.

Curriculum objectives

1. Describe the *indications* for sonography for HPS
   - The sonographic evaluation for pyloric stenosis should be considered in young infants with non-bilious emesis.
2. Describe the *limitations* of the pyloric examination
   - Difficulty with pyloric visualization may arise from gastric over-distention, which may displace the pylorus posteriorly.
   - Gastric air or bowel gas may cause shadowing artifact over the area of interest.
3. Describe the *relevant anatomy* to be identified in the examination of the pylorus
   - The pyloric muscle is in continuity with the gastric wall and arises to the right of midline. Using the liver as a sonographic window, the gastric wall is identified overlaying a gas and/or fluid-filled stomach. The gastric wall is then traced caudally to the right of midline along the lesser curvature of the stomach until it meets the pyloric antrum.
   - The beginning of the pyloric antrum is identified by the incisura angularis, which appears like a notch in the gastric wall's serosal surface.
   - The distal end of the pylorus is identified by the interface between the pyloric sphincter and the first portion of the duodenum or duodenal cap. The appearance is dependent on whether the pyloric sphincter and/or channel muscles are relaxed or contracted. However, the thicker muscle wall of the pylorus is easily recognized in contrast to the thinner-walled duodenum. Another notch in the wall, the duodenal pyloric constriction, may also be noted at this junction.
   - Diagnostic measurements include the pyloric muscle thickness and the pyloric channel length. A pyloric muscle thickness of less than 2 mm is considered normal, between 2 and 2.9 mm seen in both normal and pylorospasm, and greater than 3 mm considered diagnostic of HPS [285, 286, 290, 291]. The channel length may be difficult to measure in a normal patient and is less consistent than the more easily appreciated pyloric muscle thickness. The channel length is considered abnormal if it is greater than 15 mm [290, 292–294]. Both measurements should occur in tandem, and caution would be prudent if only a thickness or length measurement was abnormal.
   - A normal pylorus allows gastric contents to pass through the relaxed pyloric canal with gastric peristalsis. The normal pylorus may also be transiently thickened, but returns to normal thickness after muscular contraction in contrast to HPS, where the pylorus is continuously thickened. These observations may require viewing the pylorus for 5–10 min. Wall relaxation and distention with passage of gastric contents are not seen with pyloric stenosis.
   - In addition to the abnormal measurements, other sonographic signs seen in HPS include the "antral nipple" sign seen in long-axis view where the opposed mucosa layers project back into the antrum, the "shoulder" sign, created by the circular pyloric muscle similarly projecting into the antrum, and the "donut" or "target" sign seen when the pylorus is viewed in cross section. In addition, there is failure of gastric contents to pass through the pyloric channel when visualized in real time.
4. Recognize specific *pitfalls* involved in POCUS of the pylorus.
   Pitfalls to avoid when performing the pyloric examination include the following:
   - Pylorospasm and/or normal pyloric peristaltic contraction may mimic HPS findings. With borderline measurements, the area should be observed for 5–10 min to observe for pyloric relaxation and passage of gastric contents (thereby excluding HPS).
   - Misidentification of gastric or duodenal wall for the pyloric wall may result in a false-negative exam.
   - Tangential measurements may erroneously exaggerate pyloric thickness.
   - Non-visualization of the pylorus secondary to gastric air, or a posterior position from gastric distention may prevent an effective evaluation. Positioning the patient in a right or left decubitus oblique position (respectively) may facilitate imaging.

- A struggling or crying infant makes examination much more challenging. Gel should be at ambient temperature and a pacifier dipped in sucrose-water solution may be helpful. The patient may be examined in the arms of family

Reporting Guideline for Ultrasound Evaluation for Pyloric Stenosis

Patient Demographics:

Patient Name:
Patient Gender: ☐Male ☐Female

DOB: _/_/__
MR#:
Date & Time: _/_/__ _:_
Examination Demographics:

☐Initial Exam
☐Repeat Exam

Operator Name(s): ________

Operator Training: ☐Attending ☐Fellow ☐Resident ☐Medical Student
☐Other: ________

☐Patient consents to these images being used for educational purposes
☐Patient consents to these images being used for research purposes

Indication(s) for exam:

☐ Projectile non-bilious vomiting ☐ Progressive vomiting
☐ Vomiting with weight loss ☐ Educational ☐ Other: ____________

Views:

Pylorus short axis:	☐Adequate	☐Limited	☐Not obtained
Pylorus long axis:	☐Adequate	☐Limited	☐Not obtained

Findings:

Pylorus	☐Visualized	☐Not Visualized	
Muscle wall thickness > 3 mm	☐Absent	☐Present	☐Indeterminate
Fluid moving through channel	☐Absent	☐Present	☐Indeterminate
Peristalsis through channel	☐Absent	☐Present	☐Indeterminate
Channel length > 15 mm	☐Absent	☐Present	☐Indeterminate

Interpretation:

☐Normal exam ☐Hypertrophic Pyloric Stenosis

Quality assurance:

Image Quality: ☐Adequate ☐Inadequate

Accuracy of interpretation: ☐Agree ☐Disagree ☐Unable to assess

Accuracy of interpretation as compared to a gold standard: ☐Not performed ☐TP ☐TN ☐FP ☐FN

Comments:

Ultrasound evaluation of the soft tissue

Evidence

1. Summary/brief explanation of indications
   - Differentiating between cellulitis and abscess can be difficult based on clinical examination alone, as there are overlapping features of both. Soft tissue POCUS can be utilized to identify the presence, location, and size of an abscess.
   - POCUS can localize soft tissue foreign bodies. This is of particular utility if there is concern for a radiolucent object.

2. Relevant adult-specific literature
   - *Skin and soft tissue infections* POCUS in adult patients is more accurate than clinical examination alone. One study demonstrated clinical examination sensitivity for identifying an abscess of 86 % (95 % CI 76, 93 %), specificity of 70 % (95 % CI 55, 82 %). Sensitivity when POCUS was added to the clinical examination was 98 % (95 % CI 93, 100 %), and specificity was 88 % (95 % CI 76, 96 %) [295].
   - POCUS can be performed with accuracy even among novice sonographers. The accuracy of novice sonographer identification of abscess by POCUS had a sensitivity of 97 % (95 % CI 83, 100 %) and a specificity of 67 % (95 % CI 24, 94 %) as compared to clinical exam which had a sensitivity of 76 % (95 % CI 58, 89 %) and a specificity of 83 % (95 % CI 36, 99 %) [296].
   - POCUS can help guide management interventions in cases of skin soft tissue infections. In one study, ultrasound altered physician intervention in 50 % of cases. The addition of ultrasound either assisted with identification of clinically occult abscesses or helped avoid invasive procedures in cases of cellulitis without abscess [297].
   - A recent pilot study described a clinical decision rule for ultrasound diagnosis of Methicillin Resistant Staphylococcus Aureus (MRSA) abscesses. The findings of a lack of a well-defined abscess edge, small volume and an irregular shape together were seven times more likely to be culture positive for MRSA. The decision rule demonstrated a sensitivity of 89 % (95 % CI 85, 93 %) and specificity of 44 % (95 % CI 41, 48 %) [298].
   - *Soft tissue foreign bodies* The authors have cited wide ranges in diagnostic accuracy for detection of foreign bodies in simulation-based studies. For example, chicken thighs, beef cubes and cadaveric models have been used, with sensitivities for localization ranging from 43–98 % and specificities ranging from 59–98 % [299–301].
   - In several case series of radiology ultrasound and POCUS, ultrasound was able to correctly identify the presence of a retained foreign body [302–305].

3. Relevant pediatric-specific literature
   - *Skin and soft tissue infections* Clinical examination has been shown to be an unreliable method of distinguishing cellulitis from abscess requiring drainage among pediatric EM physicians [306, 307]. One prospective pediatric study found POCUS to be 90 % sensitive (95 % CI 77, 100 %) and 83 % specific (95 % CI 66, 94 %) for distinguishing abscess from cellulitis, as compared to clinical suspicion, which had a sensitivity of 75 % (95 % CI 70, 97 %) and a specificity of 80 % (95 % CI 66, 94 %) [308]. In that study, POCUS resulted in a change in management in 22 % of cases.
   - Another prospective study of 65 children with clinical examination findings consistent with a skin and soft tissue infection sought to compare the test characteristics of clinical examination to those with the addition of POCUS. In this study, the sensitivity of clinical examination for the detection of abscess was 78 % (95 % CI 71, 84 %) with a specificity of 66 % (95 % CI 47, 81 %). The addition of POCUS resulted in statistically significant improvement in sensitivity to 97 % (95 % CI 90, 99 %) but not of specificity (69 %; 95 % CI 57, 72 %) [309].
   - A third study demonstrated that POCUS did not improve upon the already optimal test characteristics of clinical examination alone when physicians were certain of their diagnosis; however, POCUS may be of use in cases of clinical uncertainty [310].
   - Soft tissue POCUS is a skill that is easily mastered after even a short period of instruction. One study demonstrated that after a 6-h instructional period, novice pediatric emergency medicine fellows and attendings were able to perform adequate scans and their interpretations agreed with an expert sonologist (kappa 0.8) [311].
   - *Soft tissue foreign bodies* A pediatric study of 131 wounds compared the diagnostic accuracy of radiographs to POCUS alone, and to ultrasound plus patient perception of a tissue foreign body [312]. There was no statistically significant difference in the diagnostic accuracy of radiographs as compared to ultrasound alone for the diagnosis of tissue foreign body. However, the specificity of POCUS when combined with patient perception [76.5 % (95 % CI 66.9, 84.5)] was lower than that of radiography [88 % (95 % CI 80.8, 94.3)].

- One pediatric case report described how easily POCUS can be incorporated into the clinical evaluation of wounds that have a high probability of tissue foreign body. In this report, a wood splinter was clearly visualized under ultrasound and ultrasound further assisted in guiding foreign body removal [313].

4. Voids in the literature
   - *Skin and soft tissue infections* There are no published reports regarding the impact that POCUS has on emergency department outcome measures (including morbidity, length of stay, cosmetic results, and cost effectiveness).
   - To date, no studies have looked at emergency provider performed ultrasound for the management of soft tissue neck masses.
   - *Soft tissue foreign bodies* There is a paucity of pediatric literature evaluating ultrasound for the diagnosis and management of foreign bodies.
   - There have been no published pediatric prospective studies comparing outcomes of foreign body removal using ultrasound guidance compared to blind removal after radiographic or sonographic localization.
   - Currently, there are no published reports on ultrasound training for pediatric emergency providers for localization of foreign bodies either in vivo or with a simulation-based design.

Curriculum objectives

1. Describe the *indications* for soft tissue POCUS
   Indications for skin and soft tissue ultrasound include:
   - Suspicion for a soft tissue infection or lymphadenitis such as the presence of a tender, fluctuant, erythematous lesion.
   - Concern for a retained foreign body such as with a history of a soft tissue infection not improving with appropriate treatment, or a history of trauma with the potential for foreign body exposure.

2. Describe the *limitations* of soft issue POCUS
   - Ultrasound cannot differentiate between infectious and inflammatory fluid collections [314].
   - The development of an abscess in an area of cellulitis can make the distinction between abscess with cellulitis and cellulitis alone challenging [315].
   - In the evaluation of tissue foreign body, any introduction of air, whether from the trauma itself, or from the manipulation of the wound, can obscure the identification of the foreign body on ultrasound or prompt the misdiagnosis of a foreign body when there is none actually there [315].

3. Describe the *relevant anatomy* to be identified with soft tissue POCUS
   - Normal soft tissue architecture consists of layers of epidermis and dermis overlying muscle, tendons, and ligaments. Vessels and nerves may also be seen. The most important anatomic landmark for evaluation of soft tissue infections and foreign bodies is the superficial muscle fascia (or tendon or bone in areas without muscle). This distinguishes superficial processes from deeper ones which require complex management.
   - "Cobblestoning" (lobular appearance of the subcutaneous fat) is the classic sonographic finding with cellulitis, and is secondary to the interstitial edema within the tissue.
   - An anechoic (dark) fluid-filled irregularly shaped lesion with posterior acoustic enhancement is consistent with an abscess. Gentle downward pressure on the lesion may demonstrate internal movement of pus. Color Doppler can be used to confirm that the lesion is not a vessel or lymph node.
   - A loculated abscess will have internal echoes and septations within the fluid-filled space.
   - A lymph node will appear as well-circumscribed structure with a hypoechoic cortex and hyperechoic medulla. With color Doppler, internal flow will be seen, and there may be surrounding hyperemia.
   - Both radiopaque and radiolucent foreign bodies appear hyperechoic on ultrasound, often with posterior acoustic shadowing which may assist in the detection of the foreign body [306–310]. Other sonographic findings include reverberation (or "comet tails") artifact, and a hypoechoic halo. The latter is caused by an inflammatory reaction, which will be more common with organic foreign bodies, and those that are less acute (present for more than 24–48 h).

4. Recognize specific *pitfalls* involved with soft tissue POCUS
   - Mistaking a vessel, hematoma, or lymph node for an abscess.
   - Mistaking subcutaneous edema for a drainable fluid collection.
   - Failure to increase the depth appropriately, such that a deep tissue abscess is not recognized. Conversely, a superficial abscess can be missed if there is insufficient gel or if the depth is too great [315].
   - While an abscess often appears anechoic or hypoechoic, it can also appear as an isoechoic or hypere-

choic collection. Optimal gain settings, recognition of posterior acoustic enhancement, and identification of the to-and-fro motion of pus with probe pressure may be needed to detect such abscesses.

- Small and deep foreign bodies can be challenging to identify.
- Foreign bodies may only be identifiable by the reverberation and/or shadowing artifacts that they cause.
- A foreign body can easily be confused with normal soft tissue structures, such as fibrous septations, muscle fascia, bones, and cartilage, especially in the hands and feet. As with foreign bodies, these structures appear hyperechoic and may cause shadowing [308].
- Care must be taken to scan through entire tissue area systematically and in two orthogonal planes so as not to miss the presence of a foreign body.
- When using color Doppler, appropriate attention to color flow gain and scale is necessary.

*Discussion of ultrasound-guided abscess drainage can be found in the procedures section.

Reporting Guideline for Ultrasound Evaluation of the Soft Tissue

Patient Demographics:

Patient Name:
Patient Gender: ☐Male ☐Female

DOB: _/_/__
MR#:
Date & Time: _/_/__ _:_

Examination Demographics:

☐Initial Exam
☐Repeat Exam

Operator Name(s): ________

Operator Training: ☐Attending ☐Fellow ☐Resident ☐Medical Student ☐Other: ________

☐Patient consents to these images being used for educational purposes
☐Patient consents to these images being used for research purposes

Indication(s) for exam:

☐ Swelling ☐ Redness ☐ Mass ☐ Fever
☐ Foreign body ☐ Pain ☐ Educational ☐ Educational
☐ Other: ____________

Views:

Soft tissue at area of interest:	☐Adequate	☐Limited	☐Not obtained
Doppler at area of interest:	☐Adequate	☐Limited	☐Not obtained

Findings:

Cobblestone appearance: ☐Absent ☐Present ☐Indeterminate

Fluid collection: ☐Absent ☐Present ☐Indeterminate

Size: x:____cm y:____cm z:____cm

Doppler pattern: ☐No flow ☐ Internal color flow present

Subcutaneous gas: ☐Absent ☐Present ☐Indeterminate

Fascial plane edema: ☐Absent ☐Present ☐Indeterminate

Foreign body: ☐Absent ☐Present ☐Indeterminate

Other:_______________

Interpretation:

☐Normal exam ☐Cellulitis ☐Abscess ☐Necrotizing fasciitis
☐Foreign body ☐Lymph node ☐Other:____

Technique:

Procedural guidance: ☐ No procedure performed ☐ Static ☐ Dynamic

Outcome:

Pus: ☐ Obtained ☐ Not obtained

Complication(s):_____________
Other:_____________

Quality assurance:

Image Quality: ☐Adequate ☐Inadequate

Accuracy of interpretation: ☐Agree☐Disagree ☐Unable to assess

Accuracy of interpretation as compared to a gold standard: ☐Not performed ☐TP ☐TN ☐FP ☐FN

Comments:

Ultrasound evaluation of the testicles

Evidence

1. Summary/brief explanation of indication
   - The evaluation of acute testicular pain is a time-sensitive clinical challenge requiring accurate diagnosis.
   - POCUS is indicated for patients with clinical findings suggestive of an acute process that require immediate management (i.e., testicular torsion, traumatic hematomas and incarcerated hernias). These need to be distinguished from less urgent entities such as epididymitis, epididymo-orchitis, and a hydrocele.
2. Relevant literature in adult patients
   - In 2001, Blaivas et al. performed a retrospective study of POCUS in the evaluation of 36 ED patients presenting with acute testicular pain. To date, this is the only emergency physician-performed ultrasound study of its kind. They accurately diagnosed multiple testicular entities with a sensitivity and specificity of 95 and 94 %, respectively. All possible pathologies were included and there were no missed cases of testicular torsion [316].
   - In 2013, Cannis et al. presented a case report of a 22-year-old male for which the use of POCUS facilitated early diagnosis of a ruptured testicle and allowed for prompt urological consultation and timely surgical repair [317].
   - In 2009, Bomann et al. reported the use of POCUS by an emergency physician to diagnosis torsion in a 26-year old with successful detorsion [318].
3. Relevant pediatric literature
   - In 2000, Blaivas et al. presented a case report of a 14-year-old boy found to have testicular torsion by a POCUS examination that led to rapid diagnosis and subsequent successful salvage of the affected testicle [319].
   - There are also case reports in the literature of POCUS identification of testicular teratoma [320] and testicular dislocation secondary to trauma [321].
4. Outstanding questions to be answered/voids in the literature to date
   - The use of POCUS by pediatric emergency physicians in pediatric patients has not been studied other than case reports.
   - Prospective ED studies are needed to assess the impact of POCUS in pediatric patients presenting with acute scrotum.
   - Research is needed into the feasibility of teaching testicular POCUS imaging to pediatric emergency physicians and exploring how to achieve and assess competence.

Curriculum objectives

1. Describe the *indications* for testicular POCUS
   - For clinicians with expertise in POCUS evaluation of the testicle, the exam is indicated for patients with acute scrotal or inguinal pain, swelling, or trauma.
2. Describe the *limitations* of testicular POCUS
   - Studies have shown that the identification of flow in the normal pre-pubertal testis may be difficult or impossible, making the diagnosis of torsion on the contralateral, symptomatic side more challenging.
   - Intermittent torsion may present with relatively normal to increased flow, thus making definitive diagnosis difficult. Serial ultrasound examinations are not likely to be of benefit and the patient needs to be evaluated by urology for possible orchiopexy.
3. Describe the *relevant anatomy* to be identified with testicular POCUS
   - Relevant anatomy includes the testicular skin, tunica vaginalis (with or without hydrocele), capsule (tunica albuginea), spermatic cord, testicular vein and artery, appendix testes, epididymis, and testicle.
   - While performing bilateral testicular B-mode sonography, continuous clips through the entire organ in the longitudinal and transverse planes are ideal. If recording in still images, necessary views include central, medial, and lateral views in the longitudinal plane, and superior, mid, and inferior views in the transverse plane. The "raphe" view, a comparison of both testes in transverse orientation, evaluates the size, echogenicity, vascularity of each testis in a side-by-side image. Color and/or spectral Doppler are needed to evaluate flow to the testicle and epididymis. Having the patient perform a Valsalva maneuver may help identify varicoceles.
   - A torsed appendix testis will appear as a 5 mm or larger, spherical or round appendage with variable echogenicity, increased periappendiceal blood flow, and no blood flow within the torsed appendage.
   - Epididymitis will appear as an enlarged epididymis with variable echotexture and increased blood flow. There may be scrotal wall thickening and an associated reactive hydrocele.
   - Orchitis may present sonographically only as asymmetric or bilateral hypervascularity on color Doppler. The testicle(s) may be diffusely enlarged and have variable echogenicity. A reactive hydrocele and scrotal wall edema may further support the diagnosis.

- A hydrocele will appear as an anechoic fluid collection adjacent to the testis, and is common with all testicular pathology.
- A hernia will appear as a fluid-filled structure within the inguinal canal, spermatic cord, and/or scrotal sac. Depending on whether there is incarceration/strangulation, there may be peristalsis and mucosal blood flow identified by color Doppler.

4. Recognize specific *pitfalls* involved in testicular POCUS
   - Failing to use proper color flow and Doppler gain settings may lead to a false interpretation of torsion due to the low velocity flow within the intratesticular vessels.
   - Mistaking extratesticular blood flow for intratesticular flow may lead to a false-negative interpretation of torsion.
   - The presence of increased paratesticular flow may occur with chronic torsion, intermittent torsion, or orchitis.
   - Failure to recognize the presence of detorsion. After detorsion, there may be increased testicular blood flow mimicking epididymitis or orchitis or there may be normal testicular blood flow. These patients are at high risk for retorsion and require urological evaluation.
   - A scrotal pearl is a benign calcification that can be seen and is idiopathic in nature. It appears as a hyperechoic lesion with acoustic shadowing and may be mistaken for pathology.
   - Relying on a diagnosis of torsion of the appendix testis, orchitis, or epididymitis before ruling out testicular torsion which can lead to false-negative exams

Reporting Guideline for Ultrasound Evaluation of the Testicles

Patient Demographics:

Patient Name:
Patient Gender: ☐Male ☐Female

DOB: _/_/__
MR#:
Date & Time: _/_/__ _:_

Examination Demographics:

☐Initial Exam
☐Repeat Exam

Operator Name(s): ________

Operator Training: ☐Attending ☐Fellow ☐Resident ☐Medical Student ☐Other: ________

☐Patient consents to these images being used for educational purposes
☐Patient consents to these images being used for research purposes

Indication(s) for exam:

☐Scrotal Pain ☐Scrotal swelling/mass
☐Scrotal Trauma ☐Inguinal pain or swelling
☐Educational ☐ Other: ____________

Views:

Transverse bilateral testis	☐Adequate	☐Limited	☐Not obtained
Transverse bilateral testis with Doppler	☐Adequate	☐Limited	☐Not obtained

Right Testicle:

Transverse view	☐Adequate	☐Limited	☐Not obtained
Transverse with Doppler	☐Adequate	☐Limited	☐Not obtained
Sagittal View	☐Adequate	☐Limited	☐Not obtained
Sagittal with Doppler	☐Adequate	☐Limited	☐Not obtained

Left Testicle:

Transverse view	☐Adequate	☐Limited	☐Not obtained
Transverse with Doppler	☐Adequate	☐Limited	☐Not obtained
Sagittal view	☐Adequate	☐Limited	☐Not obtained
Sagittal with Doppler	☐Adequate	☐Limited	☐Not obtained

Findings:

Right Testicle:

Appearance:	☐Homogeneous	☐ Heterogeneous	☐Indeterminate	
Testicular Blood Flow:	☐Absent	☐Present	☐Increased	☐Indeterminate
Epididymal Blood Flow:	☐Absent	☐Present	☐Increased	☐Indeterminate
Fluid Collection:	☐Absent	☐Present	☐Indeterminate	

Other:____

Left Testicle:

Appearance:	☐Homogeneous	☐ Heterogeneous		☐Indeterminate
Testicular Blood Flow:	☐Absent	☐Present	☐Increased	☐Indeterminate
Epididymal Blood Flow:	☐Absent	☐Present	☐Increased	☐Indeterminate
Fluid Collection:	☐Absent	☐Present	☐Indeterminate	

Other:____

Interpretation:

☐Normal Exam	☐Testicular Torsion	☐ Epididymitis
☐ Orchitis	☐ Hematoma	☐ Fractured Testicle
☐ Hydrocele	☐ Inguinal Hernia	☐ Tumor
☐ Scrotal Abscess	☐ Other:___________	☐Indeterminate

Quality assurance:

Image Quality: ☐Adequate ☐Inadequate

Accuracy of interpretation: ☐Agree☐Disagree ☐Unable to assess

Accuracy of interpretation as compared to a gold standard: ☐Not performed ☐TP ☐TN ☐FP ☐FN

Comments:

Ultrasound evaluation of the urinary tract

Evidence

1. Summary/brief explanation of indications
   - POCUS can be used to evaluate the kidneys, collecting systems, and bladder in pediatric patients to assess for hydronephrosis, the presence of renal calculi, abscesses, and cysts.
2. Relevant adult-specific literature
   - *Renal colic/hydronephrosis* Several studies have looked at the ability of POCUS to detect hydronephrosis in the setting of renal colic. Results show a sensitivity between 76 and 87 %, and a specificity between 78 and 83 %, using CT as the gold standard [322–325]. The absence of hydronephrosis on ultrasound predicts easier passage of calculi, thereby mitigating the clinical need for further evaluation [326]. There are varying reports on the potential for POCUS to identify the actual calculi, partly dependent on size and location of the stone, with a sensitivity between 61 and 100 %. The size of the calculi identified on ultrasound tends to be overestimated [327–329]. POCUS can be the only imaging acquired in the initial assessment of a patient with suspected nephrolithiasis, with no increase in serious adverse events, return ED visits or hospitalizations [330].
   - *UTI/pyelonephritis* POCUS may detect complications such as renal abscesses [331].
   - *Renal cysts* POCUS is helpful in diagnosing and evaluating renal cysts [332, 333].
3. Relevant pediatric-specific literature
   - *Renal colic/hydronephrosis* Although much less common in pediatric patients, the incidence of urolithiasis is increasing, with some accounts reporting as much as an 86 % increase in children diagnosed with renal colic in the past decade [334–336]. Ultrasound is less sensitive than CT in identifying urolithiasis, especially ureteric stones [337].
   - *UTI/pyelonephritis* The majority of pediatric patients diagnosed with a UTI do not require imaging in the acute setting. However, for those patients who fail to respond to standard treatment and present to the emergency department, POCUS may assist in identifying abnormalities such as renal or perirenal abscesses or hydronephrosis. Further alternative imaging may be necessary to evaluate for renal scarring or reflux, as ultrasound has been shown to be less sensitive and specific than other modalities such as DMSA in these settings [338–343].
   - *Renal cysts* Renal cysts are congenital or acquired. They are uncommonly seen in the pediatric population, but the incidence increases with age. Cysts may be noted especially in at-risk patients with a family history of polycystic kidney disease [344–346].
4. Outstanding questions to be answered/voids in the literature to date
   - There are currently minimal data on the use of POCUS in the pediatric emergency department for assessing the urinary tract. It is limited to reports on bladder assessment, and a few emerging studies on POCUS for suspected renal colic.
   - Since the test characteristics of ultrasound in the assessment of pediatric urinary tract ailments are currently unknown, it is unclear in which patients a bedside renal ultrasound should be performed, and how the results of the ultrasound should be incorporated into medical decision making.

Curriculum objectives

1. Describe the *indications* for POCUS of the urinary tract
   - Indications for performing POCUS of the urinary tract include the following: flank pain, hematuria, dysuria and unexplained renal failure, depending on the clinical context. POCUS may be used to evaluate for hydronephrosis, the presence of renal calculi, cysts or tumors.
2. Describe the *limitations* of POCUS of the urinary tract
   - Identification of obstructing ureteral calculi is beyond the skill of most point-of-care sonologists.
   - Normal ureters are not visualized on ultrasound.
   - Ultrasound is not useful in the diagnosis of pyelonephritis; however, it may assist in identifying underlying causes or complications.
   - Ultrasound is not sensitive or specific for diagnosing renal scarring.
   - The examination may be technically limited by bowel gas, abdominal pain, the patient having an empty bladder as well as large body habitus.
3. Describe the *relevant anatomy* to be identified in the POCUS examination of the urinary tract
   - The urinary tract should be evaluated by visualizing both kidneys and the collecting systems, together with the bladder. Each kidney needs to be scanned in the longitudinal and transverse orientation, ensuring that the entire kidney together with the collecting system is evaluated. Each kidney is enclosed in a layer of fascia (Gerota's fascia). Between this fascia and the fibrous renal capsule, there is a layer of perinephric fat. The kidneys

themselves are divided into the outer cortex, an inner medulla and the renal sinus, which include the renal collecting system, blood supply and adipose tissue. The renal pelvis refers to the part of the collecting system between the convergence of the calyces and the transition into the proximal ureter. In healthy individuals, these cannot be seen on ultrasound. The bladder is an anechoic structure, surrounded by an echogenic wall. It should be evaluated in both the transverse (when it can appear trapezoid in shape) and longitudinal orientation. Ureteral jets can also be viewed with the application of color Doppler in the transverse orientation.

4. Recognize specific pitfalls involved in POCUS of the urinary tract.

   Pitfalls to avoid when evaluating the urinary tract include the following:

- Incorrectly ascribing hydronephrosis to obstruction in a patient with a full bladder or one who is over hydrated. Ideally patients undergoing evaluation of the urinary tract should be well hydrated, but not overly so, and have a partly filled, but not distended bladder.
- Conversely, dehydration may prevent the formation of hydronephrosis, thereby masking obstruction.
- Incorrectly ruling out a renal stone in the absence of hydronephrosis. Small stones may not cause hydronephrosis.
- Incorrectly ruling out ureterolithiasis, if no stone is visible. Mistaking renal cysts for hydronephrosis. The two can be distinguished with systematic real-time scanning through the entire kidney.
- Mistaking renal pyramids, which can be prominent in pediatric patients, for hydronephrosis. Their location is outside the renal sinus in contrast to hydronephrosis, which always occurs inside the renal sinus.
- Failure to identify unilateral absence of a kidney or horseshoe kidney. Both these conditions have important implications for the patient, and may affect acute management. Further diagnostic testing is likely to be indicated in such circumstances.
- Failure to visualize the entire kidney bilaterally and to evaluate the bladder

Reporting Guideline for Ultrasound Evaluation of the Urinary Tract

Patient Demographics:

Patient Name:
Patient Gender: ☐Male ☐Female

DOB: __/__/____
MR#:
Date & Time: __/__/____ __:__

Examination Demographics:

☐Initial Exam
☐Repeat Exam

Operator Name(s): ________

Operator Training: ☐Attending ☐Fellow ☐Resident ☐Medical Student ☐Other: ________

☐Patient consents to these images being used for educational purposes
☐Patient consents to these images being used for research purposes

☐Billed exam

Indication(s) for exam:

☐Abdominal pain	☐Renal failure	☐Flank pain	☐Anuria
☐Back pain	☐Post-void	☐Dysuria	☐Fever
☐Hematuria	☐Educational	☐Other:________	

Views:

Right kidney long axis:	☐Adequate	☐Limited	☐Not obtained
Right kidney short axis:	☐Adequate	☐Limited	☐Not obtained
Left kidney long axis:	☐Adequate	☐Limited	☐Not obtained
Left kidney short axis:	☐Adequate	☐Limited	☐Not obtained
Transverse bladder:	☐Adequate	☐Limited	☐Not obtained
Sagittal bladder:	☐Adequate	☐Limited	☐Not obtained
Other: _______			

Findings:

Right Kidney

Hydronephrosis:	☐Normal	☐Moderate	☐Severe
Hydroureter:	☐Absent	☐Present	☐Indeterminate
Kidney stone(s):	☐Absent	☐Present	☐Indeterminate
Cyst(s):	☐Absent	☐Present	☐Indeterminate
☐Other:_______			

Left Kidney

Hydronephrosis:	☐Normal	☐Moderate	☐Severe
Hydroureter:	☐Absent	☐Present	☐Indeterminate
Kidney stone(s):	☐Absent	☐Present	☐Indeterminate
Cyst(s):	☐Absent	☐Present	☐Indeterminate
☐Other:_______			

Bladder

Bladder Volume Estimate:___________

Right ureteral jet:	☐Present	☐Absent
Left ureteral jet:	☐Present	☐Absent
☐Other:________		

Interpretation:

☐Normal exam ☐Hydronephrosis ☐Hydroureter
☐Nephrolithiasis ☐Renal cysts
☐Other:_______

Quality assurance:

Image Quality: ☐Adequate ☐Inadequate

Accuracy of interpretation: ☐Agree ☐Disagree ☐Unable to assess

Accuracy of interpretation as compared to a gold standard: ☐Not performed ☐TP ☐TN ☐FP ☐FN

Comments:

Ultrasound-guided procedures

A unified reporting/quality assurance sheet for all procedures is presented at the end of the section.

Ultrasound guidance for arthrocentesis

Evidence

1. Summary/brief explanation of indications (hip and knee)
   - Arthrocentesis, also known as joint aspiration, is most commonly utilized to differentiate septic joint fluid from other types of joint effusions.
   - In children who present with pain, limping or the inability to bear weight, ultrasound can assist arthrocentesis and result in more rapid diagnosis and treatment.
   - Occasionally arthrocentesis may be done for therapeutic indications to relieve pain, either with medication injection or fluid removal.
   - Dynamic ultrasound guidance uses real-time imaging to aid the procedure, with direct visualization of the needle into the joint space.
   - Static technique is used to identify the location of the effusion relative to the skin surface and to mark an optimal location for needle insertion. The actual procedure is performed without ultrasound.
2. Relevant adult-specific literature
   - Multiple studies demonstrate emergency physician success in using ultrasound to diagnose and aspirate hip effusions [213, 347–349].
   - POCUS leads to greater fluid aspiration in knee arthrocentesis [350] and is better at identifying knee effusion than clinical examination alone [351].
3. Relevant pediatric-specific literature
   - There are case reports of POCUS-guided arthrocentesis in pediatric patients [211, 241, 352].
4. Outstanding questions to be answered/voids in the literature to date
   - POCUS-guided arthrocentesis in pediatric patients requires further investigation, specifically, the evaluation of success rates compared with landmark approaches, as well as evidence-based guidelines for training.
   - Static versus dynamic technique is currently utilized based on operator preference.

Curriculum objectives (hip and knee)

1. Describe the *indications* for POCUS for arthrocentesis
   - POCUS-guided arthrocentesis may be used for diagnostic or therapeutic aspiration of a joint effusion.
2. Describe the *limitations* of POCUS for arthrocentesis.
   Limitations include the following:
   - The examination and procedure are dependent on both operator expertise and patient size/cooperation.
3. Describe the *relevant anatomy* to be identified during POCUS for arthrocentesis
   - Hip:
     - During imaging of the joint, the femoral head, femoral neck, acetabulum and iliopsoas muscle should be identified [353].
     - Joint fluid will appear hypoechoic or anechoic in the anterior synovial space.
     - The location of the femoral vessels should be identified sonographically prior to arthrocentesis.
     - For those with experience in its use, the addition of color Doppler allows the provider to locate and avoid the femoral vessels during needle insertion [354].
   - Knee:
     - A joint effusion is detected with distension of the suprapatellar recess. Hypoechoic or anechoic fluid is within this recess [355].
     - The effusion will appear as a hypoechoic fluid collection separated from the brightly echogenic femoral cortex by a thin layer of hyperechoic pre-femoral fat.
4. Recognize specific *pitfalls* involved in POCUS for arthrocentesis
   - Incorrectly ruling out a septic joint due to lack of effusion, as infection may be present in the "normal" amount of joint fluid or only in the synovial tissue.
   - Artifact induced false-positive effusions due to anisotropy of the muscles of the hip joint and lack of provider expertise [356].
   - Misdiagnosing hypoechoic articular cartilage as an effusion, especially in hips of infants [357].
   - Misdiagnosing a prepatellar bursitis as a joint effusion.
   - Failure to observe the usual precautions and recommendations applicable to arthrocentesis whether performed with or without ultrasound guidance.

*Discussion of musculoskeletal ultrasound can be found in the diagnostic indications section.

Ultrasound guidance for arterial catheter placement

Evidence

1. Summary/brief explanation of indications
   - An arterial catheter is typically placed in critically ill or injured patients who require continuous hemodynamic monitoring and/or frequent laboratory testing.
   - The radial and femoral arteries are frequently chosen for cannulation.
   - The smaller size of these arteries in infants and children makes performing the procedure blindly more difficult.
   - Ultrasound guidance may facilitate successful placement of arterial catheters.
2. Relevant adult-specific literature
   - A randomized trial of 60 patients compared palpation to POCUS assistance for arterial cannulation. The ultrasound group demonstrated a shorter time to placement [107 vs. 314 s, (p = 0.004)], fewer attempts [1.2 vs. 2.2 (p = 0.001)], and fewer sites required for successful placement [1.1 vs. 1.6 (p = 0.001)] [358].
3. Relevant pediatric-specific literature
   - A randomized trial of ultrasound-guided radial artery cannulation by anesthesiology trainees demonstrated higher overall as well as first attempt success rates, shorter time to identifying the vessel, and a smaller proportion of hematomas in the ultrasound group [359].
   - A randomized trial of ultrasound-guided radial artery cannulation by pediatric anesthesiologists revealed no statistically significant difference in successful cannulation on first attempt, time to cannulation, or total number of attempts [360].
4. Outstanding questions to be answered/voids in the literature to date
   - Trials are needed in pediatric patients comparing ultrasound assistance/guidance to palpation for arterial cannulation.
   - Studies are needed to assess how many ultrasound-guided arterial catheters are needed to become proficient.
   - It is unknown to what extent training and/or proficiency in ultrasound-guided venous access translates into that for ultrasound-guided arterial catheter placement.
   - With newer, higher frequency, technology, ultrasound-guided arterial cannulation may prove more feasible.

Curriculum objectives

1. Describe the *indications* for ultrasound-assisted arterial catheter placement
   - Ultrasound-assisted arterial catheter placement is indicated when an arterial catheter is needed for hemodynamic or blood gas monitoring in critically ill patients.
2. Describe the *limitations* for ultrasound-assisted arterial catheter placement
   - User familiarity and experience with the procedure both with and without ultrasound can determine success of the procedure.
   - The small size of the artery and depth (too shallow or too deep) can also hinder cannulation.
   - Patient characteristics like movement, blood pressure, volume status, and body habitus will also pose a challenge for placement.
3. Describe the *relevant anatomy* to be identified while performing ultrasound-assisted arterial catheter placement
   - The most common sites for arterial catheter placement in pediatrics are the radial and femoral arteries.
   - A vessel can be visualized in either the short-axis (cross sectional) or the long-axis plane, along the length of the vessel.
   - The radial artery originates from the brachial artery medial to the biceps tendon and continues to the styloid process of the radius. Up to 30 % of individuals have variants in the course of the radial artery. The portion of the radial artery in the distal forearm has less anatomical variation making it the preferable site for cannulation [361].
   - The most easily accessible portion of the femoral artery is in the femoral triangle, made up of the inguinal ligament superiorly, the Sartorius muscle laterally and medially by the adductor longus muscle.
   - The relationship between the femoral vein (medial to artery) and femoral nerve (lateral to artery) should be noted in an effort to minimize accidental cannulation of or injury to adjacent structures [362].
   - If the operator is proficient in the use of Doppler, this modality can be used to distinguish the artery from veins and nerves.
4. Recognize specific *pitfalls* involved in performing ultrasound-assisted arterial catheter placement
   - Small vessels like the radial artery may be compressed and, therefore, difficult to visualize with minimal pressure from the ultrasound transducer.

- Failure to confirm that the vessel is actually an artery, not a nerve or a vein. For those proficient in the use of Doppler, this modality can be used to distinguish the artery from veins and nerves.
- As with other procedures in pediatric patients, small patient size, and lack of patient cooperation may present additional challenges to successful cannulation of the artery.
- There may be significant overlap of the femoral vein and artery in the femoral triangle. Changes in leg position may reduce this overlap, but this will require immobilizing the patient in the optimal position throughout the procedure [362, 363].
- In the short-axis view, the operator must follow the needle tip at all times to avoid damage to the posterior wall of the vessel or other structures.
- In the long-axis view, the length of the vessel and entire needle should be visualized. This may not be possible if the vessel is not straight. It may also require greater operator skill since the transducer, needle, and vessel must be visualized in the same plane throughout the procedure. It may also require more advanced skill to distinguish an adjacent artery and vein in the longitudinal plane.
- Failure to observe the usual precautions and recommendations applicable to arterial catheter placement whether performed with or without ultrasound guidance.

Ultrasound guidance for incision and drainage of soft tissue abscesses

Evidence

1. Summary/brief explanation of indications
   - After ultrasound diagnosis of an abscess, ultrasound guidance can be used to facilitate surgical drainage of an abscess. Dynamic and static techniques can be used. In both cases, ultrasound is used to determine the size, depth, and location of the abscess, and to identify surrounding structures (e.g., nerves, vessels), which need to be avoided
     - Dynamic ultrasound guidance uses real-time imaging with direct visualization of the needle or scalpel passing into the abscess.
     - Using the static technique, an optimal location for incision or needle insertion is determined by ultrasound, and the skin is marked. The actual procedure is then performed without ultrasound.
2. Relevant adult-specific literature
   - POCUS evaluation may identify surrounding vascular structures, and avoid potentially serious complications of incision and drainage [364].
   - POCUS-guided needle aspiration has been shown to be insufficient in treating abscesses, when compared with incision and drainage [365].
3. Relevant pediatric-specific literature
   - To date, there are no studies in pediatric patients specifically evaluating ultrasound-guided incision and drainage.
4. Outstanding questions to be answered/voids in the literature to date
   - It is unknown whether ultrasound-guided drainage in pediatric patients is more effective and leads to improved outcomes compared with drainage without the use of ultrasound guidance.
   - To date, there are no ultrasound studies on size and volume parameters for abscess drainage. The presence of a fluid collection on ultrasound does not necessarily indicate that drainage is needed.

Curriculum objectives

1. Describe the *indications* for ultrasound-guided incision and drainage
   - Ultrasound may assist in determining the extent of surgical drainage by revealing the depth and boundaries of abscesses (e.g., in the distinction between perianal versus perirectal abscess).
   - Ultrasound can identify the presence of infection involving deeper structures (e.g., tenosynovitis) in infections that appear to be limited to the superficial soft tissues.
   - Ultrasound may identify the presence of foreign bodies in soft tissue infections.
   - Ultrasound-guided needle aspiration may be useful in those areas where the lesion is in close proximity to vascular and nerve structures.
   - Ultrasound can help to guide surgical management (needle aspiration versus incision and drainage) in cosmetically sensitive locations (e.g., the face).
   - Ultrasound can be used to ensure that a lesion has been completely drained.
2. Describe the *limitations* of ultrasound-guided incision and drainage
   - At this time, there are no known limitations or contraindications to sonographic evaluation of soft tissue abscesses prior to surgical drainage.
   - The current literature demonstrates the inferiority of needle aspiration under ultrasound guidance compared to incision and drainage in terms of clinical resolution [365].

3. Describe the *relevant anatomy* to be identified during ultrasound-guided incision and drainage
   - An abscess is identified as a heterogeneous hypoechoic, occasionally isoechoic, irregularly shaped lesion with posterior acoustic enhancement. Gas or foreign bodies may also be seen.
   - Vessels and nerves in the region of the abscess should be positively identified prior to surgical drainage.
   - The superficial fascia of underlying musculoskeletal structures should be identified to exclude involvement of deeper structures. Color flow may be useful to identify vessels and lymph nodes.

4. Recognize specific *pitfalls* involved in ultrasound-guided incision and drainage
   - Mistaking a vessel, hematoma, or lymph node for an abscess.
   - Failure to recognize the full extent or depth of an abscess. This may be particularly challenging with perianal or gluteal infections.
   - Failure to recognize that an infection is arising from structures below the dermis.
   - Failure to observe the usual precautions and recommendations applicable to incision and drainage whether performed with or without ultrasound guidance.

*Discussion of skin and soft tissue ultrasound can be found in the diagnostic indications section.

Ultrasound guidance for lumbar puncture

Evidence

1. Summary/brief explanation of indication
   - The lumbar puncture (LP) is routinely performed in the emergency department for febrile neonates, children with a clinical suspicion for meningitis or encephalitis, and in patients with suspected or diagnosed idiopathic intracranial hypertension.
   - Ultrasound can identify the spinous processes, interspinous spaces, and guide needle placement via static or dynamic imaging.
   - Ultrasound may be particularly useful in neonates who have small interspinous spaces as well as obese patients where palpation of anatomical landmarks is difficult.
   - In neonates, the spine is largely cartilaginous allowing for visualization of the spinal canal including the level of conus medullaris. Ossification of the vertebra occurs around 1 year of age.
   - Ultrasound assistance ('static technique') is the use of ultrasound prior to lumbar puncture to determine an optimal location for needle insertion. The procedure is then performed without ultrasound.
   - Dynamic ultrasound-guidance provides direct visualization of the passage of the needle from the skin into the spinal canal.

2. Relevant adult-specific literature
   - Tuffier's line (the line between the superior portion of posterior iliac crests) is commonly used to estimate the L4 vertebra. In a study by Pysyk, ultrasound showed that Tuffier's line is not a reliable method to consistently identify a particular vertebral space [366].
   - In adult patients, POCUS has been shown to be highly effective in identifying bony landmarks for LP, even in those who are obese [367, 368].
   - In one study, the success rate of ultrasound-assisted LP was found to be 92.3 %, regardless of the subjects' body mass index (BMI) [369].
   - In a randomized controlled trial comparing POCUS with the traditional landmark approach, POCUS had a success rate of 95.8 % and was more likely to be successful (RR 1.32, 95 % CI 1.01–1.72). In obese patients, with BMI $\geq$ 30, there were fewer failed attempts in the POCUS group (RR 2.33, 95 % CI 0.99–5.49) [370].
   - Another randomized controlled trial of 80 patients found that ultrasound-assisted LP was associated with decreased procedure time, number of attempts, traumatic tap rate, and pain score during the procedure. Such benefits seem to be more prominent in those with a higher BMI [371].

3. Relevant pediatric-specific literature
   - Pediatric studies have shown that POCUS can be used to measure the interspinous space and to determine how the measurement changes in different positions [372, 373]. The interspinous space is maximized in a seated position with hip flexion. In the decubitus position, neck flexion does not change the interspinous space and, thus, the neck should not be flexed for the procedure [372].
   - Another pediatric study used POCUS to assess the angle of needle placement [374]. It demonstrated that the angle for children under 12 months was significantly less (on average 50° to the skin, directed cephalad) than that for patients above this age (on average 60°).
   - In neonates, ultrasound can be used to identify the level of conus medullaris [375, 376] as well as evaluate reasons for failed LP attempts [377].
   - In 2014, a feasibility study conducted on 19 patients found that using POCUS was associated with higher

confidence score in selecting the insertion site for the LP needle compared to the traditional landmark approach [378].
- Preliminary data ($n = 26$) from a randomized controlled trial of infants 0-12 months found no significant difference between the groups (POCUS vs. landmark approach) in terms of LP success rate, traumatic LP rate (RBC > 10,000/mm^3 on CSF analysis), number of LP attempts, or total LP duration [379].

4. Outstanding questions to be answered/voids in the literature to date
   - To date, there are no large randomized controlled trials investigating the effect of POCUS on success rates, complications, costs, patient flow, or patient satisfaction related to LPs performed in the ED.
   - Investigations are needed to determine the comparative effectiveness of static vs. dynamic techniques of ultrasound guidance.

Curriculum objectives

1. Describe the *indications* for POCUS-assisted LP
   - Patients in whom bony landmarks of the spinous processes are difficult to palpate.
   - Patients in whom the interspinous spaces are small and difficult to identify.
   - Patients in whom LP has failed using the landmark approach.
2. Describe the *limitations* of POCUS-assisted LP
   - Inability to visualize the anatomy sonographically for any reason.
   - After vertebral ossification, ultrasound is limited to visualization of the spinous processes and interspinous spaces.
   - Movement of the patient prior to needle insertion after marking by ultrasound using the static technique may alter the location of underlying structures, especially in young infants.
   - Success is dependent on the operator and the level of experience with ultrasound as well as with the LP procedure.
3. Describe the *relevant anatomy* for POCUS-assisted LP
   - It is most important to identify the spinous processes and the interspinous spaces.
   - The spinous processes will be the most superficial bony prominence that is palpated clinically and visualized sonographically.
   - In neonates, the spine is mostly cartilaginous allowing for visualization of the anatomy from the spine to the spinal canal. In this case, ultrasound can identify the skin, spinous process, interspinous space, ligaments, epidural space, dura/arachnoid, and subarachnoid space. Within the subarachnoid space, ultrasound can visualize the spinal canal, conus medullaris, cauda equina, as well as, the filum terminale.
4. Recognize specific *pitfalls* involved POCUS-assisted LP
   - Misidentifying the transverse process as the spinous process as a result of the transducer being misplaced laterally and not in the midline.
   - Mistaking the spinal cord as cerebrospinal fluid in the subarachnoid space.
   - Failure to observe the usual precautions and recommendations applicable to lumbar puncture whether performed with or without ultrasound guidance.

Ultrasound guidance for paracentesis

Evidence

1. Summary/indications
   - Ascites may be present in patients with nephrotic syndrome, malnutrition, malignancy, congestive heart failure, pancreatitis, bacterial peritonitis, nonbacterial causes of peritoneal inflammation, tuberculosis or dengue fever. Other causes of abdominal fluid collections include biliary and urinary tract injury, which may be iatrogenic in etiology.
   - POCUS can identify small amounts of free fluid in the abdominal cavity, and can be useful in its diagnosis. Symptoms of abdominal fluid collections range from asymptomatic to pain, distension and respiratory distress.
   - Using ultrasound to localize intra-abdominal fluid and to perform paracentesis involves direct visualization of fluid, as well as structures to be avoided during the procedure including bowel, the urinary bladder, and the inferior epigastric vessels.
     - Dynamic ultrasound guidance uses real-time imaging to aid paracentesis with direct visualization of the needle trajectory.
     - Static technique is used to identify anatomic landmarks and the extent of the peritoneal fluid, and to determine an optimal location for needle insertion. The actual procedure is performed without ultrasound.
2. Relevant adult-specific literature
   - In a prospective randomized study, Nazeer et al. showed that ultrasonographic guidance not only improves the rate of successful paracentesis by emergency physicians, but also helps determine the need for the procedure, thus reducing unnecessary interventions and patient discomfort [380].

- Patel et al. performed a retrospective analysis comparing blind and ultrasound-assisted paracentesis. Adverse events (post-paracentesis infection, hematoma, seroma) were lower (1.4 vs 4.7 % $p = 0.01$) as well as hospital costs in the ultrasound-assisted group [381]. An additional study also showed decreased bleeding complications and hospitalization cost [382].
- One case series suggested that ultrasound-guided, emergent paracentesis in the management of unstable, hypotensive patients assisted in the characterization of the fluid, thereby guiding patient management [383].

3. Relevant pediatric-specific literature
   - There have been no studies to date evaluating POCUS for paracentesis in pediatric patients.
4. Outstanding questions to be answered/voids in the literature to date
   - There are currently no published investigations of the relative benefits and risks of ultrasound-guided paracentesis compared to traditional technique with respect to complication rates, patient satisfaction, pain, or other outcomes. However, the infrequent need for paracentesis in pediatric patients would make design of such studies difficult. Under such circumstances, it may be justifiable to generalize the favorable risk:benefit profile demonstrated in adult patients to the pediatric setting.
   - It is unclear how much training and how many procedures are required to attain competency.

Curriculum objectives

1. Describe the *indications* for POCUS for paracentesis
   - POCUS for paracentesis should be used in those patients with suspected free intra-abdominal fluid in order to diagnose ascites, assist with fluid sampling for diagnosis, and for symptomatic relief.
   - Once intraabdominal fluid is identified, POCUS is indicated to identify the largest pocket of fluid and intra-abdominal structures that need to be avoided during the procedure. Additionally, with color Doppler, POCUS may assist in the identification and location of the inferior epigastric vessels.
2. Describe the *limitations* of POCUS for paracentesis
   - As with all ultrasound procedures, use is operator dependent and requires training.
   - Ultrasound usually cannot differentiate between types of free fluid.
   - Even with optimal technique, bowel can move within the abdomen, and therefore, perforation is still possible particularly when the static technique is used.
3. Describe the *relevant anatomy* to be identified with POCUS for paracentesis
   - The first step is to identify pockets of free fluid. The technique is similar to the one used during the FAST examination. It consists of examination of bilateral upper and lower quadrants, the hepatorenal and splenorenal spaces, and the pelvis. The peritoneal lining is hyperechoic and pockets of ascites are anechoic or hypoechoic.
   - When free fluid is identified, the area should be interrogated to assure that there is a direct unobstructed line from the skin to the target fluid collection. Intra-abdominal organs and vessels need to be identified to avoid them during puncture. The inferior epigastric vessels arise from the external iliac vessels immediately superior to the femoral canal and course superiorly along the approximate line of the lateral margin of the rectus abdominis muscle. They are located immediately deep to the abdominal muscle layers and superficial to the peritoneum. These should be identified and their trajectory and course drawn on the patient's skin, designating an area to avoid. Color Doppler should be used to identify the inferior epigastric vessels, with the threshold set low.
   - It is important to recognize that a full bladder might simulate free fluid. If a Foley catheter is not placed prior to performing the procedure, the sonologist should make positive identification of the dome of the bladder prior to the procedure.
   - Once the fluid collection and surrounding structures are identified, it is important to maintain the patient's position, in order to avoid shifts in fluid and structures.
4. Recognize the specific *pitfalls* involved in POCUS for paracentesis
   - Movement of the patient after fluid mapping may lead to a shift in the fluid or bowel, especially if the static technique is used.
   - Failure to visualize the largest pocket of fluid.
   - Insertion of the needle in close proximity to bowel.
   - Mistaking the bladder or cystic masses for ascites.
   - Failure to observe the usual precautions and recommendations applicable to paracentesis whether performed with or without ultrasound guidance.

Ultrasound guidance for pericardiocentesis

Evidence

1. Summary/brief explanation of indications
   - Pericardiocentesis is the aspiration of fluid, blood, or pus, from the space between the visceral and parietal pericardium.

- Use of ultrasound guidance to perform pericardiocentesis has been described since 1979, and has fewer complications than performing the procedure blindly [384].
- Indications for a therapeutic pericardiocentesis are impending or current cardiac tamponade. In children, this usually occurs post-cardiac surgery or from traumatic injury.
  - Dynamic ultrasound guidance uses real-time imaging to aid the procedure with direct visualization of the needle into the pericardial space.
  - Static technique is used to identify the location of the effusion relative to the chest wall and to mark an optimal location for needle insertion. The actual procedure is performed without ultrasound.

2. Relevant adult-specific literature
   - There are several case reports which describe ultrasound-assisted pericardiocentesis [385–387].
   - An in-plane approach has been described [388].

3. Relevant pediatric-specific literature
   - To date, there are no studies evaluating pediatric emergency physician-performed POCUS for pericardiocentesis.

4. Outstanding questions to be answered/voids in the literature to date
   - Pericardial tamponade is a very rare condition, particularly in pediatric patients. This is likely the reason for the paucity of literature describing ultrasound-guided pericardiocentesis.
   - Given the infrequency with which it is performed, it is not clear what method is best (e.g., simulation, animal models) for achieving competence with the procedure.

Curriculum objectives

1. Describe the *indications* for ultrasound-assisted pericardiocentesis
   - The only indication for emergent ultrasound-assisted pericardiocentesis is life-threatening cardiac tamponade.
   - The non-emergent indication is the need for sampling pericardial fluid for diagnostic purposes.

2. Describe the *limitations* of ultrasound-assisted pericardiocentesis
   - Success is largely dependent on operator comfort and experience with the procedure.
   - Transducer placement and site of needle entry may be limited by the small size of the child.

3. Describe the *relevant anatomy* to be identified during ultrasound-assisted pericardiocentesis
   - The heart, specifically the right and left ventricles, liver, pericardium and pericardial space are all structures that must be identified prior to beginning the procedure.
   - A pericardial effusion will appear as an anechoic (black) space surrounding the heart contained by the bright echogenic pericardium.
   - Tamponade is demonstrated by poor filling and/or diastolic collapse of the right side of the heart (right atria or right ventricle).
   - Tamponade can occur with as little as 50 ml of fluid, if the fluid rapidly accumulates such as with blood from trauma. Tamponade can also occur with considerably more fluid if the accumulation is more gradual, such as in rheumatologic or oncologic conditions [389].
   - Images can be obtained in the parasternal long, apical, or subxiphoid view, in order to determine best placement of the needle based on where the effusion is closest to the transducer.

4. Recognize specific *pitfalls* involved in ultrasound-assisted pericardiocentesis
   - As with other ultrasound-guided procedures, the procedure may be complicated by patient characteristics, including body habitus, and movement during the procedure.
   - Failure to determine the appropriate needle entry site and trajectory while avoiding vital structures and accessing the largest fluid accumulation closest to body surface [384].
   - Failing to recognize and avoid the internal mammary artery (3–5 cm lateral to the lower sternal boarder) and the neurovascular bundles that run below each rib [389].
   - Laceration of myocardial tissue or vessels due to side-to-side needle manipulation during entry through the heart.
   - Failure to observe the usual precautions and recommendations applicable to pericardiocentesis whether performed with or without ultrasound guidance.

*Discussion of cardiac ultrasound can be found in the diagnostic indications section.

Ultrasound guidance for regional anesthesia

Evidence

1. Summary/brief explanation of indications

- Use of ultrasound to guide regional anesthesia in patients has greatly improved the ability to deliver safe and effective analgesia.
- The majority of the literature surrounds anesthesiologist-performed ultrasound for this indication.
  - Dynamic ultrasound guidance uses real-time imaging to perform the nerve blockade, with direct visualization of the needle path to the nerve bundle.
  - Static technique is used to identify the location of the nerve and surrounding vessels to avoid, and to mark an optimal location for needle insertion. The actual procedure is performed without ultrasound.

2. Relevant adult literature
   - A small study of emergency department (ED) patients demonstrated that emergency physicians could easily learn ultrasound-guided nerve blockade, and perform the procedure effectively and without complications [390].
   - In another small study of patients assigned to either procedural sedation or ultrasound-guided supraclavicular brachial plexus nerve blockade, the mean ED length of stay was nearly 3 h shorter in the nerve blockade group [391].

3. Relevant pediatric literature
   - Anesthesiologist-performed ultrasound allows for visualization of peripheral nerves and their surrounding anatomy in real time, thereby enabling reliable drug delivery to the target nerve while avoiding mechanical nerve injury, local and systemic drug toxicity, or injection into adjacent structures in pediatric patients [392–394].
   - A retrospective study of pediatric emergency physician-performed ultrasound-guided femoral nerve blocks showed that patients had longer duration of analgesia, required fewer doses of analgesic medications, and needed fewer nursing interventions than those receiving analgesic medication alone [395].
   - A feasibility study of pediatric emergency physician-performed ultrasound-guided forearm nerve blocks showed effective analgesia, minimized iatrogenic risk and procedure time ideal for emergency department workflow [396].

4. Outstanding questions to be answered/voids in the literature to date
   - There are limited data to compare pediatric emergency physician-performed ultrasound-guided regional anesthesia to traditional methods of pain control or anesthesia.
   - Further study may include novel techniques, anesthesia agents, and target nerves that are pediatric-specific.
   - Scientific information is needed to determine the costs and benefits of ultrasound-guided regional anesthesia with respect to success rates, complications, costs, ED length of stay, and patient satisfaction.

Curriculum objectives

1. Describe the *indications* for ultrasound-guided regional anesthesia
   - The indication for ultrasound-guided regional anesthesia includes any pain control scenario in which analgesia in the distribution of a peripheral nerve or nerves is desired for pain control or anesthesia. Examples include: fractures, dislocations, burns, abscess incision and drainage, foreign body removal, and laceration repair.

2. Describe the *limitations* of ultrasound-guided regional anesthesia
   - An uncooperative patient can limit successful nerve blockade. Patients may benefit from topical anesthesia and anxiolytic adjuncts to minimize pain with needle entry and patient anxiety during the procedure. Limiting patient movement using age-appropriate restraints may also be necessary.
   - The inability to visualize a target nerve or deliver the anesthetic agent to the perineural area due to patient anatomy should prompt alternative pain control measures.

3. Define the *relevant anatomy* associated with commonly used nerve blocks including: interscalene, supraclavicular, forearm, intercostal, femoral, and popliteal nerve blocks
   - Depending on the size of the patient's limb and the footprint of the transducer, the target nerve can be visualized in cross section or longitudinally. Where both views are available, many sonologists prefer to view the nerve in cross section, allowing for demonstration of anesthetic solution surrounding the nerve.
   - Regardless of the scanning plane with respect to the nerve, most sonologists prefer to introduce the needle in the plane of the ultrasound transducer. The in-plane approach allows for visualization of the entire length of the needle, and with injection, the anesthetic should be seen surrounding the target nerve, creating a halo.
   - Interscalene block—The brachial plexus trunks should be identified, as well as the middle and ante-

rior scalene muscles and the sternocleidomastoid muscle.

- Supraclavicular block—The brachial plexus divisions should be identified as well as the subclavian artery, the first rib and the pleural line.
- Forearm nerve block—The radial, median and ulnar nerves should be identified as well as the radial and ulnar arteries.
- Intercostal nerve block—The intercostal space should be identified at the intended level of the block as well as the inferior margin of the rib and the pleural line.
- Femoral nerve block—The femoral nerve should be identified as well as the femoral artery, fascia lata and fascia iliacus.
- Popliteal nerve block—The popliteal, tibial and common peroneal nerves, and their points of bifurcation should be identified as well as the popliteal artery and vein.

4. Recognize the *pitfalls* associated with ultrasound-guided regional anesthesia
   - Failure to maintain continuous visualization of the needle tip in-plane during entry and injection.
   - Complications to be avoided include: neuronal injury by direct mechanical trauma, vascular puncture and vascular injection of anesthesia agent.
   - Pneumothorax is a rare potential complication for regional anesthesia of the brachial plexus and intercostal nerves.
   - Failure to observe the usual precautions and recommendations applicable to regional anesthesia whether performed with or without ultrasound guidance.

Ultrasound guidance for suprapubic bladder aspiration

Evidence

1. Summary/brief explanation of indications
   - In addition to assessing for adequate bladder volume prior to catheterization, POCUS may be used to assist in performing suprapubic bladder aspiration (SPA).
     - Dynamic ultrasound guidance uses real-time imaging to aid SPA with direct visualization of the needle trajectory.
     - Static technique is used to identify the size and location of the bladder and to mark an optimal location for needle insertion. The actual procedure is performed without ultrasound.
2. Relevant adult-specific literature
   - There are few studies in adult patients, since suprapubic aspiration is uncommonly performed in adult patients.
3. Relevant pediatric-specific literature
   - The failure rate of SPA without ultrasound guidance is reported as 8 % or higher [397].
   - When ultrasound was performed prior to SPA to evaluate for the presence of sufficient urine in the bladder, first attempt success was shown to be 100 %, when compared with 36 % without prior ultrasound evaluation [398].
   - Ultrasound-guided SPA has been shown to be more successful compared to blind SPA [399, 400].
   - The use of the bladder scan which is a portable ultrasound device prior to suprapubic aspiration has been shown to have success rates of 53 %, which is lower than reported success rates of real-time ultrasound [401].
4. Outstanding questions to be answered/voids in the literature to date
   - Given the frequency with which urethral catheterization is performed today, in lieu of SPA, it is not clear what method is best (e.g., simulation, animal models) for training and demonstrating competence with the procedure.

Curriculum objectives

1. Describe the *indications* for POCUS for suprapubic aspiration
   - Indications for performing bladder ultrasound include patients in whom a sterile urine specimen is needed and who are unable to voluntarily provide a specimen (i.e., children less than 2 years of age, or those who have limited mobility), or in whom urethral catheterization is unsuccessful.
2. Describe the *limitations* of POCUS for suprapubic aspiration or urethral catheterization.
   - Success is dependent on operator comfort and their level of experience with suprapubic aspiration, which is uncommon in many settings.
3. Describe the *relevant anatomy* to be identified in the POCUS examination for suprapubic aspiration or urethral catheterization
   - The bladder is recognized as an anechoic structure with a surrounding thin echogenic line, indicating its wall.
   - Imaging in the sagittal plane and introducing the needle in the plane of the ultrasound beam are preferred for ultrasound guidance, to visualize the entire length of the needle.
4. Recognize specific *pitfalls* involved in POCUS for suprapubic aspiration or urethral catheterization

- An empty (i.e., collapsed) bladder may not be identified by ultrasound examination.
- Other fluid-filled structures, e.g., loops of bowel with ileus, must be distinguished from bladder.
- Not following the full trajectory of the needle may result in penetration of other structures (e.g., bowel).
- Failure to observe the usual precautions and recommendations applicable to suprapubic or urethral catheterization whether performed with or without ultrasound guidance.

*Discussion of bladder ultrasound can be found in the diagnostic indications section.

Ultrasound guidance for thoracentesis

Evidence

1. Summary/indications
   - Lung ultrasound allows timely recognition, characterization and precise localization of pleural effusions. Ultrasound allows visualization of structures to be avoided during the procedure such as the diaphragm and lung parenchyma.
   - Ultrasound-guided thoracentesis has been shown to reduce iatrogenic complications and to increase the success of thoracentesis.
     - Dynamic ultrasound guidance uses real-time imaging to aid thoracentesis with direct visualization of the needle trajectory.
     - Static technique is used to identify anatomic landmarks and the extent of the pleural effusion, and to mark an optimal location for needle insertion. The procedure is then performed without real-time ultrasound guidance.
2. Relevant adult-specific literature
   - Ultrasound-guided thoracentesis reduces rates of pneumothorax [382, 402–408], increases rates of success [382, 402, 404–408] and reduces complications such as the need for subsequent tube thoracostomy [403, 404, 406–408].
   - Additional studies suggest that ultrasound-guided thoracentesis is associated with lower hospital length of stay, costs, and a lower incidence of pneumothoraces [382, 407].
3. Relevant pediatric-specific literature
   - There have been no studies to date evaluating POCUS for thoracentesis in pediatric patients.
4. Outstanding questions to be answered/voids in the literature to date
   - As no randomized controlled trials of POCUS for thoracentesis in pediatric patients exist, it is unknown whether there is a benefit in procedure duration, complication rate, patient/parent satisfaction, pain, or outcome. The favorable risk:benefit profile demonstrated in some studies of adult patients may be translated to the pediatric setting.

Curriculum objectives

1. Describe the *indications* for POCUS for thoracentesis
   - POCUS for thoracentesis should be used whenever a thoracentesis is to be performed, especially when a difficult procedure is anticipated.
2. Describe the *limitations* of POCUS for thoracentesis
   - Thoracentesis is an invasive procedure with potential complications such as pneumothorax and injury of solid organs or the diaphragm.
3. Describe the *relevant anatomy* to be identified in the ultrasound for thoracentesis
   - The optimal site for drainage of a non-loculated pleural effusion is usually on the posterior axillary line above the diaphragm. POCUS can confirm this or prompt the choice of an alternative location. The hemithorax of interest should be scanned from the inferior border of the scapula to the upper lumbar region and the costophrenic sulcus should be evaluated from the paravertebral region posteriorly to the parasternal region anteriorly.
   - Structures such as the diaphragm, subdiaphragmatic organs (spleen and liver) and thoracic organs (lung, heart and ribs) should be identified before the procedure. Ideally, a rib-space above and below the site of thoracentesis and a pocket at least 15 mm deep should be identifiable throughout the respiratory cycle at the site selected for thoracentesis.
   - In loculated effusions, a space, usually anechoic, is identified in the costophrenic sulcus between the parietal and visceral pleura. Fluid moves with patient positioning and will accumulate in the most dependent areas of the hemithorax; thus, the upright position is optimal.
   - The presence of septations and/or fibrinous strands usually suggests an exudate and/or a loculated collection. A loculated effusion may appear as multiple pockets of fluid separated by septations. It will not be mobile and, therefore, may not be dependent.
4. Recognize the specific *pitfalls* involved in POCUS for thoracentesis

- Free fluid in the abdominal cavity could be misidentified as a pleural effusion if the diaphragm is not identified, especially when there is an elevated hemidiaphragm.
- The patient should not move after the effusion is mapped, as fluid can shift.
- Not visualizing the lung and diaphragm through all phases of the respiratory cycle may result in organ injury.
- Recommendations regarding safe volumes for evacuation during a single thoracentesis are beyond the scope of this document.
- Failure to observe the usual precautions and recommendations applicable to thoracentesis whether performed with or without ultrasound guidance.

*Discussion of lung ultrasound can be found in the diagnostic indications section.

Ultrasound guidance for vascular access

Evidence

1. Summary/brief explanation of indications
   - Venous access can be a life-saving procedure for many children who present to the emergency department.
   - Smaller children, especially those with extensive medical histories, and volume-depleted patients pose particular difficulties with venous access.
   - Ultrasound guidance may facilitate peripheral intravenous (IV) access, thereby avoiding central catheter placement or intraosseous needle placement, which can be associated with complications.
   - There are international recommendations regarding the use of ultrasound for central and peripheral venous access [409]/
     - Dynamic ultrasound guidance uses real-time imaging with direct visualization of the needle passing into the vessel. Most of this information that follows relates to the dynamic technique.
     - Using static ultrasound guidance, an optimal location for needle insertion is determined by ultrasound, and the skin is marked. The actual procedure is then performed without real-time ultrasound guidance. This technique is useful for practitioners who have not developed skill in dynamic ultrasound-guided vascular access.
2. Relevant adult-specific literature
   - *Central venous access* Ultrasound has been shown to facilitate central venous access in adult patients. When compared with the landmark method, ultrasound guidance was shown to have a lower overall and first attempt failure rate [410].
   - Compared with traditional landmark-guided approaches, ultrasound guidance results in fewer complications, mean insertion attempts, and placement failures [411, 412].
   - A randomized study of three different approaches to internal jugular venous cannulation evaluated the success of the landmark approach compared to dynamic and static ultrasound guidance. Dynamic guidance 54 times the odds of successful cannulation compared to the landmark approach and the static approach had three times the odds of success compared to the landmark approach [413].
   - A 2015 Cochrane systematic review of 35 studies (31 of adult patients) of ultrasound guidance for internal jugular vein cannulation concluded that ultrasound offered "gains" in both safety and quality compared with an anatomical landmark technique [414]. The Cochrane review of 13 studies (11 of adult patients) of ultrasound guidance for femoral and subclavian cannulation concluded that there were only "small gains" in safety and quality compared with an anatomical landmark method [415].
   - The Institute of Medicine recommends ultrasound guidance as standard of care in the placement of all central catheters to improve patient safety [416]. The use of ultrasound guidance for central venous cannulation is listed as one of the top 11 methods to improve patient safety by the Agency for Healthcare Research and Quality [417].
   - *Peripheral venous access* When compared with traditional cannulation techniques, ultrasound-guided peripheral intravenous catheter placement has greater success rates, fewer skin punctures, decreased time for intravenous catheter placement, and fewer complications [418, 419].
   - The use of ultrasound-guided peripheral intravenous catheter placement is associated with decreased use of central venous catheter use [420].
   - *Intraosseous placement* One study in eight cadaveric legs demonstrated the ability of ultrasound using color power Doppler to accurately assess placement of intraosseous needles [421].
3. Relevant pediatric-specific literature
   - *Central venous access* Ultrasound has been show to facilitate central venous access in pediatric patients. In surgical patients, the overall success rate for ultrasound guidance was 91.5 % compared with 72.5 % in the landmark-guided group. However, in children less than 1 year of age and less than 10 kg,

the success rates were not statistically different [422].

- In pediatric patients, surgeon-performed central venous access was more successful with ultrasound guidance than the landmark approach, with first attempt success in 65 % patients in the US group, compared with 45 % in the landmark group ($p = 0.02$); success was achieved within three attempts in 95 % of the ultrasound group vs. 74 % of the landmark group ($p < 0.001$) [423].
- When evaluating the femoral vessels with ultrasound, it was found that external landmarks were not always predictive of internal anatomy. The femoral vein may be completely or partially overlapped by the femoral artery in 12 % of patients. Therefore, visualization by ultrasound is recommended prior to femoral vein catheterization [424].
- Additional confirmation of proper central catheter placement in children involves flushing the central catheter with agitated saline solution [425].
- *Peripheral venous access* One study of ultrasound for procedural-guidance revealed no change in overall success rates, but decreased time to placement, decreased number of attempts, and decreased number of needle redirections [426].
- *Intraosseous placement* One case series of five critically ill patients describes the use of ultrasound with color Doppler to correctly identify proper and improperly positioned intraosseous needles [427].

4. Outstanding questions to be answered/voids in the literature to date
   - Further investigation is needed in pediatric patients to address the overall success rate of ultrasound-guided peripheral IV access compared with blind insertion.
   - It is unclear how much training and how many ultrasound-guided catheter placements should be required to become competent in the procedure.

Curriculum objectives

1. Describe the *indications* for ultrasound-guided vascular access
   - Those patients with a history of difficult access, or who at the time of presentation have had failed attempts at access by traditional methods.
2. Describe the *limitations* of ultrasound guidance for vascular access.

   Limitations of vascular access ultrasound include the following:
   - Success of ultrasound-guided vascular access is largely dependent on the operator and his/her level of experience.
   - Regardless of whether ultrasound is used for vascular access, there are still some intrinsic difficulties with the veins themselves: valves, collapsing and rolling.
   - Smaller diameter vessels, and deeper vessels are often more difficult to cannulate [428].
3. Describe the *relevant anatomy* to be identified when using ultrasound for vascular access
   - Vessels should be "pre-scanned" in longitudinal and transverse planes to identify important surrounding structures, anatomic anomalies, and to determine the optimal site(s) for cannulation.
   - The most common sites for central catheter placement include the femoral vein, internal jugular vein, and subclavian vein.
   - Peripheral venous cannulations are commonly performed in the basilic, brachial, cephalic, and saphenous veins.
   - Vessels may be cannulated in the short-axis ("out of plane"), or in the long-axis ("in plane").
4. Recognize specific *pitfalls* involved in ultrasound-*guided vascular access*
   - Procedural ultrasound may be complicated by patient characteristics, including large body habitus and movement during the procedure or after marking during a static procedure.
   - When utilizing the short-axis technique, errors in placement of the needle or positioning of the transducer may lead to erroneous positioning of the needle in relation to the vessel.
   - Using the short-axis technique, the most common error is failure to maintain constant localization of the needle tip. The needle tip should be guided in real time into the lumen of the vessel.
   - The long-axis technique allows for visualization of the entire path of the needle, but is technically more challenging since the transducer, needle, and vessel need to remain continuously in the same plane.
   - "Flashback" of blood into the needle chamber occurs as the bevel of the needle enters the vessel lumen. Advancing the catheter over the needle at this point will result in failure of cannulation. The needle and catheter should be advanced together for several millimeters after "flashback" in order for the catheter to enter the vessel.
   - Veins must be distinguished from nerves and arteries with which they frequently travel. Nerves are non-compressible and will demonstrate internal echoes when the scanning plane is exactly perpendicular to the nerve.
   - Arteries may compress and be difficult to distinguish from veins, resulting in arterial cannulation. This is especially common in younger children. The

operator should look for arterial pulsations or Doppler color flow to further distinguish arteries from veins. It may be particularly difficult to distinguish an artery from a vein in a patient in shock.

- Failure to observe the usual precautions and recommendations applicable to regional anesthesia whether performed with or without ultrasound guidance

Reporting Guidelines for Ultrasound-Guided Procedures

Patient Demographics:

Patient Name:
Patient Gender: ☐Male ☐Female

DOB: _/_/__

MR#:
Date & Time: _/_/__ _:_

Procedure:

☐ Arthrocentesis ☐ Arterial catheter placement ☐ Abscess incision and drainage

☐ Lumbar puncture ☐ Paracentesis ☐ Pericardiocentesis

☐ Regional anesthesia ☐ Suprapubic bladder aspiration ☐ Thoracentesis

☐ Venous access

Examination Demographics:

Operator Name(s): ____________________

Operator Training: ☐Attending ☐Fellow ☐Resident ☐Medical Student ☐Other: ____________

Indication(s):

Anatomic location(s):

Number of attempts:

Outcome:

Complications:

Comments:

Authors' contributions

JRM and REL conceived the idea for the manuscript, all authors participated in drafting sections ofthe manuscript. All authors read and approved the final manuscript.

Author details

[1] Children's Hospital of Pittsburgh, 4401 Penn Ave, AOB Suite 2400, Pittsburgh, PA 15224, USA. [2] Children's National Medical Center, Washington DC, USA. [3] Maimonides Medical Center, Brooklyn, NY, USA. [4] New York Methodist Hospital, Brooklyn, NY, USA. [5] Hospital for Sick Children, Toronto, Ontario, Canada. [6] Boston Children's Hospital, Boston, MA, USA. [7] Queens Medical Center, Honolulu, HI, USA. [8] University of California-Davis, Sacramento, CA, USA. [9] Morgan Stanley Children's Hospital, New York, NY, USA. [10] University of California-San Diego, San Diego, CA, USA. [11] Dell Children's Medical Center, Austin, USA. [12] Boston Medical Center, Boston, MA, USA. [13] Massachusetts General Hospital, Boston, MA, USA. [14] Boston University Medical Center, Boston, NY, USA. [15] Columbia University Medical Center, New York, NY, USA. [16] St. Lukes-Roosevelt Hospital, New York, NY, USA. [17] Montefiore Medical Center, Bronx, NY, USA. [18] Newark Beth Israel Medical Center, Newark, NJ, USA. [19] Mount Sinai Hospital, New York, NY, USA. [20] Cohen Children's Medical Center, New Hyde Park, USA. [21] Weill Cornell Medical Center, New York, NY, USA. [22] University of Colorado, Aurora, CO, USA.

Acknowledgements

None.

References

1. Moore CL, Copel JA (2011) Point-of-care ultrasonography. N Engl J Med 364(8):749–757
2. Gregory S, Kuntz K, Sainfort F, Kharbanda A (2016) Cost-effectiveness of integrating a clinical decision rule and staged imaging protocol for diagnosis of appendicitis. Value Health 19(1):28–35
3. Becker DM, Tafoya CA, Becker SL, Kruger GH, Tafoya MJ, Becker TK (2016) The use of portable ultrasound devices in low- and middle-income countries: a systematic review of the literature. Trop Med Int Health 21(3):294–311
4. Kearl YL, Claudius I, Behar S, Cooper J, Dollbaum R, Hardasmalani M, Hardiman K, Rose E, Santillanes G, Berdahl C (2016) Accuracy of magnetic resonance imaging and ultrasound for appendicitis in diagnostic and nondiagnostic studies. Acad Emerg Med 23(2):179–185
5. Zouari M, Jallouli M, Louati H, Kchaou R, Chtourou R, Kotti A, Dhaou MB, Zitouni H, Mhiri R (2016) Predictive value of C-reactive protein, ultrasound and Alvarado score in acute appendicitis: a prospective pediatric cohort. Am J Emerg Med 34(2):189–192
6. Basile V, Di Mauro A, Scalini E, Comes P, Lofù I, Mostert M, Tafuri S, Manzionna MM (2015) Lung ultrasound: a useful tool in diagnosis and management of bronchiolitis. BMC Pediatr 15:63
7. Chen L, Kim Y, Moore CL (2007) Diagnosis and guided reduction of forearm fractures in children using bedside ultrasound. Pediatr Emerg Care 23(8):528–531
8. Glover CD, Paek JS, Patel N, Manyang P, McKay SD, Watcha M (2015) Postoperative pain and the use of ultrasound-guided regional analgesia in pediatric supracondylar humerus fractures. J Pediatr Orthop B 24(3):178–183
9. Mathews JD, Forsythe AV, Brady Z, Butler MW, Goergen SK, Byrnes GB, Giles GG, Wallace AB, Anderson PR, Guiver TA, McGale P, Cain TM, Dowty JG, Bickerstaffe AC, Darby SC (2013) Cancer risk in 680,000 people exposed to computed tomography scans in childhood or adolescence: data linkage study of 11 million Australians. BMJ 346:f2360
10. American College of Emergency Physicians (2001) American college of emergency physicians emergency ultrasound guidelines. Ann Emerg Med 38(4):470–481
11. Fagley RE, Haney MF, Beraud AS, Comfere T, Kohl BA, Merkel MJ, Pustavoitau A, von Homeyer P, Wagner CE, Wall MH (2015) Critical care basic ultrasound learning goals for american anesthesiology critical care trainees: recommendations from an expert group. Anesth Analg 120(5):1041–1053
12. Lewiss RE, Pearl M, Nomura JT, Baty G, Bengiamin R, Duprey K, Stone M, Theodoro D, Akhtar S (2013) CORD-AEUS: consensus document for the emergency ultrasound milestone project. Acad Emerg Med 20(7):740–745
13. Marin JR, Lewiss RE, American Academy of Pediatrics Committee on Pediatric Emergency Medicine, Society for Academic Emergency Medicine Academy of Emergency Ultrasound, American College of Emergency Physicians Pediatric Emergency Medicine Committee, World Interactive Network Focused on Critical Ultrasound (2015) Policy statement: point-of-care ultrasonography by pediatric emergency physicians. Ann Emerg Med 65(4):472–478
14. Marin JR, Lewiss RE, American Academy of Pediatrics Committee on Pediatric Emergency Medicine, Society for Academic Emergency Medicine Academy of Emergency Ultrasound, American College of Emergency Physicians Pediatric Emergency Medicine Committee, World Interactive Network Focused on Critical Ultrasound (2015) Technical report: point-of-care ultrasonography by pediatric emergency medicine physicians. Pediatrics 135(4):e113–e122
15. Doria AS, Moineddin R, Kellenberger CJ, Epelman M, Beyene J, Schuh S, Babyn PS, Dick PT (2006) US or CT for diagnosis of appendicitis in children and adults? A meta-analysis. Radiology 241:83–94
16. Rosen MP, Ding A, Blake MA, Baker ME, Cash BD, Fidler JL, Grant TH, Greene FL, Jones B, Katz DS, Lalani T, Miller FH, Small WC, Spottswood S, Sudakoff GS, Tulchinsky M, Warshauer DM, Yee J, Coley BD (2011) ACR appropriateness criteria (R) right lower quadrant pain-suspected appendicitis. J Am Coll Radiol: JACR 8:749–755
17. Chen SC, Wang HP, Hsu HY, Huang PM, Lin FY (2000) Accuracy of ED sonography in the diagnosis of acute appendicitis. Am J Emerg Med 18:449–452
18. Fox JC, Solley M, Anderson CL, Zlidenny A, Lahham S, Maasumi K (2008) Prospective evaluation of emergency physician performed bedside ultrasound to detect acute appendicitis. Eur J Emerg Med 15:80–85
19. Mallin M, Craven P, Ockerse P, Steenblik J, Forbes B, Boehm K, Youngquist S (2015) Diagnosis of appendicitis by bedside ultrasound in the ED. Am J Emerg Med 33:430–432
20. Taylor GA (2004) Suspected appendicitis in children: in search of the single best diagnostic test. Radiology 231:293–295
21. Bachur RG, Dayan PS, Bajaj L, Macias CG, Mittal MK, Stevenson MD, Dudley NC, Sinclair K, Bennett J, Monuteaux MC, Kharbanda AB (2012) The effect of abdominal pain duration on the accuracy of diagnostic imaging for pediatric appendicitis. Ann Emerg Med 60:582–590
22. Frei SP, Bond WF, Bazuro RK, Richardson DM, Sierzega GM, Reed JF (2008) Appendicitis outcomes with increasing computed tomographic scanning. Am J Emerg Med 26:39–44
23. Martin AE, Vollman D, Adler B, Caniano DA (2004) CT scans may not reduce the negative appendectomy rate in children. J Pediatr Surg 39:886–890 **(discussion 886–890)**
24. Krishnamoorthi R, Ramarajan N, Wang NE, Newman B, Rubesova E, Mueller CM, Barth RA (2011) Effectiveness of a staged US and CT protocol for the diagnosis of pediatric appendicitis: reducing radiation exposure in the age of ALARA. Radiology 259:231–239
25. Ramarajan N, Krishnamoorthi R, Barth R, Ghanouni P, Mueller C, Dannenburg B, Wang NE (2009) An interdisciplinary initiative to reduce radiation exposure: evaluation of appendicitis in a pediatric emergency department with clinical assessment supported by a staged ultrasound and computed tomography pathway. Acad Emerg Med 16:1258–1265
26. Garcia Pena BM, Cook EF, Mandl KD (2004) Selective imaging strategies for the diagnosis of appendicitis in children. Pediatrics 113(1 Pt 1):24–28
27. Wan MJ, Krahn M, Ungar WJ, Caku E, Sung L, Medina LS, Doria AS (2009) Acute appendicitis in young children: cost-effectiveness of US versus CT in diagnosis—a Markov decision analytic model. Radiology 250:378–386
28. Sivitz A, Cohen S, Tejani C (2014) Evaluation of acute appendicitis by pediatric emergency physician sonography. Ann Emerg Med 64(358–364):e4

29. Elikashvili I, Tay ET, Tsung JW (2014) The effect of point-of-care ultrasonography on emergency department length of stay and computed tomography utilization in children with suspected appendicitis. Acad Emerg Med 21:163–170
30. Kim C, Kang BS, Choi HJ, Lim TH, Oh J, Chee Y (2015) Clinical application of real-time tele-ultrasonography in diagnosing pediatric acute appendicitis in the ED. Am J Emerg Med 33:1354–1359
31. Rettenbacher T, Hollerweger A, Macheiner P, Rettenbacher L, Tomaselli F, Schneider B, Gritzmann N (2001) Outer diameter of the vermiform appendix as a sign of acute appendicitis: evaluation at US. Radiology 218:757–762
32. Goldin AB, Khanna P, Thapa M, McBroom JA, Garrison MM, Parisi MT (2011) Revised ultrasound criteria for appendicitis in children improve diagnostic accuracy. Pediatr Radiol 41:993–999
33. Sulowski C, Doria AS, Langer JC, Man C, Stephens D, Schuh S (2011) Clinical outcomes in obese and normal-weight children undergoing ultrasound for suspected appendicitis. Acad Emerg Med 18:167–173
34. Sivit CJ (1993) Diagnosis of acute appendicitis in children: spectrum of sonographic findings. AJR Am J Roentgenol 161:147–152
35. Quillin SP, Siegel MJ, Coffin CM (1992) Acute appendicitis in children: value of sonography in detecting perforation. AJR Am J Roentgenol 159:1265–1268
36. Tulin-Silver S, Babb J, Pinkney L, Strubel N, Lala S, Milla SS, Tomita S, Fefferman NR (2015) The challenging ultrasound diagnosis of perforated appendicitis in children: constellations of sonographic findings improve specificity. Pediatr Radiol 45:820–830
37. Puylaert JB (1986) Acute appendicitis: US evaluation using graded compression. Radiology 158:355–360
38. Rettenbacher T, Hollerweer A, Macheiner P, Gritzmann N, Daniaux M, Schwamberger K, Ulmer H, zur Nedden D (2003) Ovoid shape of the vermiform appendix: a criterion to exclude acute appendicitis–evaluation with US. Radiology 226:95–100
39. Kaneko K, Tsuda M (2004) Ultrasound-based decision making in the treatment of acute appendicitis in children. J Pediatr Surg 39:1316–1320
40. Bailet PV, Connors RH, Tracy TF, Sotelo-Avila C, Lewis JE, Weber TR (1989) Changing spectrum of cholelithiasis and cholecystitis in infants and children. Am J Surg 158:585–588
41. CDC Division of Nutrition, physical activity, and obesity. http://www.cdc.gov/obesity/childhood/. Accessed 20 Sept 2011
42. van Rijn RR, Nievelstein RA (2014) Paediatric ultrasonography of the liver, hepatobiliary tract and pancreas. Eur J Radiol 83:1570–1581
43. Kendall JL, Shimp RJ (2001) Performance and interpretation of limited right upper quadrant ultrasound by emergency physicians. J Emerg Med 21:7–13
44. Miller AH, Pepe PE, Brockman CR, Delaney KA (2006) ED ultrasound in hepatobiliary disease. J Emerg Med 30:69–74
45. Blaivas M, Harwood RA, Lambert MJ (1999) Decreasing length of stay with emergency ultrasound examination of the gallbladder. Acad Emerg Med 6:1020–1023
46. Conway D (2011) Emergency Department patients evaluated by bedside biliary ultrasonography: does radiology ultrasonography alter disposition? Ann Emerg Med 58:S195
47. Roy S (2002) Hepatobiliary. In: Ma OJ, Mateer JE (eds) Emergency ultrasound. McGraw Hill, Columbus
48. Gaspari RJ, Dickman E, Blehar D (2009) Learning curve of bedside ultrasound of the gallbladder. J Emerg Med 37:51–56
49. Bloch A (2010) Patient satisfaction with bedside ultrasonography in the emergency department. Ann Emerg Med 56:S117
50. Tsung JW, Raio CC, Ramirez-Shrempp D, Blaivas M (2010) Point-of-care ultrasound diagnosis of pediatric cholecystitis in the ED. Am J Emerg Med 28:338–342
51. Jang TB (2010) The learning curve of resident physicians using emergency ultrasonography for cholelithiasis and cholecystitis. Acad Emerg Med 17:1247–1252
52. Wheeler J, O'Riordan M, Allareddy V, Speicher D (2015) Would the use of bedside bladder ultrasound decrease the necessity of invasive bladder catheterization in the pediatric intensive care unit? Clin Pediatr 54:800–802
53. Selius BA, Subedi R (2008) Urinary retention in adults: diagnosis and initial management. Am Fam Physician 77:643–650
54. Chan H (1993) Noninvasive bladder volume measurement. J Neurosci Nurs 25:309–312
55. Milling TJ Jr, Van Amerongen R, Melville Santiago L, Gaeta T, Birkhahn R, Melniker L (2005) Use of ultrasonography to identify infants for whom urinary catheterization will be unsuccessful because of insufficient urine volume: validation of the urinary bladder index. Ann Emerg Med 45:510–513
56. Chen L, Hsiao AL, Moore CL, Dziura JD, Santucci KA (2005) Utility of bedside bladder ultrasound before urethral catheterization in young children. Pediatrics 115:108–111
57. Witt M, Baumann BM, McCans K (2005) Bladder ultrasound increases catheterization success in pediatric patients. Acad Emerg Med 12:371–374
58. Price DP, Peterson MA (2003) Pediatric applications. In: Ma OJ, Mateer JR (eds) Emergency ultrasound. McGraw-Hill Companies, Columbus
59. Hiraoka M, Tsukahara H, Tsuchida S, Hori C, Sudo M (1993) Ultrasonographic evaluation of bladder volume in children. Pediatr Nephrol 7:533–535
60. Burnside PR, Brown MD, Kline JA (2008) Systematic review of emergency physician-performed ultrasonography for lower-extremity deep vein thrombosis. Acad Emerg Med 15:493–498
61. Theodoro D, Blaivas M, Duggal S, Snyder G, Lucas M (2004) Real-time B-mode ultrasound in the ED saves time the diagnosis of deep vein thrombosis (DVT). Am J Emerg Med 22:197–200
62. Magazzini S, Vanni S, Toccafondi S, Paladini B, Zanobetti M, Giannazzo G, Federico R, Grifoni S (2007) Duplex ultrasound in the emergency department for the diagnostic management of clinically suspected deep vein thrombosis. Acad Emerg Med 14:216–220
63. Jolly BT, Massarin E, Pigman EC (1997) Color Doppler ultrasonography by emergency physicians for the diagnosis of acute deep venous thrombosis. Acad Emerg Med 4:129–132
64. Bernardi E, Camporese G, Büller HR, Siragusa S, Imberti D, Berchio A, Ghirarduzzi A, Verlato F, Anastasio R, Prati C, Piccioli A, Pesavento R, Bova C, Maltempi P, Zanatta N, Cogo A, Cappelli R, Bucherini E, Cuppini S, Noventa F, Prandoni P, Erasmus Study Group (2008) Serial 2-point ultrasonography plus D-dimer vs whole-leg color-coded Doppler ultrasonography for diagnosing suspected symptomatic deep vein thrombosis: a randomized controlled trial. JAMA 300:1653–1659
65. Tay ET, Stone MB, Tsung JW (2012) Emergency ultrasound diagnosis of deep venous thrombosis in the pediatric emergency department. Pediatr Emerg Care 28:90–95
66. Dean AJ, Ku BS (2008) Deep vein thrombosis In: Sonoguide. http://www.sonoguide/dvt.html. Accessed 1 Aug 2010
67. Blaivas M (2000) Bedside emergency department ultrasonography in the evaluation of ocular pathology. Acad Emerg Med 7:947–950
68. Blaivas M, Theodoro D, Sierzenski PR (2002) A study of bedside ocular ultrasonography in the emergency department. Acad Emerg Med 9:791–799
69. Vrablik ME, Snead GR, Minnigan HJ, Kirschner JM, Emmett TW, Seupaul RA (2015) The diagnostic accuracy of bedside ocular ultrasonography for the diagnosis of retinal detachment: a systematic review and meta-analysis. Ann Emerg Med 65(199–203):e1
70. Geeraerts T, Merceron S, Benhamou D, Vigué B, Duranteau J (2008) Non-invasive assessment of intracranial pressure using ocular sonography in neurocritical care patients. Intensive Care Med 34(11):2062–2067
71. Tayal VS, Neulander M, Norton HJ, Foster T, Saunders T, Blaivas M (2007) Emergency department sonographic measurement of optic nerve sheath diameter to detect findings of increased intracranial pressure in adult head injury patients. Ann Emerg Med 49:508–514
72. Blaivas M, Theodoro D, Sierzenski PR (2003) Elevated intracranial pressure detected by bedside emergency ultrasonography of the optic nerve sheath. Acad Emerg Med 10:376–381
73. Major R, Girling S, Boyle A (2011) Ultrasound measurement of optic nerve sheath diameter in patients with a clinical suspicion of raised intracranial pressure. Emerg Med J 28:679–681
74. Buzzard AK, Linklater DR (2009) Pediatric retinal detachment due to Coats' disease diagnosed with bedside emergency department ultrasound. J Emerg Med 37:390–392
75. Braun A, Doniger SJ (2014) Point-of-care ultrasonography for the identification of 2 children with optic disc drusen mimicking papilledema. Pediatr Emerg Care 30:505–507

76. Presley BC, Flannigan MJ (2013) Emergency department bedside ultrasound diagnosis of retinoblastoma in a child. Pediatr Emerg Care 29:1128–1131
77. Riggs BJ, Trimboli-Heidler C, Spaeder MC, Miller M, Dean NP, Cohen JS (2015) The use of ophthalmic ultrasonography to identify retinal injuries associated with abusive head trauma. Ann Emerg Med 67(5):620–624
78. Korber F, Scharf M, Moritz J, Dralle D, Alzen G (2005) Sonography of the optical nerve—experience in 483 children. Rofo 177:229–235
79. Driessen C, Bannink N, Lequin M, van Veelen ML, Naus NC, Joosten KF, Mathijssen IM (2011) Are ultrasonography measurements of optic nerve sheath diameter an alternative to funduscopy in children with syndromic craniosynostosis? J Neurosurg Pediatr 8:329–334
80. Ballantyne J, Hollman AS, Hamilton R, Bradnam MS, Carachi R, Young DG, Dutton GN (1999) Transorbital optic nerve sheath ultrasonography in normal children. Clin Radiol 54:740–742
81. Newman WD, Hollman AS, Dutton GN, Carachi R (2002) Measurement of optic nerve sheath diameter by ultrasound: a means of detecting acute raised intracranial pressure in hydrocephalus. Br J Ophthalmol 86:1109–1113
82. Malayeri AA, Bavarian S, Mehdizadeh M (2005) Sonographic evaluation of optic nerve diameter in children with raised intracranial pressure. J Ultrasound Med 24:143–147
83. Le A, Hoehn ME, Smith ME, Spentzas T, Schlappy D, Pershad J (2009) Bedside sonographic measurement of optic nerve sheath diameter as a predictor of increased intracranial pressure in children. Ann Emerg Med 53:785–791
84. Tsung JW, Blaivas M, Cooper A, Levick NR (2005) A rapid noninvasive method of detecting elevated intracranial pressure using bedside ocular ultrasound: application to 3 cases of head trauma in the pediatric emergency department. Pediatr Emerg Care 21:94–98
85. Hall MK, Spiro DM, Sabbaj A, Moore CL, Hopkins KL, Meckler GD (2013) Bedside optic nerve sheath diameter ultrasound for the evaluation of suspected pediatric ventriculoperitoneal shunt failure in the emergency department. Childs Nerv Sys 29:2275–2280
86. McAuley D, Paterson A, Sweeney L (2009) Optic nerve sheath ultrasound in the assessment of paediatric hydrocephalus. Childs Nerv Syst 25:87–90
87. Yoonessi R, Hussain A, Jang TB (2010) Bedside ocular ultrasound for the detection of retinal detachment in the emergency department. Acad Emerg Med 17:913–917
88. Berg C, Doniger SJ, Zaia B, Williams SR (2015) Change in intraocular pressure during point-of-care ultrasound. Wes J Emerg Meds 16:263–268
89. Stengel D, Rademacher G, Ekkernkamp A, Güthoff C, Mutze S (2015) Emergency ultrasound-based algorithms for diagnosing blunt abdominal trauma. Cochrane Database Syst Rev 9:CD004446
90. Melniker LA, Leibner E, McKenney MG, Lopez P, Briggs WM, Mancuso CA (2006) Randomized controlled clinical trial of point-of-care, limited ultrasonography for trauma in the emergency department: the first sonography outcomes assessment program trial. Ann Emerg Med 48(3):227–235
91. Rose JS, Levitt MA, Porter J, Hutson A, Greenholtz J, Nobay F, Hilty W (2001) Does the presence of ultrasound really affect computed tomographic scan use? A prospective randomized trial of ultrasound in trauma. J Trauma 51(3):545–550
92. Ma OJ, Mateer JR, Ogata M, Kefer MP, Wittmann D, Aprahamian C (1995) Prospective analysis of a rapid trauma ultrasound examination performed by emergency physicians. J Trauma 38(6):879–885
93. Rozycki GS, Ballard RB, Feliciano DV, Schmidt JA, Pennington SD (1998) Surgeon-performed ultrasound for the assessment of truncal injuries: lessons learned from 1540 patients. Ann Surg 228(4):557–567
94. Rozycki GS, Ochsner MG, Jaffin JH, Champion HR (1993) Prospective evaluation of surgeons' use of ultrasound in the evaluation of trauma patients. J Trauma 34(4):516–526 **(discussion 526–517)**
95. Kern SJ, Smith RS, Fry WR, Helmer SD, Reed JA, Chang FC (1997) Sonographic examination of abdominal trauma by senior surgical residents. Am Surg 63(8):669–674
96. Shackford SR, Rogers FB, Osler TM, Trabulsy ME, Clauss DW, Vane DW (1999) Focused abdominal sonogram for trauma: the learning curve of nonradiologist clinicians in detecting hemoperitoneum. J Trauma 46(4):553–562 **(discussion 562–554)**
97. Smith RS, Kern SJ, Fry WR, Helmer SD (1998) Institutional learning curve of surgeon-performed trauma ultrasound. Arch Surg 133(5):530–535 **(discussion 535–536)**
98. Volpicelli G, Elbarbary M, Blaivas M, Lichtenstein DA, Mathis G, Kirkpatrick AW, Melniker L, Gargani L, Noble VE, Via G et al (2012) International evidence-based recommendations for point-of-care lung ultrasound. Intensive Care Med 38(4):577–591
99. Ma OJ, Mateer JR, Blaivas M (2008) Emergency ultrasound, 2nd edn. McGraw-Hill Professional, Columbus, pp 77–108
100. Fox JC, Boysen M, Gharahbaghian L, Cusick S, Ahmed SS, Anderson CL, Lekawa M, Langdorf MI (2011) Test characteristics of focused assessment of sonography for trauma for clinically significant abdominal free fluid in pediatric blunt abdominal trauma. Acad Emerg Med 18(5):477–482
101. Holmes JF, Gladman A, Chang CH (2007) Performance of abdominal ultrasonography in pediatric blunt trauma patients: a meta-analysis. J Pediatr Surg 42(9):1588–1594
102. Holmes JF, Brant WE, Bond WF, Sokolove PE, Kuppermann N (2001) Emergency department ultrasonography in the evaluation of hypotensive and normotensive children with blunt abdominal trauma. J Pediatr Surg 36(7):968–973
103. Scaife ER, Rollins MD, Barnhart DC, Downey EC, Black RE, Meyers RL, Stevens MH, Gordon S, Prince JS, Battaglia D et al (2013) The role of focused abdominal sonography for trauma (FAST) in pediatric trauma evaluation. J Pediatr Surg 48(6):1377–1383
104. Sola JE, Cheung MC, Yang R, Koslow S, Lanuti E, Seaver C, Neville HL, Schulman CI (2009) Pediatric FAST and elevated liver transaminases: an effective screening tool in blunt abdominal trauma. J Surg Res 157(1):103–107
105. Menaker J, Blumberg S, Wisner DH, Dayan PS, Tunik M, Garcia M, Mahajan P, Page K, Monroe D, Borgialli D et al (2014) Use of the focused assessment with sonography for trauma (FAST) examination and its impact on abdominal computed tomography use in hemodynamically stable children with blunt torso trauma. J Trauma Acute Care Surg 77(3):427–432
106. Ng C, Tsung JW (2014) Point-of-care ultrasound for assisting in needle aspiration of spontaneous pneumothorax in the pediatric ED: a case series. Am J Emerg Med 32(5):488 **(e483–e488)**
107. Holmes JF, Lillis K, Monroe D, Borgialli D, Kerrey BT, Mahajan P, Adelgais K, Ellison AM, Yen K, Atabaki S et al (2013) Identifying children at very low risk of clinically important blunt abdominal injuries. Ann Emerg Med 62(2):107–116 **(e102)**
108. Rozycki GS, Ochsner MG, Feliciano DV, Thomas B, Boulanger BR, Davis FE, Falcone RE, Schmidt JA (1998) Early detection of hemoperitoneum by ultrasound examination of the right upper quadrant: a multicenter study. J Trauma 45(5):878–883
109. Nance ML, Mahboubi S, Wickstrom M, Prendergast F, Stafford PW (2002) Pattern of abdominal free fluid following isolated blunt spleen or liver injury in the pediatric patient. J Trauma 52(1):85–87
110. Via G, Hussain A, Wells M, Reardon R, ElBarbary M, Noble VE, Tsung JW, Neskovic AN, Price S, Oren-Grinberg A, Liteplo A, International Conference of Focused Cardiac UltraSound (IC-FoCUS) (2014) International evidence-based recommendations for focused cardiac ultrasound. J Am Soc Echocardiogr 27:683-e1 **(e33)**
111. Labovitz AJ, Noble VE, Bierig M, Goldstein SA, Jones R, Kort S, Porter TR, Spencer KT, Tayal VS, Wei K (2010) Focused cardiac ultrasound in the emergent setting: a consensus statement of the American Society of Echocardiography and American College of Emergency Physicians. J Am Soc Echocardiogr 23:1225–1230
112. Lai WW, Geva T, Shirali GS, Frommelt PC, Humes RA, Brook MM, Pignatelli RH, Rychik J, Committee Writing (2006) Guidelines and standards for performance of a pediatric echocardiogram: a report from the task force of the Pediatric Council of the American Society of Echocardiography. J Am Soc Echocardiogr 19:1413–1430
113. Mertens L, Seri I, Marek J, Arlettaz R, Barker P, McNamara P, Moon-Grady AJ, Coon PD, Noori S, Simpson J, Lai WW (2011) Targeted neonatal echocardiography in the Neonatal Intensive Care Unit: practice guidelines and recommendations for training. Writing group of the American Society of Echocardiography (ASE) in collaboration with the European Association of Echocardiography (EAE) and the Association for European Pediatric Cardiologists (AEPC). J Am Soc Echocardgr 24:1057–1078

114. Joseph MX, Disney PJ, Da Costa R, Hutchison SJ (2004) Transthoracic echocardiography to identify or exclude cardiac cause of shock. Chest 126:1592–1597
115. Rozycki GS, Feliciano DV, Ochsner MG, Knudson MM, Hoyt DB, Davis F, Hammerman D, Figueredo V, Harviel JD, Han DC, Schmidt JA (1999) The role of ultrasound in patients with possible penetrating cardiac wounds: a prospective multicenter study. J Trauma 46:543–552
116. Plummer D, Brunette D, Asinger R, Ruiz E (1992) Emergency department echocardiography improves outcome in penetrating cardiac injury. Ann Emerg Med 21:709–712
117. Schiavone WA, Ghumrawi BK, Catalano DR, Haver DW, Pipitone AJ, L'Hommedieu RH, Keyser PH, Tsai AR (1991) The use of echocardiography in the emergency management of nonpenetrating traumatic cardiac rupture. Ann Emerg Med 20:1248–1250
118. Baxa MD (1991) Cardiac rupture secondary to blunt trauma: a rapidly diagnosable entity with two-dimensional echocardiography. Ann Emerg Med 20:902–904
119. Mandavia DP, Hoffner RJ, Mahaney K, Henderson SO (2001) Bedside echocardiography by emergency physicians. Ann Emerg Med 38:377–382
120. Mayron R, Gaudio FE, Plummer D, Asinger R, Elsperger J (1988) Echocardiography performed by emergency physicians: impact on diagnosis and therapy. Ann Emerg Med 17:150–154
121. Kleinman ME, de Caen AR, Chameides L, Atkins DL, Berg RA, Berg MD, Bhanji F, Biarent D, Bingham R, Coovadia AH, Hazinski MF (2010) Part 10: pediatric basic and advanced life support. Focused echocardiogram to detect reversible causes of cardiac arrest section. Circulation 122:466–515
122. Moore CL, Rose GA, Tayal VS, Sullivan DM, Arrowood JA, Kline JA (2002) Determination of left ventricular function by emergency physician echocardiography of hypotensive patients. Acad Emerg Med 9:186–193
123. Randazzo MR, Snoey ER, Levitt MA et al (2003) Accuracy of emergency physician assessment of left ventricular ejection fraction and central venous pressure using echocardiography. Acad Emerg Med 10:973–977
124. Salen P, O'Connor R, Sierzenski P, Passarello B, Pancu D, Melanson S, Arcona S, Reed J, Heller M (2001) Can cardiac sonography and capnography be used independently and in combination to predict resuscitation outcomes? Acad Emerg Med 8:610–615
125. Blaivas M, Fox JC (2001) Outcome in cardiac arrest patients found to have cardiac standstill on the bedside emergency department echocardiogram. Acad Emerg Med 8:616–621
126. Breitkreutz RF, Walcher F, Seeger FH (2007) Focused echocardiographic evaluation in resuscitation management: concept of an advanced life support-conformed algorithm. Crit Care Med 35:150–161
127. Breitkreutz R, Price S, Steiger HV, Seeger FH, Ilper H, Ackermann H, Rudolph M, Uddin S, Weigand MA, Müller E, Walcher F (2010) Focused echocardiographic evaluation in life support and peri-resuscitation of emergency patients: a prospective trial. Resuscitation 81:1527–1533
128. Tsung JW, Blaivas M (2008) Feasibility of correlating the pulse check with focused point-of-care echocardiography during pediatric cardiac arrest: a case series. Resuscitation 77:264–269
129. Akilli B, Bayir A, Kara F, Ak A, Cander B (2010) Inferior vena cava diameter as a marker of early hemorrhagic shock: a comparative study. Ulus Travma Acil Cerrahi Derg 16:113–138
130. Gunst M, Ghaemmaghami V, Sperry J, Robinson M, O'Keeffe T, Friese R, Frankel H (2008) Accuracy of cardiac function and volume status estimates using the bedside echocardiographic assessment in trauma/critical care. J Trauma 65:509–516
131. Duvekot JJ, Cheriex EC, Tan WD, Heidendal GA, Peeters LL (1994) Measurement of anterior–posterior diameter of inferior vena cava by ultrasonography: a new non-invasive method to assess acute changes in vascular filling state. Cardiovasc Res 28:1269–1272
132. Yanagawa Y, Nishi K, Sakamoto T, Okada Y (2005) Early diagnosis of hypovolemic shock by sonographic measurement of inferior vena cava in trauma patients. J Trauma 58:825–829
133. Lee Christopher WC, Kory Pierre D, Arntfield Robert T (2016) Development of a fluid resuscitation protocol using inferior vena cava and lung ultrasound. J Crit Care 31:96–100
134. Fields JM, Lee PA, Jenq KY, Mark DG, Panebianco NL, Dean AJ (2011) The interrater reliability of inferior vena cava ultrasound by bedside clinician sonographers in emergency department patients. Acad Emerg Med 18:96–101
135. Chamberlain MC, Reid SR, Madhok M (2011) Utilization of emergency ultrasound in pediatric emergency departments. Pediatr Emerg Care 27:628–632
136. Milner D, Losek JD, Schiff J, Sicoli R (2003) Pediatric pericardial tamponade presenting as altered mental status. Pediatr Emerg Care 19:35–37
137. Steiger HV, Rimbach K, Müller E, Breitkreutz R (2009) Focused emergency echocardiography: lifesaving tool for a 14 year old girl suffering out-of-hospital pulseless ecectrical activity because of cardiac tamponade. Eur J Emerg Med 16:103–105
138. Pershad J, Chin T (2003) Early detection of cardiac disease masquerading as acute bronchospasm: the role of bedside limited echocardiography by the emergency physician. Pediatr Emerg Care 19:e1–e3
139. Bramante RM, Cirilli A, Raio CC (2010) Point-of-care sonography in the emergency department diagnosis of acute H1N1 influenza myocarditis. J Ultrasound Med 29:1361–1364
140. Sivitz A, Nagdev A (2012) Heart failure secondary to dilated cardiomyopathy: a role for emergency bedside ultrasonography. Pediatr Emerg Care 28:163–166
141. Cheng AB, Levine DA, Tsung JW, Phoon CK (2012) Emergency physician diagnosis of pediatric infective endocarditis by point-of-care echocardiography. Am J Emerg Med 30:386-e1
142. Spurney CF, Sable CA, Berger JT, Martin GR (2005) Use of a hand carried ultrasound device by critical care physicians for the diagnosis of pericardial effusions, decreased cardiac function, and left ventricular enlargement in pediatric patients. J Am Soc Echocardiogr 18:313–319
143. Gaspar HA, Morhy SS, Lianza AC, de Carvalho WB, Andrade JL, do Prado RR, Schvartsman C, Delgado AF (2014) Focused cardiac ultrasound: a training course for pediatric intensivists and emergency physicians. BMC Med Educ 14:1
144. Pershad J, Myers S, Plouman C, Rosson C, Elam K, Wan J, Chin T (2004) Bedside limited echocardiography by the emergency physician is accurate during evaluation of the critically ill patient. Pediatrics 114:e667–e671
145. Longjohn M, Wan J, Joshi V, Pershad J (2011) Point of care echocardiography by pediatric emergency physicians. Pediatr Emerg Care 27:693–696
146. Levine AC, Shah SP, Umulisa I, Munyaneza M, Richard B, Dushimiyimana JM, Stegmann K, Musavuli J, Ngabitsinze P, Stulac S, Epino HM (2010) Ultrasound assessment of severe dehydration in children with diarrhea and vomiting. Acad Emerg Med 17:1035–1041
147. Chen L, Hsiao A, Langhan M, Riera A, Santucci KA (2010) Use of bedside ultrasound to assess degree of dehydration in children with gastroenteritis. Acad Emerg Med 17:1042–1047
148. Chen L, Kim Y, Santucci KA (2007) Use of ultrasound measurement of the inferior vena cava diameter as an objective tool in the assessment of children with clinical dehydration. Acad Emerg Med 14:841–845
149. Perera P, Mailhot T, Riley D, Mandavia D (2010) The RUSH exam: rapid ultrasound in shock in evaluation of the critically Ill. Emerg Med Clin N Am 28:29–56
150. Otto CA, Shemenski R, Drudi L (2012) Real-time tele-echocardiography: diagnosis and management of a pericardial effusion secondary to pericarditis at an Antarctic Research Station. Telemed J E Health 18:521–524
151. Barbier P, Dalla Vecchia L, Mirra G, Di Marco S, Cavoretto D (2012) Near real-time echocardiography teleconsultation using low bandwidth and MPEG-4 compression: feasibility, image adequacy and clinical implications. J Telemed Telecare 18:204–210
152. Liteplo AS, Noble VE, Attwood B (2010) Real-time video transmission of ultrasound images to an iPhone. Crit Ultrasound J 1(3):105–110
153. Levitov A, Marik PE (2012) Echocardiographic assessment of preload responsiveness in critically ill patients. Cardiol Res Pract 2012:819696
154. Lin E, Chen AE, Panebianco N, Conlon T, Ju NR, Carlson D, Kopenitz J, Nishisaki A (2016) Effect of inhalational anesthetics and positive-pressure ventilation on ultrasound assessment of the great vessels: a prospective study at a Children's hospital. Anesthesiology 124(4):870–877
155. Nagdev A, Stone MB (2011) Point-of-care ultrasound evaluation of pericardial effusions: does this patient have cardiac tamponade? Resuscitation 82:671–673

156. Cross KP, Santucci KA (2006) Transitional medicine: will emergency medicine physicians be ready for the growing population of adults with congenital heart disease? Pediatr Emerg Care 22:775–781
157. Dean AJ, Lafferty K, Villanueva TC (2003) Emergency medicine bedside ultrasound diagnosis of intussusception in a patient with chronic abdominal pain and unrecognized Peutz-Jeghers syndrome. J Emerg Med 24:203–210
158. Burke LF, Clark E (1977) Ileocolic intussusception—a case report. J Clin Ultrasound 5:346–347
159. Ko HS, Schenk JP, Troger J, Rohrschneider WK (2007) Current radiological management of intussusception in children. Eur Radiol 17:2411–2421
160. Applegate KE (2009) Intussusception in children: evidence-based diagnosis and treatment. Pediatr Radiol 39(Suppl 2):S140–S143
161. Verschelden P, Filiatrault D, Garel L, Grignon A, Perreault G, Boisvert J, Dubois J (1992) Intussusception in children: reliability of US in diagnosis—a prospective study. Radiology 184:741–744
162. Daneman A, Navarro O (2004) Intussusception. Part 2: an update on the evolution of management. Pediatr Radiol 34:97–108 **(quiz 187)**
163. Navarro O, Daneman A (2004) Intussusception. Part 3: diagnosis and management of those with an identifiable or predisposing cause and those that reduce spontaneously. Pediatr Radiol 34:305–312 **(quiz 369)**
164. Eshed I, Gorenstein A, Serour F, Witzling M (2004) Intussusception in children: can we rely on screening sonography performed by junior residents? Pediatr Radiol 34:134–137
165. Riera A, Hsiao AL, Langhan ML et al (2012) Diagnosis of intussusception by physician novice sonographers in the emergency department. Ann Emerg Med 60(3):264–268
166. Swischuk LE, John SD, Swischuk PN (1994) Spontaneous reduction of intussusception: verification with US. Radiology 192:269–271
167. del-Pozo G, Gonzalez-Spinola J, Gomez-Anson B, Serrano C, Miralles M, Gonzales-delOrbe G, Cano I, Martinez A (1996) Intussusception: trapped peritoneal fluid detected with US–relationship to reducibility and ischemia. Radiology 201:379–383
168. Hryhorczuk AL, Strouse PJ (2009) Validation of US as a first-line diagnostic test for assessment of pediatric ileocolic intussusception. Pediatr Radiol 39:1075–1079
169. Swischuk LE, Stansberry SD (1991) Ultrasonographic detection of free peritoneal fluid in uncomplicated intussusception. Pediatr Radiol 21:350–351
170. Kong MS, Wong HF, Lin SL, Chung JL, Li JN (1997) Factors related to detection of blood flow by color Doppler ultrasonography in intussusception. J Ultrasound Med 16:141–144
171. Weihmiller SN, Buonomo C, Bachur R (2011) Risk stratification of children being evaluated for intussusception. Pediatrics 127:e296–e303
172. Kuppermann N, O'Dea T, Pinckney L, Hoecker C (2000) Predictors of intussusception in young children. Arch Pediatr Adolesc Med 154:250–255
173. Saxton V, Katz M, Phelan E, Beasley SW (1994) Intussusception: a repeat delayed gas enema increases the nonoperative reduction rate. J Pediatr Surgy 29:588–589
174. Gorenstein A, Raucher A, Serour F, Witzling M, Katz R (1998) Intussusception in children: reduction with repeated, delayed air enema. Radiology 206:721–724
175. Friedman L, Tsung JW (2011) Extending the focused assessment with sonography for trauma examination in children. Clin Ped Emerg Med 12(1):2–17
176. Lichtenstein DA (2009) Ultrasound examination of the lungs in the intensive care unit. Pediatr Crit Care Med 10(6):693–698
177. Blaivas M, Lyon M, Duggal S (2005) A prospective comparison of supine chest radiography and bedside ultrasound for the diagnosis of traumatic pneumothorax. Acad Emerg Med 12(9):844–849
178. Lichtenstein D, Maziere G, Biderman P, Gepner A (1999) The comet-tail artifact, an ultrasound sign ruling out pneumothorax. Intensive Care Med 25:383–388
179. Kirkpatrick AW, Sirois M, Laupland KB, Liu D, Rowan K, Ball CG, Hameed SM, Brown R, Simons R, Dulchavsky SA, Hamilton DR, Nicolaou S (2004) Hand-held thoracic sonography for detecting post-traumatic pneumothoraces: the extended focused assessment with sonography for trauma (EFAST). J Trauma 57(2):288–295
180. Zhang M, Liu ZH, Yang JX, Gan JX, Xu SW, You D, Jiang GY (2006) Rapid detection of pneumothorax by ultrasonography in patients with multiple traumas. Crit Care 10(4):R112
181. Lichtenstein DA, Meziere G, Lascolis N, Biderman P, Courret JP, Gepner A, Goldstein I, Tenoudji-Cohen M (2005) Ultrasound diagnosis of occult pneumothorax. Crit Care Med 33(6):1231–1238
182. Lichtenstein D, Hulot JS, Rabiller A, Tostivint I, Meziere G (1999) Feasibility and safety of ultrasound-aided thoracentesis in mechanically ventilated patients. Intensive Care Med 25:955–958
183. Lichtenstein D, Goldstein I, Mourgeon E, Cluzel P, Grenier P, Rouby JJ (2004) Comparative diagnostic performances of auscultation, chest radiography, and lung ultrasonography in ARDS. Anesthesiology 100:9–15
184. Lichtenstein D, Lasols N, Meziere G, Gepner A (2004) Ultrasound diagnosis of alverolar consolidation in the critically ill. Intensive Care Med 30:276–281
185. Parlamento S, Copetti R, Bartolomeo SD (2009) Evaluation of lung ultrasound for the diagnosis of pneumonia in the ED. Am J Emerg Med 27:379–384
186. Copetti R, Cattarossi L (2008) Ultrasound diagnosis of pneumonia in children. Radiol Med 113(2):190–198
187. Iuri D, De Candia A, Bazzocchi M (2009) Evaluation of the lung in children with suspected pneumonia: usefulness of ultrasonography. Radiol Med 14(2):321–330
188. Caulio VA, Gargani L, Caiulo S, Fisiciaro A, Moramarco F, Latini G, Picano E, Mele G (2013) Lung ultrasound characteristics of community acquired pneumonia in hospitalized children. Pediatr Pulmonol 48(3):280–287
189. Shah VP, Tunik MG, Tsung JW (2013) Prospective evaluation of point-of-care ultrasonography for the diagnosis of pneumonia in children and young adults. JAMA Pediatr 167(2):119–125
190. Reali F, Sferrazza Papa GF, Carlucci P, Fracasso P, Di Marco F, Mandelli M, Soldi S, Riva E, Centanni S (2014) Can lung ultrasound replace chest radiography for the diagnosis of pneumonia in hospitalized children? Respiration 88(2):112–115
191. Pereda MA, Chavez MA, Hooper-Miele CC, Gilman RH, Steinhoff MC, Ellington LE, Gross M, Price C, Tielsch JM, Checkley W (2015) Lung ultrasound for the diagnosis of pneumonia in children, a meta-analysis. Pediatrics 135(4):714–722
192. Daswani DD, Shah VP, Avner JR, Manwani DG, Kurian J, Rabiner JE (2016) Accuracy of point-of-care lung ultrasonography for diagnosis of acute chest syndrome in pediatric patients with sickle cell disease and fever. Acad Emerg Med 23(8):932–940
193. Jones BP, Tay ET, Eliskashvili E, Sanders JE, Paul AZ, Nelson BP, Spina LA, Tsung JW (2016) Feasibility and safety of substituting lung ultrasonography for chest radiography when diagnosing pneumonia in children: a randomized controlled trial. Chest 150(1):131–138
194. Chavez MA, Naithani N, Gilman RH, Tielsch JM, Khatry S, Ellington LE, Miranda JJ, Gurung G, Rodrigeuz S, Checkley W (2015) Agreement between the World Health Organization algorithm and lung consolidation identified by point-of-care ultrasound for the diagnosis of childhood pneumonia by general practitioners. Lung 193(4):531–583
195. Caiulo VA, Gargani L, Caiulo S, Fisicaro A, Moramarco F, Latini G, Picano E (2011) Lung ultrasound in bronchiolitis-comparison with chest x-ray. Eur J Pediatr 11:1427–1433
196. Tsung JW, Kessler DO, Shah VP (2012) Prospective application of clinician-performed lung ultrasonography during the 2009 H1N1 influenza A pandemic: distinguishing viral from bacterial pneumonia. Crit Ultrasound J 4:16–25
197. Hajalioghli P, Nemati M, Dinprast Saleh L, Fouladi DF (2016) Can chest computed tomography be replaced by lung ultrasonography with or wihtout plain chest radiography in pediatric pneumonia? J Thorac Imaging 31(4):247–252
198. Catarossi L, Copetti R, Brusa G (2016) Pintaldi S. Lung ultrasound diagnostic accuracy in neonatal pneumothorax. Can Respir J 2016:6515069
199. Raimondi F, Rodriguez Fanjul J, Aversa S, Chirico G, Yousef N, De Luca D, Corsini I, Dani C, Grappone L, Orfeo L, Migliario F, Vallone G, Capasso L (2016) Lung ultrasound for diagnosing pneumothorax in the critically ill neonate. J Pediatr 175(74–78):e1

200. Migliaro F, Sodano A, Capasso L, Raimondi F (2014) Lung ultrasound-guided emergency pneumothorax needle aspiration in a very preterm infant. BMJ Case Rep 14:2014
201. Lichtenstein D, Meziere G, Biderman P, Gepner A (1998) The "lung point": an ultrasound sign specific to pneumothorax. Intensive Care Med 24(12):1331–1334
202. Vergine M, Copetti R, Brusa G, Cattarossi L (2014) Lung ultrasound accuracy in respiratory distress syndrome and tranisent tachypnea of the newborn. Neonatalogy 106(2):87–93
203. Stone M, Secko M (2009) Bedside Ultrasound Diagnosis of pulmonary contusion. Pediatric Emerg Care 25(12):854–855
204. Vazquez M, Paul AZ, Tay ET, Tsung JW (2016) Evaluation and monitoring of a child with hydrocarbon pneumonitis using point-of-care lung ultrasound in the pediatric emergency department. Pediatr Emerg Care 32(9):642–644
205. Varshney T, Mok E, Shapiro AJ, Li P, Dubrovsky AS (2016) Point-of-care lung ultrasound in young children with respiratory tract infctions and wheeze. Emerg Med J. doi:10.1136/emermed-2015-205302
206. Marshburn TH, Legome E, Sargsyan A, Li SM, Noble VA, Dulchavsky SA, Sims C, Robinson D (2004) Goal-directed ultrasound in the detection of long-bone fractures. J Trauma 57:329–332
207. Hurley ME, Keye GD, Hamilton S (2004) Is ultrasound really helpful in the detection of rib fractures? Injury 35:562–566
208. Griffith JF, Rainer TH, Ching AS, Law KL, Cocks RA, Metreweli C (1999) Sonography compared with radiography in revealing acute rib fracture. AJR Am J Roentgenol 173:1603–1609
209. Platon A, Poletti PA, Van Aaken J, Fusetti C, Della Santa D, Beaulieu JY, Becker CD (2011) Occult fractures of the scaphoid: the role of ultrasonography in the emergency department. Skeletal Radiol 40:869–875
210. Smith SW (1999) Emergency physician-performed ultrasonography-guided hip arthrocentesis. Acad Emerg Med 1999:84–86
211. Tsung JW, Blaivas M (2008) Emergency department diagnosis of pediatric hip effusion and guided arthrocentesis using point-of-care ultrasound. J Emerg Med 35:393–399
212. Roy S, Dewitz A, Paul I (1999) Ultrasound-assisted ankle arthrocentesis. Am J Emerg Med 17:300–301
213. Freeman K, Dewitz A, Baker WE (2007) Ultrasound-guided hip arthrocentesis in the ED. Am J Emerg Med 25:80–86
214. Tezel O, Kaldirim U, Bilgic S, Deniz S, Eyi YE, Ozyurek S, Durusu M, Tezel N (2014) A comparison of suprascapular nerve block and procedural sedation analgesia in shoulder dislocation reduction. Am J Emerg Med 32:549–552
215. Graf D (2008) Ultrasound-guided interscalene block for shoulder dislocation reduction in the ED. Am J Emerg Med 26:1061
216. LaRocco BG, Zlupko G, Sierzenski P (2008) Ultrasound diagnosis of quadriceps tendon rupture. J Emerg Med 35:293–295
217. Nesselroade RD, Nickels LC (2010) Ultrasound diagnosis of bilateral quadriceps tendon rupture after statin use. West J Emerg Med 11(4):306–309
218. Phillips K, Costantino TG (2014) Diagnosis of patellar tendon rupture by emergency ultrasound. J Emerg Med 47:204–206
219. Berg K, Peck J, Boulger C, Bahner DP (2013) Patellar tendon rupture: an ultrasound case report. BMJ Case Rep 2013. doi:10.1136/bcr-2012-008189
220. Sisson C, Nagdev A, Tirado A, Murphy M, Suner S (2011) Ultrasound diagnosis of traumatic partial triceps tendon tear in the emergency department. J Emerg Med 40:436–438
221. Blaivas M, Lyon M, Brannam L, Duggal S, Sierzenski P (2004) Water bath evaluation technique for emergency ultrasound of painful superficial structures. Am J Emerg Med 22:589–593
222. Adhikari S, Marx J, Crum T (2012) Point-of-care ultrasound diagnosis of acute Achilles tendon rupture in the ED. Am J Emerg Med 30(634):e3–e4
223. Hübner U, Schlicht W, Outzen S, Barthel M, Halsband H (2000) Ultrasound in the diagnosis of fractures in children. J Bone Joint Surg Br 82(8):1170–1173
224. Williamson D, Watura R, Cobby M (2000) Ultrasound imaging of forearm fractures in children: a viable alternative? J Accid Emerg Med 17:22–24
225. Lewis D, Logan P (2000) Sonographic diagnosis of toddler's fracture in the emergency department. J Clin Ultrasound 34:190–194
226. Weinberg ER, Tunik MG, Tsung JW (2010) Accuracy of clinician-performed point-of-care ultrasound for the diagnosis of fractures in children and young adults. Injury 41:862–868
227. Barata I, Spencer R, Suppiah A, Raio C, Ward MF, Sama A (2012) Emergency ultrasound in the detection of pediatric long-bone fractures. Pediatr Emerg Care 28:1154–1157
228. Durston W, Swartzentruber R (2000) Ultrasound guided reduction of pediatric forearm fractures in the ED. Am J Emerg Med 18:72–77
229. Patel DD, Blumberg SM, Crain EF (2009) The utility of bedside ultrasonography in identifying fractures and guiding fracture reduction in children. Pediatr Emerg Care 25:221–225
230. Chen L, Kim Y, Moore CL (2007) Diagnosis and guided reduction of forearm fractures in children using bedside ultrasound. Pediatr Emerg Care 23:528–531
231. Dubrovsky AS, Kempinska A, Bank I, Mok E (2015) Accuracy of ultrasonography for determining successful realignment of pediatric forearm fractures. Ann Emerg Med 65:260–265
232. Rabiner JE, Khine H, Avner JR, Friedman LM, Tsung JW (2013) Accuracy of point-of-care ultrasonography for diagnosis of elbow fractures in children. Ann Emerg Med 61:9–217
233. Cross KP, Warkentine FH, Kim IK, Gracely E, Paul RI (2010) Bedside ultrasound diagnosis of clavicle fractures in the pediatric emergency department. Acad Emerg Med 17:687–693
234. Chien M, Bulloch B, Garcia-Filion P, Youssfi M, Shrader MW, Segal LS (2011) Bedside ultrasound in the diagnosis of pediatric clavicle fractures. Pediatr Emerg Care 27:1038–1041
235. Chaar-Alvarez FM, Warkentine F, Cross K, Herr S, Paul RI (2011) Bedside ultrasound diagnosis of nonangulated distal forearm fractures in the pediatric emergency department. Pediatr Emerg Care 27:1027–1032
236. Tessaro MO, McGovern TR, Dickman E, Haines LE (2015) Point-of-care ultrasound detection of acute scaphoid fracture. Pediatr Emerg Care 31:222–224
237. Ramirez-Schrempp D, Vinci RJ, Liteplo AS (2011) Bedside ultrasound in the diagnosis of skull fractures in the pediatric emergency department. Pediatr Emerg Care 27:312–314
238. Rabiner JE, Friedman LM, Khine H, Avner JR, Tsung JW (2013) Accuracy of point-of-care ultrasound for diagnosis of skull fractures in children. Pediatrics 131:e1757–e1764
239. Parri N, Crosby BJ, Glass C, Mannelli F, Sforzi I, Schiavone R, Ban KM (2013) Ability of emergency ultrasonography to detect pediatric skull fractures: a prospective, observational study. J Emerg Med 44:135–141
240. Shavit I, Eidelman M, Galbraith R (2006) Sonography of the hip-joint by the emergency physician: its role in the evaluation of children presenting with acute limp. Pediatr Emerg Care 22:570–573
241. Vieira RL, Levy JA (2010) Bedside ultrasonography to identify hip effusions in pediatric patients. Ann Emerg Med 55:284–289
242. Rabiner JE, Khine H, Avner JR, Tsung JW (2015) Ultrasound findings of the elbow posterior fat pad in children with radial head subluxation. Pediatr Emerg Care 31:327–330
243. Dohi D (2013) Confirmed specific ultrasonographic findings of pulled elbow. J Pediatr Orthop 33:829–831
244. Breslin K, Boniface K, Cohen J (2014) Ultrasound-guided intra-articular lidocaine block for reduction of anterior shoulder dislocation in the pediatric emergency department. Pediatr Emerg Care 30:217–220
245. Carr JC, Hanly S, Griffin J, Gibney R (2001) Sonography of the patellar tendon and adjacent structures in pediatric and adult patients. AJR Am J Roentgenol 176:1535–1539
246. Bialik V, Farhoud F, Eidelman M, Katzman A, Bialik GM (2007) Achilles tendon length in children evaluated sonographically. J Pediatr Orthop B 16:281–286
247. Goldenstein C, McCauley R, Troy M, Schaller JG, Szer IS (1989) Ultrasonography in the evaluation of wrist swelling in children. J Rheumatol 16:1079–1987
248. Hashimoto BE, Kramer DJ, Wiitala L (1999) Applications of musculoskeletal sonography. J Clin Ultrasound 27:293–318
249. Yabunaka K, Ohue M, Morimoto N, Kitano N, Shinohara K, Takamura M, Gotanda T, Sanada S (2012) Sonographic measurement of transient synovitis in children: diagnostic value of joint effusion. Radiol Phys Technol 5:15–19
250. Tayal VS, Crean CA, Norton HJ, Schulz CJ, Bacalis KN, Bliss S (2008) Prospective comparative trial of endovaginal sonographic bimanual

examination versus traditional digital bimanual examination in non-pregnant women with lower abdominal pain with regard to body mass index classification. J Ultrasound Med 27:1171–1177
251. Adhikari S, Blaivas M, Lyon M (2008) Role of bedside transvaginal ultrasonography in the diagnosis of tubo-ovarian abscess in the emergency department. J Emerg Med 34:429–433
252. Zeger W, Holt K (2003) Gynecologic infections. Emerg Med Clin North Am 21:631–648
253. Lee DC, Swaminathan AK (2011) Sensitivity of ultrasound for the diagnosis of tubo-ovarian abscess: a case report and literature review. J Emerg Med 40:170–175
254. Morton MJ, Masterson M, Hoffman B (2013) Case report: ovarian torsion in pregnancy—diagnosis and management. J Emerg Med 45:348–351
255. Johnson S, Fox JC, Koenig KL (2006) Diagnosis of ovarian torsion in a hemodynamically unstable pediatric patient by bedside ultrasound in the ED. Am J Emerg Med 24(4):496–497
256. Vijayaraghavan SB (2004) Sonographic whirlpool sign in ovarian torsion. J Ultrasound Med 23:1643–1649 **(quiz 1650–1651)**
257. Peña JE, Ufberg D, Cooney N, Denis AL (2000) Usefulness of Doppler sonography in the diagnosis of ovarian torsion. Fertil Steril 73:1047–1050
258. Semlali S, Atmane M, Chellaoui M, Chat L, Achaaban F, Alami D, Najid A, Etteybi F, Dafiri R (2004) Emergency ultrasound diagnosis of ovarian torsion in children: nine case reports. Arch Pediatr 11(4):304–307
259. Jang TB, Ruggeri W, Dyne P, Kaji AH (2010) Learning curve of emergency physicians using emergency bedside sonography for symptomatic first-trimester pregnancy. J Ultrasound Med 29:1423–1428
260. McRae A, Edmonds M, Murray H (2009) Diagnostic accuracy and clinical utility of emergency department targeted ultrasonography in the evaluation of first-trimester pelvic pain and bleeding: a systematic review. CJEM 11:355–364
261. Blaivas M, Sierzenski P, Plecque D, Lambert M (2000) Do emergency physicians save time when locating a live intrauterine pregnancy with bedside ultrasonography? Acad Emerg Med 7:988–993
262. Panebianco NL, Shofer F, Fields JM, Anderson K, Mangili A, Matsuura A, Dean AJ (2015) The utility of transvaginal ultrasound in the ED evaluation of complications of first trimester pregnancy. Am J Emerg Med 30:743–748
263. Stein JC, Wang R, Adler N, Boscardin J, Jacoby VL, Won G, Goldstein R, Kohn MA (2010) Emergency physician ultrasonography for evaluating patients at risk for ectopic pregnancy: a meta-analysis. Ann Emerg Med 56:674–683
264. Moore C, Todd WM, O'Brien E, Lin H (2007) Free fluid in morison's pouch on bedside ultrasound predicts need for operative intervention in suspected ectopic pregnancy. Acad Emerg Med 13:755–758
265. Tayal VS, Cohen H, Norton HJ (2004) Outcome of patients with an indeterminate emergency department first-trimester pelvic ultrasound to rule out ectopic pregnancy. Acad Emerg Med 11:912–917
266. Bloch AJ, Bloch SA, Lyon M (2013) Correlation of β-human chorionic gonadotropin with ultrasound diagnosis of ectopic pregnancy in the ED. Am J Emerg Med 31:876–877
267. Counselman FL, Shaar GS, Heller RA et al (1998) Quantitative b-hCG levels less than 1000 mIU/mL in patients with ectopic pregnancy: pelvic ultrasound still useful. J Emerg Med 16:699
268. Dart RG, Kaplan B, Cox C (1997) Transvaginal ultrasound in patients with low beta-human chorionic gonadotropin values: how often is the study diagnostic? Ann Emerg Med 30:135
269. Dimarchi JN, Kosasa TS, Hale RW (1989) What is the significance of human gonadotropin value in ectopic pregnancy? Obstet Gynecol 74:851
270. Avitabile NC, Kaban NL, Siadecki SD, Lewiss RE, Saul T (2015) Two cases of heterotopic pregnancy: review of the literature and sonographic diagnosis in the emergency department. J Ultrasound Med 34:527–530
271. Adhikari S, Blaivs M, Lyon M (2007) Diagnosis and management of ectopic pregnancy using bedside transvaginal ultrasonography in the ED: a 2-year experience. Am J Emerg Med 25:591–596
272. Lewiss RE, Shaukat NM, Saul T (2014) The endomyometrial thickness measurement for abnormal implantation evaluation by pelvic sonography. J Ultrasound Med 33:1143–1146
273. Durston WE, Carl ML, Guerra W, Easton A, Ackerson LM (2000) Ultrasound availability in the evaluation of ectopic pregnancy in the ED: comparison of quality and cost-effectiveness with different approaches. Am J Emerg Med 18:408–417
274. Thamburaj R, Sivitz A (2013) Does the Use of bedside pelvic ultrasound decrease length of stay in the emergency department? Pediatr Emerg Care 29:67–70
275. Chen EA, Luks FI, Gilchrist BF, Wesselhoeft CW Jr, DeLuca FG (1996) Pyloric stenosis in the age of ultrasonography: fading skills, better patients? J Pediatr Surg 31:829–830
276. Macdessi J, Oates RK (1993) Clinical diagnosis of pyloric stenosis: a declining art. BMJ 306:553–555
277. Glatstein M, Carbell G, Boddu SK, Bernardini A, Scolnik D (2011) The changing clinical presentation of hypertrophic pyloric stenosis: the experience of a large, tertiary care pediatric hospital. Clin Pediatr 50:192–195
278. Hulka F, Campbell TJ, Campbell JR, Harrison MW (1997) Evolution in the recognition of infantile hypertrophic pyloric stenosis. Pediatrics 100:E9
279. Papadakis K, Chen EA, Luks FI, Lessin MS, Wesselhoeft CW Jr, DeLuca FG (1999) The changing presentation of pyloric stenosis. Am J Emerg Med 17:67–69
280. Teele RL, Smith EH (1977) Ultrasound in the diagnosis of idiopathic hypertrophic pyloric stenosis. N Engl J Med 296:1149–1150
281. Malcom GE 3rd, Raio CC, Del Rios M, Blaivas M, Tsung JW (2009) Feasibility of emergency physician diagnosis of hypertrophic pyloric stenosis using point-of-care ultrasound: a multi-center case series. J Emerg Med 37:283–286
282. Copeland DR, Cosper GH, McMahon LE, Boneti C, Little DC, Dassinger MS, Kokoska ER, Jackson RJ, Smith SD (2009) Return of the surgeon in the diagnosis of pyloric stenosis. J Pediatr Surg 44:1189–1192
283. McVay MR, Copeland DR, McMahon LE, Cosper GH, McCallie TG, Kokoska ER, Jackson RJ, Smith SD (2009) Surgeon-performed ultrasound for diagnosis of pyloric stenosis is accurate, reproducible, and clinically valuable. J Pediatr Surg 44:169–171
284. Sivitz A, Tejani C, Cohen S (2013) Evaluation of hypertrophic pyloric stenosis by pediatric emergency physician sonography. Acad Emerg Med 20:646–651
285. Leaphart CL, Borland K, Kane TD, Hackam DJ (2008) Hypertrophic pyloric stenosis in newborns younger than 21 days: remodeling the path of surgical intervention. J Pediatr Surg 43:998–1001
286. Hernanz-Schulman M (2003) Infantile hypertrophic pyloric stenosis. Radiology 227:319–331
287. Houben CH, Rudolf O, Misra D (1999) Diagnosing hypertrophic pyloric stenosis: does size matter? Eur J Pediatr Surg 9:373–375
288. Strauss S, Itzchak Y, Manor A, Heyman Z, Graif M (1981) Sonography of hypertrophic pyloric stenosis. AJR 136:1057–1058
289. O'Keeffe FN, Stansberry SD, Swischuk LE, Hayden CK Jr (1991) Antropyloric muscle thickness at US in infants: what is normal? Radiology 178:827–830
290. Rohrschneider WK, Mittnacht H, Darge K, Tröger J (1998) Pyloric muscle in asymptomatic infants: sonographic evaluation and discrimination from idiopathic hypertrophic pyloric stenosis. Pediatr Radiol 28:429–434
291. Demian M, Nguyen S, Emil S (2009) Early pyloric stenosis: a case control study. Pediatr Surg Int 25:1053–1057
292. Mollitt DL, Golladay ES, Williamson S, Seibert JJ, Sutterfield SL (1987) Ultrasonography in the diagnosis of pyloric stenosis. South Med J 80:47–50
293. Lund Kofoed PE, Høst A, Elle B, Larsen C (1988) Hypertrophic pyloric stenosis: determination of muscle dimensions by ultrasound. BJR 61:19–20
294. Neilson D, Hollman AS (1994) The ultrasonic diagnosis of infantile hypertrophic pyloric stenosis: technique and accuracy. Clin Radiol 49:246–247
295. Squire BT, Fox JC, Anderson C (2005) ABSCESS: applied bedside sonography for convenient evaluation of superficial soft tissue infections. Acad Emerg Med 2(7):601–606
296. Berger T, Garrido F, Green J, Lema PC, Gupta J (2012) Bedside ultrasound performed by novices for the detection of abscess in ED patients with soft tissue infections. Am J Emerg Med 30(8):1569–1573
297. Tayal VS, Hasan N, Norton HJ, Tomaszewski CA (2006) The effect of soft-tissue ultrasound on the management of cellulitis in the emergency department. Acad Emerg Med 13(4):384–388
298. Gaspari RJ, Blehar D, Polan D, Montoya A, Alsulaibikh A, Liteplo A (2014) The Massachusetts abscess rule: a clinical decision rule using

ultrasound to identify methicillin-resistant Staphylococcus aureus in skin abscesses. Acad Emerg Med 21(5):558–567
299. Nienaber A, Harvey M, Cave G (2010) Accuracy of bedside ultrasound for the detection of soft tissue foreign bodies by emergency doctors. Emerg Med Australas 22(1):30–34
300. Orlinsky M, Knittel P, Feit T, Chan L, Mandavia D (2000) The comparative accuracy of radiolucent foreign body detection using ultrasonography. Am J Emerg Med 18(4):401–403
301. Schlager D, Sanders AB, Wiggins D, Boren W (1991) Ultrasound for the detection of foreign bodies. Ann Emerg Med 20(2):189–191
302. Gilbert FJ, Campbell RS, Bayliss AP (1990) The role of ultrasound in the detection of non-radiopaque foreign bodies. Clin Radiol 41(2):109–112
303. Banerjee B, Das RK (1991) Sonographic detection of foreign bodies of the extremities. Br J Radiol 64(758):107–112
304. Mohammadi A, Ghasemi-Rad M, Khodabakhsh M (2011) Non-opaque soft tissue foreign body: sonographic findings. BMC Med Imaging 11:9
305. Budhram GR, Schmunk JC (2014) Bedside ultrasound AIDS identification and removal of cutaneous foreign bodies: a case series. J Emerg Med 47(2):e43–e48
306. Marin JR, Bilker W, Lautenbach E, Alpern ER (2010) Reliability of clinical examinations for pediatric skin and soft-tissue infections. Pediatrics 126(5):925–930
307. Giovanni JE, Dowd MD, Kennedy C, Michael JG (2011) Interexaminer agreement in physical examination for children with suspected soft tissue abscesses. Pediatr Emerg Care 27(6):475–478
308. Sivitz AB, Lam SH, Ramirez-Schrempp D, Valente JH, Nagdev AD (2010) Effect of bedside ultrasound on management of pediatric soft-tissue infection. J Emerg Med 39(5):637–643
309. Iverson K, Haritos D, Thomas R, Kannikeswaran N (2011) The effect of bedside ultrasound on diagnosis and management of soft tissue infections in a pediatric ED. Am J Emerg Med 30(8):1347–1351
310. Marin JR, Dean AJ, Bilker WB, Panebianco NL, Brown NJ, Alpern ER (2013) Emergency ultrasound-assisted examination of skin and soft tissue infections in the pediatric emergency department. Acad Emerg Med 20(6):545–553
311. Marin JR, Alpern ER, Panebianco NL, Dean AJ (2011) Assessment of a training curriculum for emergency ultrasound for pediatric soft tissue infections. Acad Emerg Med 18(2):174–182
312. Friedman DI, Forti RJ, Wall SP, Crain EF (2005) The utility of bedside ultrasound and patient perception in detecting soft tissue foreign bodies in children. Pediatr Emerg Care 21(8):487–492
313. Teng M, Doniger SJ (2012) Subungual wooden splinter visualized with bedside sonography. Pediatr Emerg Care 28(4):392–394
314. Mossa-Basha M, van Holsbeeck M (2007) Musculoskeletal infection. Ultrasound Clin 2(4):639–651
315. Ma O, Mateer JR, Blaivas M (2008) Emergency ultrasound, 2nd edn. McGraw Hill, New York
316. Blaivas M, Sierzenski P, Lambert M (2001) Emergency evaluation of patients presenting with acute scrotum using bedside ultrasonography. Acad Emerg Med 8(1):90–93
317. Cannis M, Mailhot T, Perera P (2013) Bedside ultrasound in a case of blunt scrotal trauma. West J Emerg Med 14(2):127–129
318. Bomann JS, Moore C (2009) Bedside ultrasound of a painful testicle: before and after manual detorsion by an emergency physician. Acad Emerg Med 16(4):366
319. Blaivas M, Batts M, Lambert M (2000) Ultrasonographic diagnosis of testicular torsion by emergency physicians. Am J Emerg Med 18(2):198–200
320. Thimann D, Badawy M (2014) 7-month-old male with scrotal swelling. Emerg Med J 31(6):521–522
321. Matzek BA, Linklater DR (2013) Traumatic testicular dislocation after minor trauma in a pediatric patient. J Emerg Med 45(4):537–540
322. Gaspari RJ, Horst K (2005) Emergency ultrasound and urinalysis in the evaluation of flank pain. Acad Emerg Med 12:1180–1184
323. Watkins S, Bowra J, Sharma P, Holdgate A, Giles A, Campbell L (2007) Validation of emergency physician ultrasound in diagnosing hydronephrosis in ureteric colic. Emerg Med Australas 19:188–195
324. Moak J, Lyons MS, Lindsell CJ (2012) Bedside renal ultrasound in the evaluation of suspected ureterolithiasis. Am J Emerg Med 30:218–221
325. Dalziel PJ, Noble VE (2013) Bedside ultrasound and the assessment of renal colic: a review. Emerg Med J 30:3–8
326. Goertz JK, Lotterman S (2010) Can the degree of hydronephrosis on ultrasound predict kidney stone size? Am J Emerg Med 28:813–816
327. Ray AA, Ghiculete D, Pace KT, Honey RJ (2010) Limitations to ultrasound in the detection and measurement of urinary tract calculi. Urology 76:295–300
328. Sheafor DH, Hertzberg BS, Carroll BA, Keogan MT, Paulspn EK, DeLong DM, Nelson RD (2000) Nonenhanced helical CT and US in the emergency evaluation of patients with renal colic: prospective comparison. Radiology 217:792–797
329. Ulusan S, Koc Z, Tokmak N (2007) Accuracy of sonography for detecting renal stone: comparison with CT. J Clin Ultrasound 35:256–261
330. Smith-Bindman R, Aubin C, Bailitz J, Bengiamin RN, Camargo CA Jr, Corbo J, Dean AJ, Goldstein RB, Griffey RT, Jay GD, Kang TL, Kriesel DR, Ma OJ, Mallin M, Manson W, Melnikow J, Miglioretti DL, Miller SK, Mills LD, Miner JR, Moghadassi M, Noble VE, Press GM, Stoller ML, Valencia VE, Wang J, Wang RC, Cummings SR (2014) Ultrasonography versus computed tomography for suspected nephrolithiasis. N Engl J Med 371:1100–1110
331. Chen KC, Hung SW, Seow VK, Chong CF, Wang TL, Li YC, Chang H (2011) The role of emergency ultrasound for evaluating acute pyelonephritis in the ED. Am J Emerg Med 29:721–724
332. Weber TM (2006) Sonography of benign renal cystic disease. Radiol Clin North Am 44:777–786
333. Bisceglia M, Galliani CA, Senger C, Stallone C, Sessa A (2006) Renal cystic disease. Adv Anat Pathol 13:26–56
334. Routh JC, Graham DA, Nelson CP (2010) Epidemiological trends in pediatric urolithiasis at United States freestanding pediatric hospitals. J Urol 184:1816–1822
335. Corbin Bush N, Xu L, Brown BJ, Holzer Gingrich A, Schuler B, Tong L, Baker LA (2010) Hospitalizations for pediatric stone disease in United States, 2002–2007. J Urol 183:1151–1156
336. Kairam N, Allegra JR, Eskin B (2013) Rise in emergency department visits of pediatric patients for renal colic from 1999 to 2008. Pediatr Emerg Care 29:462–464
337. Palmer JS, Donaher ER, O'Riordan MA, Dell KM (2005) Diagnosis of pediatric urolithiasis: role of ultrasound and computerized tomography. J Urol 174:1413–1416
338. Saadeh SA, Mattoo TK (2001) Managing urinary tract infections. Pediatr Nephrol 26:1967–1976
339. Finnell SME, Carroll AE, Downs SM, Subcommittee on Urinary Tract Infection (2011) Technical report—diagnosis and management of an initial UTI in febrile infants and young children. Pediatrics 128:e749–e770
340. Kawashima A, LeRoy AJ (2003) Radiologic evaluation of patients with renal infections. Infect Dis Clin N Am 17:433–456
341. Guedj R, Escoda S, Blakime P, Patteau G, Brunelle F, Cheron G (2015) The accuracy of renal point of care ultrasound to detect hydronephrosis in children with a urinary tract infection. Eur J Emerg Med 22:135–138
342. Wippermann CF, Schofer O, Beetz R, Schumacher R, Schweden F, Riedmiller H, Buttner J (1991) Renal abscess in childhood: diagnostic and therapeutic progress. Pediatr Infect Dis J 10:446–450
343. Bjerklund Johansen TE (2002) Diagnosis and imaging in urinary tract infections. Curr Opin Urol 2:39–43
344. Vester U, Kranz B, Hoyer PF (2010) The diagnostic value of ultrasound in cystic kidney diseases. Pediatr Nephrol 25:231–240
345. Reed B, Nobakht E, Dadgar S, Bekheirnia MR, Masoumi A, Belibi F, Yan XD, Cadnapaphornchai M, Schrier RW (2010) Renal ultrasonographic evaluation in children at risk of autosomal dominant polycystic kidney disease. Am J Kidney Dis 56:50–56
346. Sweeney WE, Avner ED (2011) Diagnosis and management of childhood polycystic kidney disease. Pediatr Nephrol 26:675–692
347. Smith SW (1999) Emergency physician-performed ultrasonography-guided hip arthrocentesis. Acad Emerg Med 6:84–88
348. Minardi JJ, Lander OM (2012) Septic hip arthritis: diagnosis and arthrocentesis using bedside ultrasound. J Emerg Med 43:316–318
349. Minardi J, Denne N, Miller M, Larrabee H, Lander O (2013) Acute arthritis of the hip—case series describing emergency physician performed ultrasound guided hip arthrocentesis. W V Med J 109:22–24
350. Wiler JL, Costantino TG, Filippone L, Satz W (2010) Comparison of ultrasound-guided and standard landmark techniques for knee arthrocentesis. J Emerg Med 39:76–82

351. Kane D, Balint PV, Sturrock RD (2003) Ultrasonography is superior to clinical examination in the detection and localization of knee joint effusion in rheumatoid arthritis. J Rheumatol 30:966–971
352. Moak JH, Vaughan AJ, Silverberg B (2012) Ultrasound-guided hip arthrocentesis in a child with hip pain and fever. West J Emerg Med 13:316–319
353. Lewiss RE, Saul T, Shah KH (2012) Essential emergency imaging. Lippincott Williams & Wilkins, Philadelphia, pp 50–51
354. Cavalier R, Herman M, Pizzutillo P, Geller E (2003) Ultrasound–guided aspiration of the hip in children: a new technique. Clin Orthop Relat Res (415):244–247
355. Tirado A, Wu T, Noble VE, Huang C, Lewiss RE, Martin JA, Murphy MC, Sivitz A, Cohen SG (2013) Ultrasound-guided procedures in the emergency department-diagnostic and therapeutic asset. Emerg Med Clin North Am 31:129–134
356. Valley VT, Stahmer SA (2001) Targeted musculoskeletal sonography in the detection of joint effusions. Acad Emerg Med 8:361–367
357. Miralles M, Gonzalez G, Pulpeiro JR, Millan JM, Gordillo I, Serrano C, Olcoz F, Martinez A (1989) Sonography of the painful hip in children: 500 consecutive cases. AJR 152:579–582
358. Shiver S, Blaivas M, Lyon M (2006) A prospective comparison of ultrasound-guided and blindly placed radial arterial catheters. Acad Emerg Med 13:1275–1279
359. Ishii S, Shime N, Shibasaki M, Sawa T (2013) Ultrasound-guided radial artery catheterization in infants and small children. Pediatr Crit Care Med 14(5):471–473
360. Ganesh A, Kaye R, Cahill AM, Stern W, Pachikara R, Gallagher PR, Watcha M (2009) Evaluation of ultrasound-guided radial artery cannulation in children. Pediatr Crit Care Med 10:45–48
361. Brzezinski M, Luisetti T, London M (2009) Radial artery cannulation: a comprehensive review of recent anatomic and physiologic investgations. Anesth Analg 106:1763–1781
362. Hopkins JW, Warkentine FH, Gracely E, Kim IK (2009) The anatomic relationship between the common femoral artery and common femoral vein in frog leg position versus straight leg position in pediatric patients. Acad Emerg Med 16:579–584
363. Warkentine FH, Clyde Pierce M, Lorenz D, Kim IK (2008) The anatomic relationship of femoral vein to femoral artery in euvolemic pediatric patients by ultrasonography: implications for pediatric femoral cental venous access. Acad Emerg Med 15:426–430
364. Blaivas M, Adhikari S (2011) Unexpected findings on point-of-care superficial ultrasound imaging before incision and drainage. J Ultrasound Med 30:1425–1430
365. Gaspari RJ, Resop D, Mendoza M, Kant T, Blehar D (2011) A randomized controlled trial of incision and drainage versus ultrasonographically guided needle aspiration for skin abscesses and the effect of methicillin-resistant Staphylococcus aureus. Ann Emerg Med 57:483–491
366. Pysyk CL, Persaud D, Bryson GL, Lui A (2010) Ultrasound assessment of the vertebral level of the palpated intercristal (Tuffier's) line. Can J Anaesth 57:46–49
367. Ferre RM, Sweeney TW (2007) Emergency physicians can easily obtain ultrasound images of anatomical landmarks relevant to lumbar puncture. Am J Emerg Med 25:291–296
368. Stiffler KA, Jwayyed S, Wilber ST, Robinson A (2007) The use of ultrasound to identify pertinent landmarks for lumbar puncture. Am J Emerg Med 25:331–334
369. Ferre RM, Sweeney TW, Strout TD (2009) Ultrasound identification of landmarks preceding lumbar puncture: a pilot study. Emerg Med J 26:276–277
370. Nomura JT, Leech SJ, Shenbagamurthi S (2007) A randomized controlled trial of ultrasound-assisted lumbar puncture. J Ultrasound Med 26:1341–1348
371. Mofidi M, Mohammadi M, Saidi H, Kianmehr N, Ghasemi A, Hafezimoghadam P, Rezai M (2013) Ultrasound guided lumbar puncture in emergency department: time saving and less complications. J Res Med Sci 18:303–307
372. Abo A, Chen L, Johnston P, Santucci K (2010) Positioning for lumbar puncture in children evaluated by bedside ultrasound. Pediatrics 125:e1149–e1153
373. Cadigan BA, Cydulka RK, Werner SL, Jones RA (2011) Evaluating infant positioning for lumbar puncture using sonographic measurements. Acad Emerg Med 18:215–218
374. Bruccoleri RE, Chen L (2011) Needle-entry angle for lumbar puncture in children as determined by using ultrasonography. Pediatrics 127:e921–e926
375. Kesler H, Dias MS, Kalapos P (2007) Termination of the normal conus medullaris in children: a whole- spine magnetic resonance imaging study. Neurosurg Focus 23:E7
376. Sahin F, Selcuki M, Ecin N et al (1997) Level of conus medullaris in term and preterm neonates. Arch Dis Child Fetal Neonatal Ed 77:F67–F69
377. Coley BD, Shiels WE 2nd, Hogan MJ (2001) Diagnostic and interventional ultrasonography in neonatal and infant lumbar puncture. Pediatr Radiol 31:399–402
378. Kim S, Adler DK (2014) Ultrasound-assisted lumbar puncture in pediatric emergency medicine. J Emerg Med 47:59–64
379. Lam SH, Lambert MJ (2015) In reply: ultrasound-assisted lumbar puncture in pediatric patients. J Emerg Med 48:611–612
380. Nazeer SR, Dewbre H, Miller A (2005) Ultrasound assisted paracentesis performed by emergency physicians vs the traditional technique: a prospective, randomized study. Am J Emerg Med 23:363–367
381. Patel PA, Ernst FR, Gunnarsson CL (2012) Evaluation of hospital complications and costs associated with using ultrasound guidance during abdominal paracentesis procedures. J Med Econ 15(1):1–7
382. Mercaldi CJ, Lanes S (2013) Ultrasound guidance decreases complications and improves the cost of care among patients undergoing thoracentesis and paracentesis. Chest 143:532–538
383. Blaivas M (2005) Emergency diagnostic paracentesis to determine intraperitoneal fluid identity discovered on bedside ultrasound of unstable patients. J Emerg Med 29(4):461–465
384. Tsang TS, Freeman WK, Sinak LJ, Seward JB (1998) Echocardiographically guided pericardiocentesis: evolution and state-of-the-art technique. Mayo Clin Proc 73:647–652
385. Garth AP, Hwang JQ, Schuur JD, Rosborough S (2009) Ultrasound guided pericardiocentesis of cardiac tamponade. Acad Emerg Med 16(8):811
386. Fields JM, Paziana K, Vuljaj N, Fischer J, Ku BS (2012) Emergency ultrasound guided pericardiocentesis using a high-frequency linear array transducer to improve needle tip visualization. Acad Emerg Med 19(5):e16
387. Ainsworth CD, Salehian O (2011) Echo guided pericardiocentesis: let the bubbles show the way. Circulation 123:e210–e211
388. Nagdev A, Mantuani D (2013) A novel in-plane technique for ultrasound-guided pericardiocentesis. Am J Emerg Med 31(9):1424 **(e5–9)**
389. Cosby KS, Kendall JL (2006) Practical guide to emergency ultrasound. Lippincott Williams & Wilkins, Philadelphia
390. Liebmann O, Price D, Mills C, Gardner R, Wang R, Wilson S, Gray A (2006) Feasibility of forearm ultrasonography-guided nerve blocks of the radial, ulnar, and median nerves for hand procedures in the emergency department. Ann Emerg Med 48(5):558–562
391. Stone MB, Wang R, Price DD (2008) Ultrasound-guided supraclavicular brachial plexus nerve block vs procedural sedation for the treatment of upper extremity emergencies. Am J Emerg Med 26:706–710
392. Amiri HR, Espandar R (2010) Upper extremity surgery in younger children under ultrasound-guided supraclavicular brachial plexus block: a case series. J Child Orthop 4(4):315–319
393. Ivani G, Mossetti V (2009) Pediatric regional anesthesia. Minerva Anestesiol 75:1–6
394. van Geffen GJ, Pirotte T, Gielen MJ, Scheffer G, Bruhn J (2010) Ultrasound-guided proximal and distal sciatic nerve blocks in children. J Clin Anesth 22(4):241–245
395. Turner AL, Stevenson MD, Cross KP (2014) Impact of ultrasound-guided femoral nerve blocks in the pediatric emergency department. Pediatr Emerg Care 30(4):227–229
396. Frenkel O, Liebmann O, Fischer JW (2015) Ultrasound-guided forearm nerve blocks in kids: a novel method for pain control in the treatment of hand-injured pediatric patients in the emergency department. Pediatr Emerg Care 31(4):255–259
397. Saccharow L, Pryles C (1969) Further experience with the use of percutaneous suprapubic aspiration of the urinary bladder. Bacteriologic studies in 654 infants and children. Pediatrics 43(6):1018–1024
398. O'Callaghan C, McDougall P (1987) Successful suprapubic aspiration of urine. Arch Dis Child 62(10):1072–1073

399. Gochman R, Karasic R, Heller M (1991) Use of portable ultrasound to assist urine collection by suprapubic aspiration. Ann Emerg Med 20(6):631–635
400. Kiernan S, Pinckert T, Keszler M (1993) Ultrasound guidance of suprapubic bladder aspiration in neonates. J Pediatr 123(5):789–791
401. Buntsma D, Stock A, Bevan C, Babi FE (2012) Success rate of BladderScan-assisted suprapubic aspiration. Emerg Med Australas 24(6):647–651
402. Feller-Kopman D (2006) Ultrasound-guided thoracentesis. Chest 129:1709
403. Barnes TW, Morgenthaler TI, Olsen EJ et al (2005) Hesley sonographically guided thoracentesis and rate of pneumothorax. J Clin Ultrasound 33:442
404. Jones PW, Moyers JP, Rogers JT, Rodriguez RM, Lee YC, Light RW (2003) Ultrasound-guided thoracentesis: is it a safer method? Chest 123:418
405. Duncan DR, Morgenthaler TI, Ryu JH, Daniels CE (2009) Reducing iatrogenic risk in thoracentesis: establishing best practice via experiential training in a zero-risk environment. Chest 135:1315
406. Cavanna L, Mordenti P, Berte R, Palladino MA, Biasini C, Anselmi E, Seghini P, Vecchia S, Civardi G, Di Nunzio C (2014) Ultrasound guidance reduces pneumothorax rate and improves safety of thoracentesis in malignant pleural effusion: report on 445 consecutive patients with advanced cancer. World J Surg Oncol 12:139
407. Patel PA, Ernst FR, Gunnarsson CL (2012) Ultrasonography guidance reduces complications and costs associated with thoracentesis procedures. J Clin Ultrasound 40:135
408. Diacon AH, Brutsche MH, Solèr M (2003) Accuracy of pleural puncture sites: a prospective comparison of clinical examination with ultrasound. Chest 123:436
409. Lamperti M, Bodenhaum AR, Pittiruti AR, Blaivas M, Augoustides JG, Elbarbary M, Pirotte T, Karakitsos D, Ledonne J, Doniger S, Scoppettuolo G, Feller-Kopman D, Schummer W, Biffi R, Desruennes E, Melniker LA, Verhese ST (2012) International evidence-based recommendations on ultrasound-guided vascular access. Intensive Care Med 38(7):1105–1117
410. Hind D, Calvert N, McWilliams R, McWilliams Richard, Davidson Andrew, Paisley Suzy, Beverley Catherine, Thomas Steven (2003) Ultrasonic locating devices for central venous cannulation: meta-analysis. BMJ 327:361–367
411. Randolph A, Cook D, Gonzales C, Pribble C (1996) Ultrasound guidance for placement of central venous catheters: a meta-analysis of the literature. Crit Care Med 24(12):2053–2058
412. Miller A, Roth B, Mills T, Woody J, Longmoor C, Foster B (2002) Ultrasound guidance versus the landmark technique for the placement of central venous catheters in the emergency department. Acad Emerg Med 9(8):800–805
413. Milling TJ, Rose J, Briggs WM, Birkhahn R, Gaeta T, Bove JJ, Melniker LA (2005) Randomized, controlled clinical trial of point-of-care limited ultrasonography assistance of central venous cannulation: the third sonography outcomes assessment program (SOAP-3) trial. Crit Care Med 33(8):1764–1769
414. Brass P, Hellmich M, Kolodziej L, Schick G, Smith AF (2015) Ultrasound guidance versus anatomical landmarks for internal jugular vein catheterization (review). Cochrane Database Syst Rev 1:CD006962
415. Brass P, Hellmich M, Kolodziej L, Schick G, Smith AF (2015) Ultrasound guidance versus anatomical landmarks for suclavian or femoral vein catheterization (review). Cochrane Database Syst Rev 1:CD011447
416. Kohn LT, Corrigan JM, Donaldson MS (2000) To err is human: building a safer health system. National Academy Press, Institute of Medicine, Washington
417. Shojania KG, Duncan BW, McDonald KM, Wachter RM, Markowitz AJ (2001) Making health care safer: a critical analysis of patient safety practices. Evid Rep Technol Asess (Summ) (43):i-x, 1–668
418. Keyes L, Frazee B, Snoey E, Simon B, Christy D (1999) Ultrasound-guided brachial and basilic vein cannulation in emergency department patients with difficult intravenous access. Ann Emerg Med 34:711–714
419. Brannam L, Blaivas M, Lyon M, Flake M (2004) Emergency nurses' utilization of ultrasound guidance for placement of peripheral intravenous lines in difficult- access patients. Acad Emerg Med 11:1361–1363
420. Shokoohi H, Boniface K, McCarthy M, Al-tiae TK, Sattarian M, Ding R, Liu YT, Pourmand A, Schoenfeld E, Scott J, Shesser R, Yadav K (2013) Ultrasound-guided peripheral intravenous access program is associated with a marked reduction in central venous catheter use in noncritically ill emergency department patients. Ann Emerg Med 61(2):198–203
421. Stone MB, Teismann NA, Wang R (2007) Ultrasonographic confirmation of intraosseous needle placement in an adult unembalmed cadaver model. Ann Emerg Med 49(4):515–519
422. Leyvi G, Taylor D, Reith E, Wasnick J (2005) Utility of ultrasound-guided central venous cannulation in pediatric surgical patients: a clinical series. Pediatr Anesth 15(11):953
423. Bruzoni M, Slater BJ, Wall J, St Peter SD, Dutta S (2013) A prospective randomized trial of ultrasound- vs landmark-guided central venous access in the pediatric population. J Am Coll Surg 216(5):939–943
424. Warkentine F, Pierce M, Lorenz D, Kim I (2008) The anatomic relationship of femoral vein to femoral artery in euvolemic pediatric patients by ultrasonography: implications for pediatric femoral central venous access. Acad Emerg Med 15(5):426–430
425. Horowitz R, Gossett JG, Balitz J, Wax D, Pierce MC (2014) The FLUSH study–flush the line and ultrasound of the heart: ultrasonographic confirmation of central femoral venous line placement. Ann Emerg Med 63:678–683
426. Doniger S, Ishimine P, Fox J, Kanegaye J (2009) Randomized controlled trial of ultrasound-guided peripheral intravenous catheter placement versus traditional techniques in difficult-access pediatric patients. Pediatr Emerg Care 25(3):154–159
427. Tsung JW, Blaivas M, Stone MB (2009) Feasibility of point-of-care Doppler ultrasound confirmation of intraosseous needle placement during resuscitation. Resuscitation 80(6):665–668
428. Panebianco NL, Fredette JM, Szyld D, Sagalyn EB, Pines JM, Dean AJ (2009) What you see (sonographically) is what you get: vein and patient characteristics associated with successful ultrasound-guided peripheral intravenous placement in patients with difficult access. Acad Emerg Med 16(12):1298–1303

3

Focused cardiopulmonary ultrasound for assessment of dyspnea in a resource-limited setting

Sachita P. Shah[1*], Sachin P. Shah[2], Reginald Fils-Aime[3], Walkens Desir[3], Joanel Joasil[3], David M. Venesy[2] and Krithika Meera Muruganandan[4]

Abstract

Background: The diagnosis and management of acutely dyspneic patients in resource-limited developing world settings poses a particular challenge. Focused cardiopulmonary ultrasound (CPUS) may assist in the emergency diagnosis and management of patients with acute dyspnea by identifying left ventricular systolic dysfunction, pericardial effusion, interstitial pulmonary edema, and pleural effusion. We sought to assess the accuracy of emergency providers performing CPUS after a training intervention in a limited-resource setting; a secondary objective was to assess the ability of CPUS to affect change of clinician diagnostic assessment and acute management in patients presenting with undifferentiated dyspnea.

Methods and results: After a training intervention for Haitian emergency providers, patients with dyspnea presenting urgently to a regional referral center in Haiti underwent a rapid CPUS examination by the treating physician. One hundred seventeen patients (median age of 36 years, 56 % female) were prospectively evaluated with a standardized CPUS exam. Blinded expert review of ultrasound images was performed by two board certified cardiologists and one ultrasound fellowship trained emergency physician. Inter-observer agreement was determined using an agreement coefficient (kappa). Sensitivity and Specificity with confidence intervals were calculated. Pre-test and post-test clinician impressions and management plans were compared to assess for a change. We enrolled 117 patients with undifferentiated dyspnea. Upon expert image review, prevalence of left ventricular systolic dysfunction was 40.2 %, and in those with systolic dysfunction, the average EF was 14 % (±9 %). The parasternal long axis (PLAX) single view was predictive of an overall abnormal echo with PPV of abnormal PLAX 95 % and NPV 93 % of normal PLAX. Weighted kappa for pericardial effusion between the Haitian physicians and two cardiology reviewers was 0.81 (95 % CI 0.75–0.87, p value <0.001) and for ejection fraction was 0.98 (95 % CI 0.98–0.99, p value <0.001). For lung ultrasound, a kappa statistic assessing agreement between the Haitian physician and the EP for pleural effusion was 0.73, and for interstitial syndrome was 0.49. Detailed test characteristics are detailed in Table 3. Overall, there was a change in treating clinician impression in 15.4 % (95 % CI 9–22 %) and change in management in 19.6 % (95 % CI 12–27 %) of patients following CPUS. A significant structural heart disease was common: 48 % of patients were noted to have abnormal right ventricular systolic function, 36 % had at least moderate mitral regurgitation, and 7.7 % had a moderate to large pericardial effusion.

Conclusions: A focused training intervention in CPUS was sufficient for providers in a limited-resource setting to accurately identify left ventricular systolic dysfunction, pericardial effusion, evidence of interstitial syndrome, and

*Correspondence: sachita.shah@gmail.com
[1] Division of Emergency Medicine, Harborview Medical Center, University of Washington School of Medicine, Box 359702, 325 9th Ave, Seattle, WA 98104, USA
Full list of author information is available at the end of the article

pleural effusions in dyspneic patients. Clinicians were able to integrate CPUS into their clinical impressions and management plans and reported a high level of confidence in their ultrasound findings.

Keywords: Heart failure, Ultrasound, Point-of-care, Resource-limited

Background

Clinicians' world-wide rise to the diagnostic challenge presented by patients with undifferentiated dyspnea, relying on both clinical acumen and diagnostic testing to determine diagnosis. The differential diagnosis of acute dyspnea in limited-resource international settings is broad, including diagnoses in which point-of-care-ultrasound findings can influence overall assessment and acute management, such as acute decompensated heart failure (ADHF), pericardial effusion with tamponade, and large pleural effusions causing respiratory distress. The burden of heart failure in particular in the developing world is likely significant, but has not been sufficiently characterized, and resource limitations in these settings impose an obstacle to early disease recognition and appropriate therapy. Cardiopulmonary ultrasound (CPUS) is a portable and reusable resource that may be useful in establishing a diagnosis in patients presenting with acute dyspnea.

Improvements in the portability and cost of ultrasound equipment have facilitated an increase in its utilization for the rapid identification of pathology in several clinical and non-clinical settings [1–8]. CPUS has been used effectively in emergency and intensive care settings in the evaluation of the dyspneic patient [9–12]. There is sufficient evidence to support the adequacy of brief focused instruction of physicians in focused cardiac ultrasound and basic lung ultrasound [7, 10, 13], however, ours is the first study to demonstrate this type of training intervention in a resource-limited setting. In addition, no prior study has addressed whether focused ultrasound findings at the point-of-care will actually influence clinicians to change their diagnosis or management plans of acutely dyspneic patients.

Ultrasound is central to the evaluation of common causes of dyspnea. While heart failure is a syndrome of clinical signs and symptoms, echocardiography is helpful in the diagnosis and further characterization of patients with suspected ADHF. Lung ultrasound is emerging as an innovative and simple tool to identify extravascular lung water (alveolar interstitial edema and pleural effusion), pneumothorax, and alveolar consolidation [14–17]. B-lines are ultrasound comet-tailed artifacts which relate to subpleural interstitial edema (Fig. 1) [11, 17–19]. Excessive B-lines have been found to correlate with a diagnosis of ADHF, chest roentgenogram findings of pulmonary edema, brain natriuretic peptide (BNP) levels, and pulmonary arterial wedge pressure [12, 20–22]. These artifacts are easily identified with lung ultrasound of the anterior and lateral chest, are quantifiable, and rapidly resolve with decongestion [23, 24].

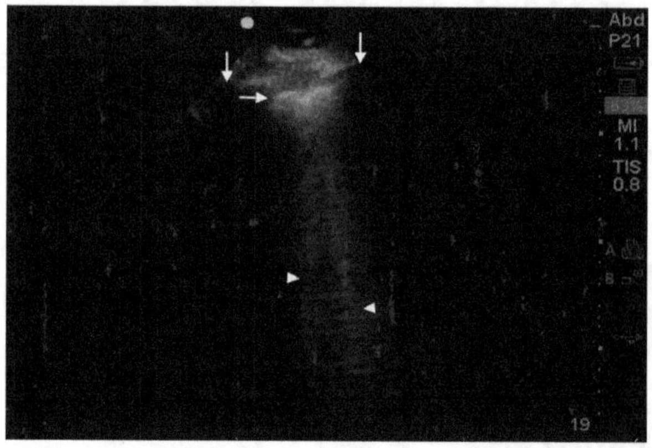

Fig. 1 Example of B-lines. The pleural line (*horizontal arrow*) is identified as an echogenic line noted about 0.5-cm deep and perpendicular to the rib shadowing (*vertical arrows*). The comet-tail or ring-down artifacts (*arrow heads*) begin at the pleural line and extend to the edge of the image

We have developed a rapid CPUS protocol to assist physicians practicing in remote, austere environments in evaluating patients presenting urgently with dyspnea. We conducted a prospective study in a single large hospital in Haiti's remote Central Plateau to characterize ability of providers to accurately perform focused cardiac and lung ultrasound after a novel training intervention, and to assess whether that information was integrated into the treating clinician's overall impression, such that a change in impression and/or management plans was initiated.

Methods

Study population

This study is a prospective cohort analysis of patients presenting with dyspnea for the urgent medical evaluation at the Hospital Bon Sauveur, a 104 bed regional referral center, in Haiti's remote Central Plateau. This study was approved by the internal review board of Zamni Lasante (Partners In Health) and all subjects provided informed consent. All adult and pediatric patients presenting to the emergency department or urgently to outpatient clinics with acute dyspnea were eligible for this study. Patients were enrolled from February to August 2012 within 24 h of presentation. Patients were excluded if they had an echocardiogram in the preceding year.

Study protocol

Patients presenting with undifferentiated dyspnea were evaluated by the treating physician with a detailed history, physical examination, and limited laboratory, and radiographic testing. A preliminary diagnosis and management plan were recorded by the treating clinician. The treating physician then performed a CPUS examination (Table 1) and recorded a post-test clinical impression and management plan. In addition, the level of confidence of the performing physician was self-reported using a five-point Likert scale. Admitted patients were followed until discharge from the hospital noting any procedures, complications, and the final discharge diagnosis.

Ultrasound training and CPUS protocol

Focused cardiac ultrasound and lung ultrasound were performed by seven Haitian physicians (internal medicine residency trained and social service residents) who underwent a 3-week ultrasound training program in point-of-care-ultrasound. The ultrasound training program entailed 10 h of structured didactic training and 20 h of supervised practice. All examinations were performed using a Sonosite Micromaxx with a phased array (P17) transducer (Sonosite Inc, Bothell, WA). The focused cardiac ultrasound included 6-second acquisitions of each the following: parasternal long axis view, parasternal short axis view at the mid-ventricular level, apical four chamber view with and without color Doppler, and subcostal four chamber view (Table 1). The treating physician was required to assess left ventricular ejection fraction (LVEF) by visual estimation, presence and size of pericardial effusion, and presence and characterization of mitral valve disease, including regurgitation using color flow and stenosis. Mitral regurgitation was defined as color flow back through the closed mitral valve during systole. The presence of mitral stenosis is difficult to assess in the absence of continuous wave Doppler, and in our study, was estimated based on visual assessment of the mitral valve in both parasternal long axis (PLAX) and parasternal short axis (PSS) view for classic findings of mitral stenosis, including valve leaflet thickening, hockey stick deformity (PLAX), fish mouth appearance (PSS), and reduced leaflet movement of both the two dimensional images, as well as prominent antegrade flow acceleration through the mitral valve during diastole using a standard Nyquist limit. The practitioners were not trained in calculating/estimating valve area or gradient based on the spectral Doppler analysis; therefore, the presence or absence of mitral stenosis was based on the above parameters and is limited to detection of severe mitral stenosis.

Lung ultrasound was performed using the same transducer. Ultrasound of the anterior and lateral chest bilaterally in the supine or recumbent position perpendicular to the ribs was performed to assess for interstitial syndrome as characterized by the presence of increased numbers of B-lines, defined as moderately hyperechoic, vertical, well-defined, dynamic lines originating from the pleural line, and extending deep to the bottom of the screen [18, 25]. Interstitial syndrome was considered present if ≥ 3 B-lines were noted in two or more rib spaces anteriorly or laterally. At least two rib spaces were scanned in each zone of the chest, and zones were upper/superior anterior, lower/inferior anterior, upper/superior lateral, and lower/inferior lateral. Ultrasound of the mid-axillary line at the level of the costophrenic recesses bilaterally was performed to evaluate for pleural effusion.

Table 1 Cardiopulmonary ultrasound protocol

Echocardiogram	
Parasternal long axis with color Doppler	Estimate LVEF Pericardial effusion Mitral valve disease
Parasternal short axis (mid-ventricle)	
Apical 4 chamber with color Doppler	
Subcostal	
Pulmonary ultrasound	
Anterior and lateral chest ultrasound, rib interspaces 2–4 on left and 2–5 on right for upper zones, and rib spaces below 5 for lower zones bilaterally	Extravascular lung water (B-lines) Pleural effusion Pneumothorax (lack of lung sliding)

LVEF left ventricular ejection fraction

Outcome measures and data interpretation

To assess our primary outcome of determining accuracy of trained health providers in Haiti using CPUS in the evaluation of dyspnea, three independent reviewers assessed the recorded ultrasound images produced by the trained subject physicians. For the focused cardiac ultrasound video clips, blinded review was conducted independently by two board certified cardiologists with experience teaching ultrasound in the developing world and specialty training in echocardiography and heart failure (HF). For the lung ultrasound recording, blinded review was conducted by an emergency ultrasound fellowship trained EP. Reviewers were blinded to the patient characteristics as well as the study physician's interpretation of the ultrasound exams.

For the quality assessment, blinded reviewers rated the ultrasound image quality using a 1–5 scale published in the American College of Emergency Physicians Emergency Ultrasound standard reporting guidelines [26]. This scale uses ratings of 1 and 2 for images with insufficient data for diagnosis, and 3–5 for images that are sufficient for diagnosis with improving image quality throughout the scale.

For accuracy assessment and establishment of test characteristics, cardiologist review of echocardiography is essential for the formal diagnosis of HF; therefore, this was considered the criterion standard for the assessment of left ventricular systolic dysfunction [27, 28]. Similarly, because several studies have established high sensitivity of emergency physician interpretation of bedside ultrasound for the diagnosis of pleural effusion, pneumothorax, and pathologic B-lines as referenced above, and due to the limited resources available at the study site (limited laboratory tests, limited plain film radiography, lack of formal ultrasound and CT), blinded review of the lung ultrasound videos was used as the criterion standard for determining presence or absence of pleural effusion, and B-lines [11, 16, 29].

Considering these criterion standards, kappas for interobserver agreement between both expert reviewers and the point-of-care study physician interpretation, as well as and performance characteristics (sensitivity SN, and specificity SP) were calculated for each ultrasound exam type, and confidence levels were evaluated. The same criteria for the diagnosis of cardiac and pulmonary sonographic abnormalities were used by the Haitian clinicians and the expert reviewers.

For the evaluation of the secondary outcome of CPUS in influencing clinicians change in management and clinical impression, pre-test and post-test diagnoses by the treating clinicians were compared, and frequency of change in the treating clinicians' impressions and management plans was calculated.

Statistical analysis

We calculated our sample size based on our primary outcome of assessing accuracy of clinicians to use CPUS at the point-of-care to accurately assess the common causes of dyspnea. Though there is a little available data on the prevalence of the top causes of dyspnea in tropical, resource-poor medical settings, we focused on powering our study to demonstrate ability of clinicians to detect left ventricular systolic dysfunction. We designed our study to include sufficient patients, such that the prevalence of LV systolic dysfunction would be not uncommon, and to demonstrate that the sensitivity to diagnose ADHF exceeded 70 %, which we defined as the minimum clinically acceptable sensitivity. Under the hypothesis that subject physicians would have 90 % sensitivity, a sample size of 40 patients with disease would have 90 % power with the exact binomial test of proportions at alpha = 0.025 (one-sided). Given a prevalence of HF in prior studies at 21–58 %, we estimated that a total of 110 dyspneic patients would be necessary to yield 40 patients with HF as a cause for their dyspnea [30–34].

Categorical data were analyzed using Fisher's exact test and continuous data using a student *t*-test. A weighted kappa measurement was calculated for assessing agreement between the physician performing the CPUS and the expert reviewer.

Results

A total of 117 patients were enrolled in the study over a 7-month period. Twenty nine (24.8 %) of the patients were children under the age of 18, the median age of the overall study cohort was 36 years (interquartile range 17–58 years). Of the pediatric patients, the average age was 3.4 years (range 2 months–17 years), and 22 of our 29 children were under 5 years old. Known comorbid conditions were not common and are detailed in Table 2. Fifty-six percent of patients were female. Most of the patients (81 %) were admitted to the hospital, with a median length of hospitalization of 8 days. Of the 95 patients admitted to the hospital, 17 (17.9 %) died during their hospitalization. There were no deaths in the hospitalized pediatric patients. The final diagnoses as determined by the treating clinicians as the charted discharge diagnosis (based on clinical presentation, laboratory studies, and chest film findings, response to treatment and ultrasound findings) of the enrolled patients are illustrated in Table 2. The most common final discharge diagnosis in adults was HF (N = 40/88), and for pediatric patients, pneumonia was the most frequent discharge diagnosis (N = 16/29).

For assessment of the primary outcome of accuracy of CPUS in a limited-resource setting, we present data on quality of images produced, and agreement compared to the criterion standard of blinded review by an expert. Of the 117 patients enrolled, all had images which were available for blinded review. One hundred eight (92.3 %) of patients had echocardiographic images considered to be of sufficient quality and 107 (91.4 %) of patients had pulmonary ultrasound images that were of sufficient quality. The average level of confidence of the performing physician (on a 5 point Likert scale, 1 = not confident and 5 = very confident) was high at 4.2.

Compared to blinded expert reviewer interpretation of ultrasound images, the treating physicians had an excellent sensitivity and specificity in detecting left ventricular (LV) systolic dysfunction (93.6 and 100 %, respectively) (Table 3), and agreement in assessing the severity of LV dysfunction was excellent (kappa = 0.98, p = <0.001). The agreement in the size of pericardial effusion (none, small, moderate, large) was excellent (kappa = 0.81, $p < 0.001$). The agreement in type of mitral valve disease (normal, regurgitation, stenosis, and mixed-valve disease) was good (kappa 0.7, $p < 0.001$).

Table 2 Demographic data, clinical findings, and outcomes

	Total patients $N = 117$	Pediatric (<18 years) $N = 29$	Adult (>18 years) $N = 88$
Female	65 (56 %)	11 (38 %)	54 (61 %)
Comorbid conditions			
Tobacco	9 (8 %)	0	9 (10 %)
Post-partum	8 (7 %)	0	8 (9 %)
Tuberculosis	5 (4 %)	0	5 (6 %)
HIV	5 (4 %)	1	4 (5 %)
Diabetes mellitus	2 (2 %)	0	2 (2 %)
Clinical findings			
Tachypnea ($n = 88$)	88 (100 %)	NA*	88 (100 %)
Tachycardia ($n = 86$)	57 (66 %)	NA*	57 (66 %)
Abnormal lung exam	83 (71 %)	27 (93 %)	56 (63 %)
Peripheral edema	44 (38 %)	0	44 (50 %)
Outcomes			
Hospitalized	95 (81 %)	28 (97 %)	67 (76 %)
Median/IQR length of hospital stay (days)	6/6 (n = 92)	6/4 ($n = 26$)	6/8 ($n = 66$)
Death during hospitalization	17 (15 %)	0	17 (19 %)

Data are reported as number of patients (percentage)

Post-partum is defined as delivery in the prior 6 months. Abnormal vital signs (tachypnea and tachycardia) are reported for adults only. Tachypnea is defined as respiratory rate >20 breaths per minute. Tachycardia is defined as heart rate >100 beats per minute. Abnormal lung exam was defined as decreased breath sounds, wheezes, crackles, and/or rhonchi, though was left to the interpretation of the treating clinician at the time of the exam. Pediatric heart rate and respiratory rate were recorded however given variability of vital signs with change in age, we did not define tachycardia/tachypnea for children

All percentages have been rounded to the nearest whole percent

HIV human immunodeficiency virus, *IQR* interquartile range, *NA* not applicable

Table 3 Cardiopulmonary ultrasound findings: prevalence and test characteristics

CPUS findings	Prevalence %	Sensitivity %	Specificity %	Kappa
Pericardial effusion	7.7 (3.8, 14.5)	88.9 (50.7, 99.4)	99.1 (94.2, 100)	0.81*
LVEF <50 %	40.2 (31.3, 49.7)	93.6 (81.4, 98.3)	100 (93.5, 100)	0.98*
MV disease	53.8 (43.2, 64.1)	86.0 (72.6, 93.7)	86.0 (71.4, 94.2)	0.696*
Pleural effusion	25.7 (20.2, 31.9)	83.1 (70.6, 91.1)	100 (97.3, 100)	0.73*
Interstitial synd.	36.3 (30.1, 43.0)	92.7 (84.2, 97.0)	97.9 (93.6, 99.5)	0.49*

Numbers are reported as a percentage (confidence interval)

CPUS cardiopulmonary ultrasound, *LVEF* left ventricular ejection fraction, *MV* mitral valve, *Interstitial synd* Interstitial Syndrome)

* $p < 0.001$

For assessment of the secondary objective of assessing integration of the new CPUS protocol into clinical impression and management decisions, we analyzed pre- and post-CPUS physician impression for comparison. An initial clinical impression of ADHF based on initial history and exam by the treating clinician was made in 49/117 (41.9 %) patients. The treating clinician's impression was changed based on the results of CPUS in 11 (22.4 %) of these patients. The remaining 68 (58.2 %) patients were clinically diagnosed with a non-heart failure cause of dyspnea. This initial assessment was changed to heart failure in 7 (10.3 %) following CPUS. Overall, the treating clinicians used their CPUS results to impact change in their clinical impression in 18 (15.4, 95 % CI 9–22 %) patients.

Change in clinical impression of the treating clinician in our pediatric population was lower as expected given the high prevalence of respiratory infections as a cause of dyspnea, and lower overall presence of HF in children world-wide. Pre-CPUS none of the 29 pediatric patients were diagnosed with ADHF as a cause of dyspnea, and after CPUS, the treating clinician's impression was changed (changed, broadened or narrowed) in 4/29 patients (13.7 %). Two children from this cohort were diagnosed with severe LV dysfunction on CPUS leading to a change in management in one patient (3.4 %).

Amongst our total study population, CPUS resulted in a change in the management strategy in 23 (19.6, 95 % CI 12–22 %) cases. One procedure (thoracentesis) was cancelled based on the ultrasound results, in the remaining 22 cases, there was a change in medical therapy. An additional 12 procedures (e.g. thoracentesis or paracentesis) were performed with the use of ultrasound guidance.

These findings suggest that not only were study clinicians able to accurately perform focused cardiac and lung ultrasound to produce high quality images, with a high level of confidence, but also that they did use this information to guide their clinical impression and management of patients at the point-of-care.

Echocardiography

For additional descriptive statistics in our patient population, we present detailed analysis of the focused cardiac ultrasound results. Of the 117 patients, 47 (40.2 %) had evidence of LV systolic dysfunction (LVEF <50 %) on CPUS. This cohort was comprised 45 adults and 2 pediatric patients found to have LV systolic dysfunction. In the subset of patients with LV systolic dysfunction, the mean EF was 14 ± 9 %, and both pediatric patients in this cohort had an EF of 10 %. Abnormal right ventricular (RV) function was noted in 56 (47.9 %) patients. Of those with RV dysfunction, the RV dysfunction was isolated (without LV dysfunction or mitral valve disease) in 12 (21.4 %) patients and was severe in 27 (48.2 %).

Mitral regurgitation could be assessed in 93 of the 117 patients, and of this 58 (62.4 %) had at least mild mitral regurgitation, of those, 42 (72.4 %) had moderate-to-severe mitral regurgitation. In 54 (93.1 % of those of with mitral regurgitation) patients, the etiology of regurgitation was considered to be functional, only four (6.9 %) of the 58 patients with any mitral regurgitation had a rheumatic deformity of the valve. A moderate or large pericardial effusion was noted in 9 (7.7 %) patients.

A single parasternal long axis view without color Doppler was reviewed for each patient in isolation and then compared to the all echocardiogram images. Patients with a normal appearing parasternal long axis image were very unlikely to have significant structural heart disease (defined as LV or RV systolic dysfunction, moderate-to-large pericardial effusion, or more than mild mitral valve disease) detected on the remaining images. The negative predictive value of normal parasternal long axis was 93 %.

Lung ultrasound

Lung ultrasound revealed pleural effusions in 30 (25.7 %) patients, all adults. B-lines as defined as ≥3 B-lines found in two or more rib spaces anteriorly or laterally were noted in 42 (35.9 %) patients, including 7 children and 35 adults. Of note, B-lines were diffuse in all lung zones in two of the pediatric patients, those found to have ADHF, and focal in the remaining five pediatric patients, all subsequently diagnosed with pneumonia as their final diagnosis. Using expert interpretation of ultrasound as the reference standard, the sensitivity and specificity of the performing physician's interpretation for pleural effusion were 83.1 and 100 %, and for B-lines was 92.7 and 97.9 %, respectively.

Discussion

Our study suggests that providers in an international, limited-resource setting can perform CPUS after a relatively brief training with a high degree of accuracy to detect sonographically evident potential causes of dyspnea, such as left ventricular systolic dysfunction and pericardial effusion. To our knowledge, this is the first study of the impact of a novel curriculum for a focused point-of-care-ultrasound protocol for dyspnea to be conducted in a limited-resource setting.

Using a similar curriculum to those used in the US emergency medicine residency programs, we developed a training intervention for focused cardiac and lung ultrasound and included not only training for common causes of dyspnea world-wide, such as HF and pericardial effusion, but also included specialized training for rheumatic valvular disease [35]. Our study training period was relatively brief, 3 weeks, but included 20 h of hands-on training, including bedside instruction on how to integrate ultrasound findings into clinical care. Our findings reflect that study physicians reported a high level of confidence in their CPUS ultrasound exams after the training, and used their CPUS exams to influence their clinical impression and management plans in a significant number of cases.

The incremental diagnostic impact of portable ultrasound has been realized for over a decade, with many, including the World Health Organization, advocating for its use in resource-limited settings [2, 36]. The concept of a hand-held ultrasound or "sonoscope" used routinely in clinical practice has recently gained support, and with limited access to other diagnostic tests, the value of ultrasound in this population is magnified [1, 37–39]. For example, though ADHF is recognized as a common cause of dyspnea with high morbidity and mortality, there are significant limitations to the physical exam in the detection of ADHF as a cause for dyspnea, and brain natriuretic peptide (BNP) and chest roentgenogram are often not available and may ultimately delay diagnosis in limited-resource settings. Previous studies have described the value of focused cardiac ultrasound, lung ultrasound, or a combined protocol in resource-rich medical environments, including evidence-based support in international consensus conferences related to both clinicians performed focused echocardiography and point-of-care lung ultrasound [25, 40, 41].

Ultrasound-enhanced diagnosis of ADHF using the conventional echocardiography performed by a cardiologist or sonographer is the mainstay of current standard of care for diagnosis, and focused cardiac ultrasound is fast becoming a useful screening tool for non-cardiologists to initiate appropriate treatment and guide referrals in emergency departments in the US. The criterion standard for establishing the presence of left ventricular dysfunction for this study was the visual estimate of left ventricular systolic function using the images provided by the study physicians, a method that has been studied previously by Moore et al. to demonstrate emergency physician competence in bedside echocardiography for detection of heart failure in hypotensive patients and is supported as an established standard for the determination of ejection fraction within the cardiology literature [28, 42, 43].

Our study physicians had a high sensitivity and specificity for the detection of systolic left ventricular dysfunction in dyspneic patients compared with expert image review. Our test characteristics for accuracy and inter-rater reliability are similar to the high level of agreement seen between EM physicians and cardiologists or between cardiologists reviewing the same images [42, 43]. In addition, expert review of a single PLAX view produced in our study shows a PPV of 95 % and NPV of 93 % which would support its use as a particularly valuable screening test in patients with acute dyspnea.

The severity and prevalence of heart disease observed in our population of dyspneic patient deserve some attention. In our study, LV systolic dysfunction was found in 39.3 %, which is similar to that found in the US-based emergency populations, for example, from the "Breathing Not Properly" study published in the New England Journal of Medicine in 2002, investigators determined that of the 1500 patients studied, 47 % of them were diagnosed with CHF, and of those 2/3rd were diagnosed with ejection fraction <45 % indicating systolic dysfunction [33]. The average EF of our study patients with LVEF <50 % was 13.6 %, suggesting not only a high prevalence of previously undiagnosed left ventricular systolic dysfunction, but also increased severity upon presentation. The marked severity of LV dysfunction may relate to the barriers in access to medical care and low health literacy in this setting which likely delays presentation until the disease process is advanced.

Our study shows physicians readily integrated their CPUS findings, translating to a high proportion of patients whose clinical management and initial treating clinician impression were altered based on the CPUS. We found that the pre-CPUS treating physician's clinical impression was changed in 15.3 % of patients, and 19.6 % of patients had an alteration in the management plan. This suggests that adoption of routine CPUS after a brief training intervention may be easy to achieve and may translate into immediate clinical impact. While focused cardiac ultrasound showing left ventricular systolic dysfunction is not equivalent to a diagnosis of the complex clinical syndrome of ADHF, the treating physicians used all available data, including history, exam findings, and other diagnostic testing to make their clinical diagnosis of heart failure [44].

Our study uniquely features a study population, including both adults and children, with pediatric patients representing 24.8 % (29/117) of our total population and 22/29 of these children were under the age of 5 years. While our CPUS protocol was the same for adults and children, we note that overall mortality rate between adults (13.7 %) and children (0 %) was different, and we found a lower clinical impact, including pediatric change in clinical impression (13.7 %) and change in management (3.4 %). While the most common discharge diagnosis for our study subjects with dyspnea in adults was ADHF (N = 40/88), for pediatric patients, pneumonia was the top cause (N = 16/29). Only two of our pediatric patients were found to have left ventricular systolic dysfunction, and both of these patients had very low ejection fractions of 10 %. Focal B-lines were seen in 5/29 children presenting with dyspnea, who went on to have a discharge diagnosis of pneumonia. Given these findings and the high prevalence of pneumonia diagnoses in our study, future research on CPUS protocols, including specific training on pneumonia, may be warranted.

Limitations

Enrollment of patients was based on the availability of the treating physician and research assistant. Patients presenting with dyspnea in the evening hours or weekends were either not included or were enrolled the following day; Therefore, the interim management may have affected the ultrasound findings. Specifically, while we believe it is unlikely that significant improvement or change would occur to affect overall LV systolic function in patients with newly diagnosed ADHF given how low the average EF of the ADHF patients identified was (14 % average), it is possible that if properly diuresed overnight, B-lines as a sign of excess lung water would not be present on evaluation within hours of initial treatment. In our study, a clinical diagnosis, such as HF, was assigned by the treating clinician both prior to and after performing a limited cardiopulmonary ultrasound protocol. These diagnoses were made by the treating clinician in real time with the available information, and were not adjudicated by expert reviewers. Therefore, it remains possible that diagnostic inaccuracies would alter the sensitivity and specificity of the ultrasound findings for any of the specific diagnoses.

Our study included data on patients with severe mitral stenosis based on visual assessment of classic features of the mitral valve; however, as we did not include the use of continuous wave Doppler in the CPUS protocol, it is possible, we were not able to diagnose mild mitral stenosis without classic features.

We enrolled a mixed cohort of adults and children in our study to maximize information available, given that this is the first study of a unique CPUS protocol in dyspneic patients conducted in a limited-resource setting. Clinical assessment of dyspnea is largely similar in both adults and pediatric patients; however, specific data regarding pediatric findings of accessory muscle use and retractions were not recorded in our study, though all routine physical exam components would be captured in the physician overall impression of diagnosis pre-CPUS for adults and pediatric patients alike. Sonographic evaluation of pneumonia, a leading killer in both adults and children, was not included in our CPUS protocol, and may be a limitation to the interpretation of pulmonary portions of the ultrasound (B-lines).

We acknowledge that our CPUS protocol included only recording of lack of lung sliding as a specific and sensitive sign for pneumothorax, and did not include lack of comet-tail artifact, though this was included in the general ultrasound training received by study clinicians. This may have limited our ability to detect pneumothorax in this study.

Patients were enrolled in a single hospital in Haiti, which may limit the external validity and generalizability to other limited-resource settings.

Conclusions

To our knowledge, this is the first prospective study of a combined cardiopulmonary ultrasound protocol in the diagnostic evaluation of patients with dyspnea in an international, limited-resource setting. Our study suggests that focused CPUS performed by general practitioners following a relatively brief training course can be performed with a high degree of accuracy and impact on the treating clinician's impression and management in a significant proportion of patients. Severe underlying structural heart disease was common in this patient population, and a single parasternal long axis image had an excellent negative predictive value in excluding significant structural heart disease. Whenever possible, portable ultrasound should be used in evaluation of the dyspneic patient in resource-limited settings.

Authors' contributions

All authors have given permission and approval for this manuscript to be published, and agree to be accountable for the accuracy and integrity of the work. Sachita PS and Sachin PS: study design, data analysis, and manuscript preparation. RFA: data collection, study design, and critical review of manuscript with revisions. WD: study design, site direction for data collection and analysis, and critical review of manuscript with revisions. JJ: study design, data collection, and critical review of manuscript with revisions. DM: data analysis and critical review of manuscript with revisions. KMM: study concept and design, data collection and analysis, manuscript authoring, and critical revisions. All authors read and approved the final manuscript.

Author details

[1] Division of Emergency Medicine, Harborview Medical Center, University of Washington School of Medicine, Box 359702, 325 9th Ave, Seattle, WA 98104, USA. [2] Division of Cardiology, Lahey Hospital and Medical Center, Burlington, MA, USA. [3] Hopital Bon Sauveur, Zanmi Lasante/Partners In Health, Central Plateau, Cange, Haiti. [4] Department of Emergency Medicine, Boston Medical Center, Boston, MA, USA.

Acknowledgements

We would also like to acknowledge Dr. Heemun Kwok of University of Washington School of Medicine for assistance with the statistical analysis.

References

1. Solomon SD, Saldana F (2014) Point-of-care ultrasound in medical education—stop listening and look. N Engl J Med 370(12):1083–1085
2. Moore CL, Copel JA (2011) Point-of-care ultrasonography. N Engl J Med 364:749–757
3. Otto C, Hamilton DR, Levine BD, Hare C, Sargsyan AE, Altshuler P, Dulchavsky SA (2009) Into thin air: extreme ultrasound on Mt. Everest. Wilderness Environ Med 20(3):283–289
4. Sargsyan AE, Hamilton DR, Jones JA, Melton S, Whiston PA, Kirkpatrick AW, Martin D, Dulchavsky SA (2005) FAST at MACH 20: clinical ultrasound aboard the International Space Station. J Trauma 58:35–39
5. Nelson BP, Chason K (2008) Use of ultrasound by emergency medical services: a review. Int J Emerg Med 1:253–259
6. Brooks AJ, Price V, Simms M (2005) FAST on operational military deployment. Emerg Med J 22:263–265
7. Beck-Razi N, Fischer D, Michaelson M, Engel A, Gaitini D (2007) The utility of focused assessment with sonography for trauma as a triage tool in multiple-casualty incidents during the second Lebanon war. J Ultrasound Med 26:1149–1156
8. Rao S, van Holsbeeck L, Musial JL, Parker A, Bouffard JA, Bridge P, Jackson M, Dulchavsky SA (2008) A pilot study of comprehensive ultrasound education at the Wayne State University School of Medicine: a pioneer year review. J Ultrasound Med 27:745–749
9. Melamed R, Sprenkle MD, Ulstad VK, Herzog CA, Leatherman JW (2009) Assessment of left ventricular function by intensivists using hand-held echocardiography. Chest 135(6):1416–1420
10. Jones AE, Tayal VS, Kline JA (2003) Focused training of emergency medicine residents in goal-directed echocardiography: a prospective study. Acad Emerg Med 10:1054–1058
11. Liteplo AS, Marill KA, Villen T, Miller RM, Murray AF, Croft PE, Capp R, Noble VE (2009) Emergency thoracic ultrasound in the differentiation of the etiology of shortness of breath (ETUDES): sonographic B lines and N-terminal pro-brain-type natriuretic peptide in diagnosing congestive heart failure. Acad Emerg Med 16:201–210
12. Gargani L, Frassi F, Soldai G, Tesorio P, Gheorghiade M, Picano E (2008) Ultrasound lung comets for the differential diagnosis of acute cardiogenic dyspnoea: a comparison with natriuretic peptides. Eur J Heart Fail 10:70–77
13. Kobal SL, Trento L, Baharami S, Tolstrup K, Naqvi TZ, Cercek B, Neuman Y, Mirocha J, Kar S, Forrester JS, Siegel RJ (2005) Comparison of effectiveness of hand carried ultrasound to bedside cardiovascular physical examination. Am J Cardiol 96:1002–1006
14. Dulchavsky SA, Schwarz KL, Kirkpatrick AW, Billica RD, Williams DR, Diebel LN, Campbell MR, Sargysan AE, Hamilton DR (2001) Prospective evaluation of thoracic ultrasound in the detection of pneumothorax. J Trauma 50:201–205
15. Kirkpatrick AW, Sirois M, Laupland KB, Liu D, Rowan K, Ball GC, Hameed SM, Brown R, Simons R, Dulchavsky SA, Hamiilton DR, Nicolaou S (2004) Hand-held thoracic sonography for detecting post-traumatic pneumothoraces: the extended focused assessment with sonography for trauma (EFAST). J Trauma 57:288–295
16. Wilkerson RG, Stone MB (2010) Sensitivity of bedside ultrasound and supine anteroposterior chest radiographs for the identification of pneumothorax after blunt trauma. 2010. Acad Emerg Med 17:11–17
17. Lichtenstein DA (2007) Ultrasound in the management of thoracic disease. Crit Care Med 35:S250–S261
18. Lichtenstein D, Meziere G, Biderman P, Gepnder A, Barre O (1997) The comet-tail artifact. An ultrasound sign of alveolar-interstitial syndrome. Am J Respir Crit Care Med 156(5):1640–1646
19. Lichtenstein D, Goldstein I, Mourgeon E, Cluzel P, Grenier P, Rouby JJ (2004) Comparative diagnostic performances of auscultation, chest radiography, and lung ultrasonography in acute respiratory distress syndrome. Anesthesiology 100(1):9–15
20. Jambrik Z, Monti S, Coppola V, Agricola E, Mottola G, Miniati M, Picano E (2004) Usefulness of ultrasound lung comets as a nonradiologic sign of extravascular lung water. Am J Cardiol 93(10):1265–1270
21. Agricola E, Bove T, Oppizzi M, Marino G, Zangrillo A, Margonato A, Picano E (2005) Ultrasound comet-tail images: a marker of pulmonary edema: a comparative study with wedge pressure and extravascular lung water. Chest 127:1690–1695

22. Lichtenstein D, Meziere G (1998) A lung ultrasound sign allowing bedside distinction between pulmonary edema and COPD: the comet-tail artifact. 198. Intensive Care Med 24:1331–1334
23. Noble VE, Murray AF, Capp R, Sylvia-Reardon MH, Steele DJR, Liteplo A (2009) Ultrasound assessment for extravascular lung water in patients undergoing hemodialysis. Time course for resolution. Chest 135:1433–1439
24. Picano E, Frassi F, Agricola E, Gilgorova S, Gargani L, Mottola G (2006) Ultrasound lung comets: a clinically useful sign of extravascular lung water. J Am Soc Echocardiogr 19:356–363
25. van Volpicelli G, Elbarbary M, Blaivas M, Lichtenstein DA, Mathis G, Kirkpatrick AW, Melniker L, Gargani L, Noble VE, Via G, Dean A, Tsung JW, Soldati G, Copetti R, Bouhemad B, Reissig A, Agricola E, Rouby JJ, Arbelot C, Liteplo A, Sargsyan A, Silva F, Hoppmann R, Breitkreutz R, Seibel A, Neri L, Storti E, Petrovic T (2012) International Liaison Committee on Lung Ultrasound (ILC-LUS) for International Consensus Conference on Lung Ultrasound (ICC-LUS). International Evidence-Based Recommendations for point-of-care lung ultrasound. Intensive Care Med 38(4):577–591
26. American College of Emergency Physicians. Emergency Ultrasound Standard Reporting Guidelines. 2011. http://www.acep.org
27. Feigenbaum H, Armstrong WF, Ryan T (2005) Feigenbaum's echocardiography, 6th edition. p138. Lippincott Williams & Wilkins, Philadelphia, p 138
28. van Royen N, Jaffe CC, Krumholz HM et al (1996) Comparison and reproducibility of visual echocardiographic and quantita- tive radionuclide left ventricular ejection fractions. Am J Cardiol 77:843–850
29. Lichenstein D, Meziere G (2008) Relevance of lung ultrasound in the diagnosis of acute respiratory failure. Chest 134:117–125
30. McCullough PA, Nowak RM, McCord J et al (2002) B-type naturietic peptide and clinical judgement in emergency diagnosis of heart failure: analysis from breathing Not Properly (BNP) multinational study. Circulation 106:416–422
31. Maisel AS, McCord J, Nowak RM et al (2003) Bedside B-type natriuretic peptide in the emergency diagnosis of heart failure with reduced or preserved ejection fraction. J Am Coll Cardiol 41(11):1210–1217
32. McCullough PA, Hollander JE, Nowak RM, Storrow AB, Duc P, Omland T, McCord J, Herrmann HC, Steg PG, Westhelm A, Knudsen CW, Abraham WT, Lamba S, Wu AH, Perez A, Clopton P, Krishnaswamy P, Kazanegra R, Maisel AS, BNP Multinational Study Investigators (2003) Uncovering heart failure in patients with a history of pulmonary disease: rationale for the early use of B-type natriuretic peptide in the emergency department. Acad Emerg Med 10(3):198–204
33. Maisel AS, Krishnaswamy P, Nowak RM, McCord J, Hollander JE, Duc P, Omland T, Storrow AB, Abraham WT, Wu AHB, Clopton P, Steg PG, Westheim A, Knudsen CW, Perez A, Kazanegra R, Herrmann HC, McCullough PA (2002) Rapid measurement of B-typenatriuretic peptide in the emergency diagnosis of heart failure. N Engl J Med 347:161–167
34. Morrison LK, Harrison BS, Krishnaswamy P, Kazanegra R, Clopton P, Maisel A (2002) Utility of a rapid B-natriuretic peptide assay in differentiating congestive heart failure from lung disease in patients presenting with dyspnea. J Am Coll Cardiol 39:202–209
35. Akhtar S, Theodoro D, Gaspari R, Tayal V, Sierzenski P, Lamantia J, Stahmer S, Raio C (2009) Resident training in emergency ultrasound: consensus recommendations from the 2008 Council of Emergency Medicine Residency Directors Conference. Acad Emerg Med 16(Suppl 2):S32–S36
36. World Health Organization. Aide-Memoire for diagnostic imaging services. http://whqlibdoc.who.int/aide-memoire/a71903.pdf
37. Liebo MJ, Israel RL, Lillie EO, Smith MR, Rubenson DS, Topol EJ (2011) Is pocket mobile echocardiography the next-generation stethoscope? A cross-sectional comparison of rapidly acquired images with standard transthoracic echocardiography. Ann Intern Med 155:33–38
38. Adler RS (2007) The use of compact ultrasound in anesthesia: friend or foe. Anesth Analg 105:1530–1532
39. Greenbaum LD (2003) It is time for the sonoscope. J Ultrasound Med 22:321–322
40. Via G, Hussain A, Wells M, Reardon R, ElBarbary M, Noble VE, Tsung JW, Neskovic AN, Price S, Oren-Grinberg A, Liteplo A, Cordioli R, Naqvi N, Rola P, Poelaert J, Gulič TG, Sloth E, Labovitz A, Kimura B, Breitkreutz R, Masani N, Bowra J, Talmor D, Guarracino F, Goudie A, Xiaoting W, Chawla R, Galderisi M, Blaivas M, Petrovic T, Storti E, Neri L, Melniker L (2014) International Liaison Committee on Focused Cardiac UltraSound (ILC-FoCUS); International Conference on Focused Cardiac UltraSound (IC-FoCUS). International Evidence-Based Recommendations for Focused Cardiac Ultrasound. J Am Soc Echocardraph 27(7):683
41. Pivetta E, Goffi A, Lupia E, Tizzani M, Porrino G, Ferreri E, Volpicelli G, Balzaretti P, Banderali A, Iacobucci A, Locatelli S, Casoli G, Stone MB, Maule MM, Baldi I, Merletti F, Cibinel GA (2015) SIMEU Group for Lung Ultrasound in the Emergency Department in Piedmont. Lung Ultrasound-Implemented Diagnosis of Acute Decompensated Heart Failure in the ED: a SIMEU Multicenter Study. Chest 148(1):202–210
42. Mueller X, Stauffer JC, Jaussi A, Goy JJ, Kappenberger L (1991) Subjective visual echocardiographic estimate of left ventric- ular ejection fraction as an alternative to conventional echo- cardiographic methods: comparison with contrast angiography. Clin Cardiol 14:898–907
43. Moore CL, Rose GA et al (2002) Determination of LV function by emergency physician echocardiography of Hypotensive patients. Academic Emergency Medicine, Vol 9. No 3
44. Yancy CW, Jessup M, Bozkurt B, Butler J, Casey DE Jr, Drazner MH, Fonarow GC, Geraci SA, Horwich T, Januzzi JL, Johnson MR, Kasper EK, Levy WC, Masoudi FA, McBride PE, McMurray JJ, Mitchell JE, Peterson PN, Riegel B, Sam F, Stevenson LW, Tang WH, Tsai EJ, Wilkoff BL (2013) American College of Cardiology Foundation; American Heart Association Task Force on practice guidelines. 2013 ACCF/AHA guideline for the management of heart failure: a report of the American College Foundation/ American Heart Association task force on practice guidelines. J Am Coll Cardiol 62(16):e147–e239

4

Point-of-care ultrasound identification of pneumatosis intestinalis in pediatric abdominal pain

Vigil James, Aswin Warier, Khai Pin Lee and Gene Yong-Kwang Ong*

Abstract

We describe a case report of an infant with intussusception who presented to a pediatric emergency department with diarrhea and increased irritability. Pneumatosis intestinalis (intra-mural air) detected on point-of-care ultrasonography (but not apparent on plain abdominal radiographs) alerted the emergency physicians towards the severity of disease process.

Background

The presence of intramural air in the bowel wall or pneumatosis intestinalis in pediatric population can be due to wide range of abdominal and non-abdominal conditions. Abdominal conditions include necrotizing enterocolitis, ileo-colic intussusception with bowel ischemia, venous occlusion of the bowel vasculature and inflammatory bowel disease [1–4]. Non-abdominal conditions that can result in pneumatosis intestinalis include asthma, bronchopulmonary dysplasia, post-bone marrow transplantation, congenital heart disease, juvenile rheumatoid arthritis, hemolytic anemia and generalized vascular hypo-perfusion [5, 6].

Children with acute intussusception present with severe abdominal pain to the emergency department (ED) [7]. For children who are appearing prostrated and sick with signs of bowel obstruction, urgent interventions towards diagnosis and management are vital to decrease morbidity and mortality. A point-of-care ultrasonography (POCUS) done by the emergency physician is shown to be associated with faster diagnosis time in a large variety of conditions [8–12] and use of POCUS to diagnose intra-abdominal pathologies is becoming more popular [13]. This case is the first description of the use of POCUS by pediatric emergency physicians to detect pneumatosis intestinalis in acute abdominal pain in children.

Case

A 3-month-old baby boy, who was previously well, presented with diarrhea for 1 day and 1 episode of blood in the stools. There was history of increased irritability, poor feeding and drawing up of the legs during the crying episodes. He was lethargic on examination with a heart rate of 152 per minute, blood pressure of 118/76 mmHg, oxygen saturation of 100%, capillary refill of 2–3 s and respiratory rate of 40 per minute. On examination, the abdomen was distended with an ill-defined mass palpable in the left hypochondrium. He had another episode of diarrhea while in the ED which also was mixed blood and mucous. The initial venous blood gas showed a pH of 7.424, PCO_2 36 mmHg, HCO_3 23 mmol/L, base excess −0.6 mmol/L, Na 132 mmol/L, K 3.7 mmol/L, iCa 1.21 mmol/L, glucose 7.7 mmol/L and lactate 1.40 mmol/L. The patient was kept nil by mouth and started on maintenance intravenous fluids. A pediatric emergency physician specialized in POCUS performed an abdominal POCUS using with the low-frequency transducer (5–2 MHz) and linear transducer (8–5 MHz). This showed the presence of doughnut or target sign on the axial sonography in the left upper quadrant (Fig. 1). Detailed sonological assessment of the area revealed

*Correspondence: geneong@yahoo.com
Children's Emergency, KK Women's and Children's Hospital, 100 Bukit Timah Road, Singapore 229899, Singapore

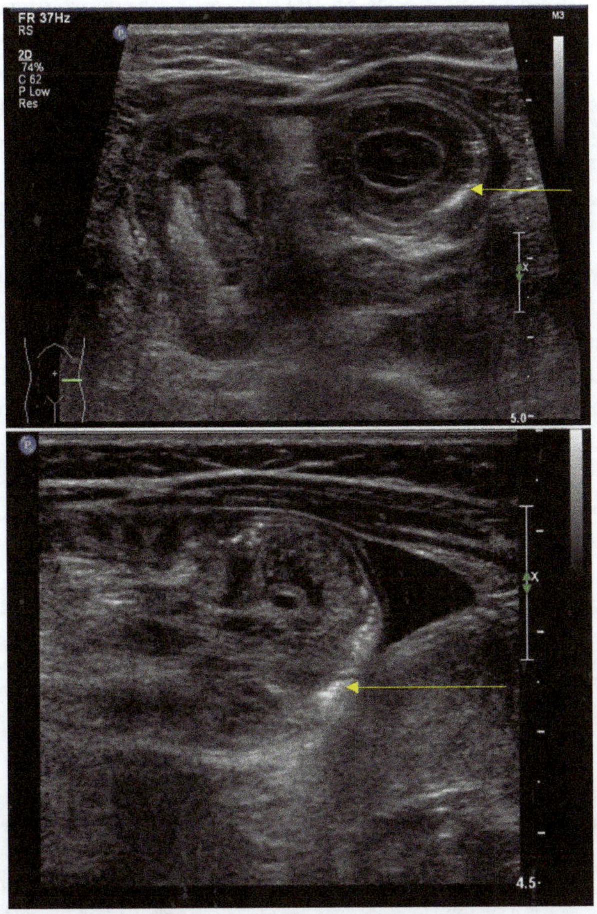

Fig. 1 Abdominal POCUS (over *left upper quadrant*): showing intramural air (*yellow arrow*) in intussusception in a 3-month-old

sub-serosal echogenic foci in the intestinal wall. This sub-serosal echogenic foci was suggestive of sonographic pneumatosis intestinalis or intramural air (Fig. 1). Abdominal X-rays done showed gasless abdominal field except in the gastric area (Fig. 2).

Comprehensive ultrasound was done by the radiologist showed ileo-colic intussusception with marked thickening of the bowel wall. Vascularity was not demonstrated on the Doppler and an echogenic foci of intramural air was also noted. A trial of pneumatic reduction was attempted which was unsuccessful. The patient then underwent laparotomy which revealed ischemic terminal ileum and caecum. A right hemicolectomy with reduction of intussusception and anastomosis of bowel was done. Histopathological evaluation revealed edematous and dusky bowel in the resected specimen. Post-operative period was uneventful and he was discharged after 5 days.

Discussion

There is a growing interest in using POCUS for diagnostic assistance for intra-abdominal pathologies in ED and critical care settings [13]. In this case, we present the first report of ultrasound application being used by pediatric emergency physicians to detect pneumatosis intestinalis in abdominal pathologies.

The diagnosis of intussusception by POCUS requires the presence of doughnut or target sign on the axial sonography or the pseudo-kidney sign on longitudinal scans [14, 15]. Ultrasound depiction of pneumatosis intestinalis in bowel wall in the form of echogenic foci or lines is a predictor of non-reducibility during air enema with a sensitivity of 47% and specificity of 96% [5]. The presence of pneumatosis intestinalis in intussusception indicates bowel ischemia [5]. The concurrent presence of sub-serosal air significantly decreased the chances of successful reduction of intussusception [5]. In our patient, the plain film done to detect pneumatosis intestinalis was negative for intramural air but the POCUS had detected the presence of intramural air. Pneumatosis intestinalis appears as echogenic dots and lines in the bowel wall and can be easily detected in the edematous, thickened bowel [5]. The detection of sub-serosal air is relatively difficult because of the presence of concurrent intraluminal air. Hence, the presence of the intramural and sub-serosal air should be confirmed on both long-axis and short-axis views of the bowel. The histopathologic diagnosis of pneumatosis intestinal can be made on the resection specimens by the presence of submucosal or sub-serosal empty spaces which is lined by histiocytes and giant cells [16].

The POCUS of the abdomen to detect the features of small and large bowel pathologies must be done with the low-frequency transducer (5–2 MHz) to begin with to get a general overview of the abdomen. This must be followed up by a systematic scanning of the bowel using the linear transducer (8–5 MHz). Use of adjuncts such as color and power Doppler can give vital information about the blood flow in the intestinal wall. The large bowel assessment is started at the right lower quadrant then proceeding upwards along the length of the ascending colon. This is then continued to the upper abdomen along the length of transverse colon and followed by the descending colon till the left lower quadrant [17]. To assess the morphology of the small bowel, the scanning must be done in the central region of the abdomen. The technique of graded compression should be used to obtain an adequate view of the small bowel by gently displacing the gas or liquid material present within the intestinal lumen [18]. The presence of intramural air must be confirmed in both short and long axis of the bowel.

The detection of pneumatosis intestinalis by POCUS done by the emergency medicine physician can alert the treating team towards the presence of an advanced stage of intussusception and bowel ischemia. These cohorts of patients' need careful risk stratification and the decision

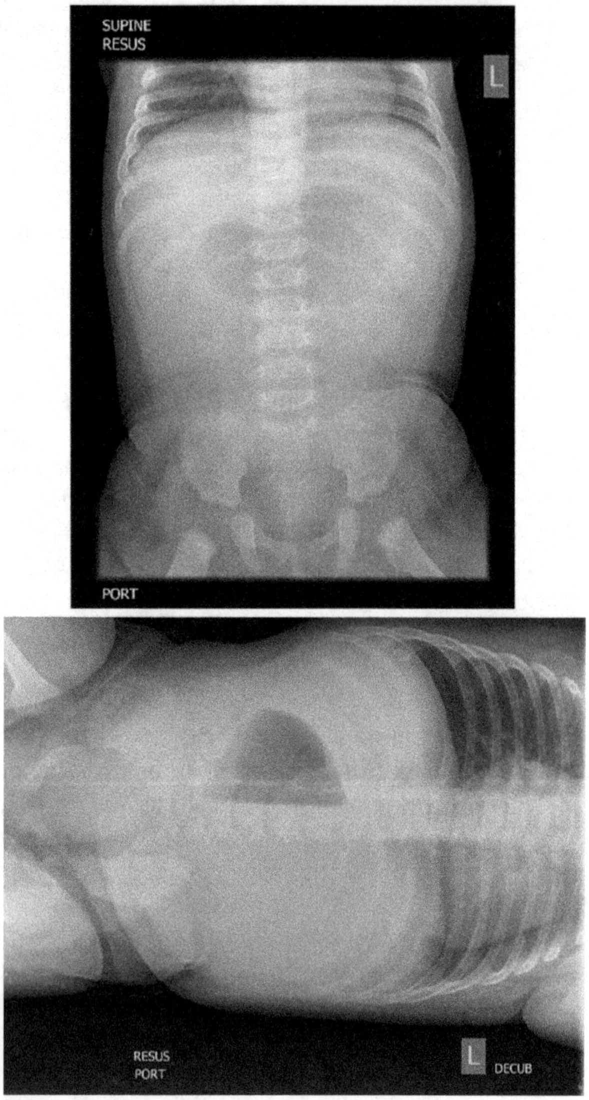

Fig. 2 Abdominal X-rays: supine and left lateral decubitus radiographs showing a gasless abdominal field except in the gastric area. There were no obvious radiographic features of peumatosis or intussusception for the infant

regarding the need for surgical intervention has to be taken at the earliest [5]. It was noted by the authors that plain abdominal radiographs (supine and left lateral decubitus) in this case study did not reveal X-Ray features of pneumatosis despite earlier detection by point-of-care ultrasound. The presence of pneumatosis intestinalis may help indicate severity in intussusception. Possible ultrasonographic risk stratification for operative reduction and unsuccessful non-surgical reduction for intussusception can be derived based on the presence of intramural air [5]. Sonologic detection of pneumatosis intestinalis in combination with other findings such as bowel wall ischemia (no flow on Doppler), peritoneal fluid and enlarged lymph nodes on the ultrasound may prognosticate failure of non-surgical reduction of intussusception. [14, 19]. Detection of pneumatosis intestinalis has also implications on early detection of enterocolitis especially in premature neonates presenting to the ED with gastrointestinal symptoms.

In this case, the POCUS result was useful in clinical decision making. Better understanding of the role of POCUS in evaluating children's acute abdominal pain and presence of pneumatosis intestinalis can help avoid radiation exposure for diagnostic purposes in this radiosensitive population. This case cannot be used to make conclusions about the epidemiology of intramural air and its significance in pediatric gastrointestinal pathologies nor the diagnostic accuracy of POCUS for detecting this condition in children, but suggests that further research into this promising modality is warranted.

Authors' contributions

VJ and AW contributed to concept and design of the study along with drafting the manuscript. LKP revised the manuscript critically for important intellectual content. GO contributed to the acquisition of data and interpretation of data, concept and design of the study, revising it critically for important intellectual content. All authors read and approved the final manuscript.

References

1. Bloom RA, Craciun E, Lebensart PD, Levy P, Ziv JB (1992) The ultrasound appearances of intramural bowel gas: the bright ring appearance and the effervescent bowel. A report of three cases. Br J Radiol 65(775):585–588
2. Oktar SO, Yücel C, Erbaş G, Ozdemir H (2006) Use of twinkling artifact in sonographic detection of intestinal pneumatosis. Abdom Imaging 31(3):293–296
3. Romano S, Lassandro F, Scaglione M, Romano L, Rotondo A, Grassi R (2006) Ischemia and infarction of the small bowel and colon: spectrum of imaging findings. Abdom Imaging 31(3):277–292
4. St Peter SD, Abbas MA, Kelly KA (2003) The spectrum of pneumatosis intestinalis. Arch Surg 138(1):68–75
5. Stranzinger E, DiPietro MA, Yarram S, Khalatbari S, Strouse PJ (2009) Intramural and subserosal echogenic foci on ultrasound in large bowel intussusception. Prognostic indicator for reducibility? Pediatr Radiol 39(1):42–46
6. West KW, Rescorla FJ, Grosfeld JL, Vane DW (1989) Pneumatosis intestinalis in children beyond the neonatal period. J Pediatr Surg 24(8):818–822
7. Kim JS (2013) Acute abdominal pain in children. Pediatr Gastroenterol Hepatol Nutr 16(4):219–224
8. Marin JR, Abo AM, Arroyo AC, Doniger SJ, Fischer JW, Rempell R et al (2016) Pediatric emergency medicine point-of-care ultrasound: summary of the evidence. Crit Ultrasound J 8(1):16
9. Menaker J, Blumberg S, Wisner DH, Dayan PS, Tunik M, Garcia M et al (2014) Use of the focused assessment with sonography for trauma (FAST) examination and its impact on abdominal computed tomography use in hemodynamically stable children with blunt torso trauma. J Trauma Acute Care Surg 77(3):427–432
10. Elikashvili I, Tay ET, Tsung JW (2014) The effect of point-of-care ultrasonography on emergency department length of stay and computed tomography utilization in children with suspected appendicitis. Acad Emerg Med 21(2):163–170
11. Sivitz AB, Tejani C, Cohen SG (2013) Evaluation of hypertrophic pyloric stenosis by pediatric emergency physician sonography. Acad Emerg Med 20(7):646–651

12. Riera A, Hsiao AL, Langhan ML, Goodman TR, Chen L (2012) Diagnosis of intussusception by physician novice sonographers in the emergency department. Ann Emerg Med 60(3):264–268
13. Kameda T, Taniguchi N (2016) Overview of point-of-care abdominal ultrasound in emergency and critical care. J Intensive Care 4:53
14. del-Pozo G, Albillos JC, Tejedor D (1996) Intussusception: US findings with pathologic correlation—the crescent-in-doughnut sign. Radiology 199(3):688–692
15. Swischuk LE, Hayden CK, Boulden T (1985) Intussusception: indications for ultrasonography and an explanation of the doughnut and pseudokidney signs. Pediatr Radiol 15(6):388–391
16. Koreishi A, Lauwers GY, Misdraji J (2007) Pneumatosis intestinalis: a challenging biopsy diagnosis. Am J Surg Pathol 31(10):1469–1475
17. Lim JH (2000) Ultrasound examination of gastrointestinal tract diseases. J Korean Med Sci 15(4):371–379
18. Worrell JA, Drolshagen LF, Kelly TC, Hunton DW, Durmon GR, Fleischer AC (1990) Graded compression ultrasound in the diagnosis of appendicitis. A comparison of diagnostic criteria. J Ultrasound Med 9(3):145–150
19. Koumanidou C, Vakaki M, Pitsoulakis G, Kakavakis K, Mirilas P (2002) Sonographic detection of lymph nodes in the intussusception of infants and young children: clinical evaluation and hydrostatic reduction. AJR Am J Roentgenol 178(2):445–450

5

A workflow task force affects emergency physician compliance for point-of-care ultrasound documentation and billing

Resa E. Lewiss[1*], Jessica Cook[2], Allison Sauler[3], Nicholas Avitabile[4], Nicole L. Kaban[5], Jeffrey Rabrich[3], Turandot Saul[3], Sebastian D. Siadecki[3] and Dan Wiener[6]

Abstract

Background: Emergency point-of-care ultrasound (POC u/s) is an example of a health information technology that improves patient care and time to correct diagnosis. POC u/s examinations should be documented, as they comprise an integral component of physician decision making. Incomplete documentation prevents coding, billing and physician group compensation for ultrasound-guided procedures and patient care. We aimed to assess the effect of directed education and personal feedback through a task force driven initiative to increase the number of POC u/s examinations documented and transferred to medical coders by emergency medicine physicians.

Methods: Three months before a chosen go-live date, departmental leadership, the ultrasound division, and residents formed a task force. Barriers to documentation were identified through brain storming and email solicitation. The total number and application-specific POC u/s examinations performed and transferred to the healthcare record and medical coders were compared for the pre- and post-task force intervention periods. Chi square analysis was used to determine the difference between the number of POC u/s examinations reported before and after the intervention.

Results: A total of 1652 POC u/s examinations were reported during the study period. Successful reporting to the patient care chart and medical coders increased from 41 % pre-task force intervention to 63 % post-intervention (*p* value 0.000). The number of scans performed during the 3-month periods (pre-intervetion, post-intervention 0–3 months, post-intervention 3–6 months) was similar (521, 594 and 537). When analyzed by specific application, the majority showed a statistically significant increase in the percentage of examinations reported, including those most critical for patient care decision making: (EFAST (41 vs. 64 %), vascular access (26 vs. 61 %), and cardiac (43 vs. 72 %); and those most commonly performed: biliary (44 vs. 61 %) and pelvic (60 vs. 66 %). Of the POC u/s studies coded and reported for reimbursement, 15.9 % were billed before intervention and 32 % were billed after intervention (*p* value: 0.000).

Conclusions: The formation of a workflow solution task force positively affected emergency physician compliance with POC u/s documentation for coding and billing over a 6-month period. Further investigation should assess the long-term effect of the intervention and whether this translates into increased revenue to the department.

Keywords: Point-of-care ultrasound, Workflow, Ultrasound workflow, Documentation compliance

Background

Health information technology is increasingly recognized as an essential tool for improving patient safety and quality of care. Emergency point-of-care ultrasound (POC u/s) is an example of a healthcare technology that improves patient care and decreases the time to making a correct diagnosis [1–4]. POC u/s examinations should be appropriately documented and the resultant emergency health records (EHRs) should accurately reflect the level of patient care provided [5]. Incomplete documentation prevents coding, billing and physician compensation for patient care

*Correspondence: resaelewiss@gmail.com
[1] Department of emergency medicine, Department of Radiology, University of Colorado Hospital, Aurora, CO, USA
Full list of author information is available at the end of the article

provided and ultrasound-guided procedures performed [6]. Prior research suggests that changing the behavior of medical providers requires active intervention based on assessment of existing barriers to change. Also, multiple simultaneous interventions are more likely to be effective than any individual intervention alone [7]. The aim of this proof-of-concept study was to evaluate if POC u/s documentation by emergency medicine attending physicians improved after the formation of a task force and the implementation of multiple specific interventional initiatives.

Methods

Study design, population and setting: This was a retrospective quality improvement project. Administrative and residency leadership faculty, two emergency ultrasound fellows, an emergency medicine resident from each class, and the lead medical coder for the emergency department formed a 13-member task force. The group met monthly for 3 months prior to a go-live date of January 1, 2014. The group recognized that the number of POC u/s examinations being performed for patient care was greater than those documented in the EHR and even greater than those subsequently coded for billing and reimbursement. Through brain storming at monthly meetings and via electronic mail communications, the task force defined and explored the suspected barriers, and sought appropriate solutions and interventions.

Based upon the barriers, the task force prioritized those for which there could timely and sustainable solutions (Table 1).

The task force met monthly and progressively introduced methods of individual and group education and personalized feedback to encourage a behavioral change in documentation compliance. Leading up to the go-live date, both resident and attending physicians received in-person and online instruction on the workflow process. A tutorial was posted online for continual review through a centralized website. Other interventions included mass electronic mail messaging, advertising of the task force initiative, and placing reminder signs on all computers at both sites to complete documentation. Emphasis was placed on performance of the ultrasound scan and documentation as one event. Daily electronic reports were generated. These listed individual attending physicians who performed an ultrasound but failed to document in the EHR or conversely, those who documented in the EHR that an ultrasound examination had been performed, but did not submit the ultrasound report itself to the medical coders for billing. The department chairman conducted individual follow-ups with the attending physicians identified in these daily reports. The task force identified physician education as the primary focus for improvement. Items for reinforcement included the definition of a patient care (diagnostic) scan, the specific steps to be completed in the workflow process, and the departmental ultrasound billing capabilities.

Table 1 Point-of-care ultrasound workflow barriers and interventions

Barriers	Interventions and solutions
Scan completed but documentation incomplete	Real-time transfer of study to image archiving software
	Direct transfer of Qpath™ report to EHR
	Attending physicians encouraged to transfer studies in real time
Q-path™ worksheet not completed real time	Emphasis on scan and documentation as a single event
Machinery upkeep	"Image of the week" email
	Consultative services, e.g. general surgery and obstetrics–gynecology educated regarding proper care of equipment
Wireless transmission delays	Biomedical engineering correspondence
	Information technology correspondence
	Hardware vendor correspondence
Q-path logout time too short	Workstation logout time increased
Provider awareness of workflow process	Faculty meeting presentation
	Resident conference presentation
	Educational module distributed to all staff
	Educational module placed on centralized website for immediate access and review
	Laminated reminder signs placed at physician workstations
Attending compliance	Daily reports generated listing attending physicians with studies performed but not documented or vice versa
	Regular follow-up from department chairman with noncompliant attending physicians

The evaluation was performed over a 9-month period (October 2013–June 2014) at an academic institution with a 3-year emergency medicine residency and an emergency POC u/s fellowship. We analyzed the existing data 3 months pre-intervention (01 October 2013 through 31 December 2013). Data collection began 01 January 2014. We then analyzed the data 3 and 6 months post-intervention. Patient data were initially known to the task force investigators involved, and then de-identified. There was no record of patient name, medical record number, or demographics included in the study. There was no funding support for the project. This study was determined exempt from institutional review board approval.

Data and analysis

Data were collected for the 3 months before and at 3 and 6 months after the study go live intervention date. SAS® 9.3 software was utilized. Chi square analysis was used to determine the difference between the total number of POC u/s examinations correctly performed and documented pre- and post-task force intervention. Application-specific data pre- and post-intervention were also analyzed.

Results

1652 total POC u/s scans were reported during the study period. The number of scans performed during the three consecutive 3-month periods pre- and post-intervention was similar (521, 594 and 537). Successful documentation increased from 41 % pre- to 63 % post-intervention (p value 0.000). When analyzed by specific application, the majority of POC u/s examinations showed a statistically significant increase in the percentage of scans documented. This included those most commonly performed on critical care patients: (EFAST (41 vs. 64 %), vascular access (26 vs. 61 %), and cardiac (43 vs. 72 %); and those most commonly performed: biliary (44 vs. 61 %) and pelvic (60 vs. 66 %) (Fig. 1).

Figure 2 illustrates a comparison of the 3-month periods: pre-intervention, first quarter of the year and second quarter of the year.

For the majority of applications, health care provider documentation increased or remained stable. For the applications, where there appeared to be a decline in documentation, the numbers were too few to be statistically significant. Of the POC u/s studies coded and reported for reimbursement, 15.9 % were billed before intervention and 32 % were billed after intervention (p value: 0.000) (Fig. 3).

The number of ocular and thoracic POC u/s examinations submitted during the study period was too few to assess for a statistical change.

Discussion

Encouraging behavioral changes in attending physicians is challenging. Attending physicians practicing in an academic environment represent a specific group of adult learners [7]. Grimshaw et al. suggest that active interventions, such as educational outreach and reminders to specific providers, are more effective than passive dissemination for changing provider behavior across a wide range of professional behavior change interventions. Additionally, multiple simultaneous interventions are more likely to be effective than any single intervention alone [7]. The formation of the ultrasound workflow solution task force was inspired by discussions with colleagues at other academic institutions and by review of relevant articles in the literature [8]. Many physicians felt the process was too time intensive, as it required logging into two software programs: the image database program and the EHR. We were able to utilize this feedback to simplify the workload of the physician as much

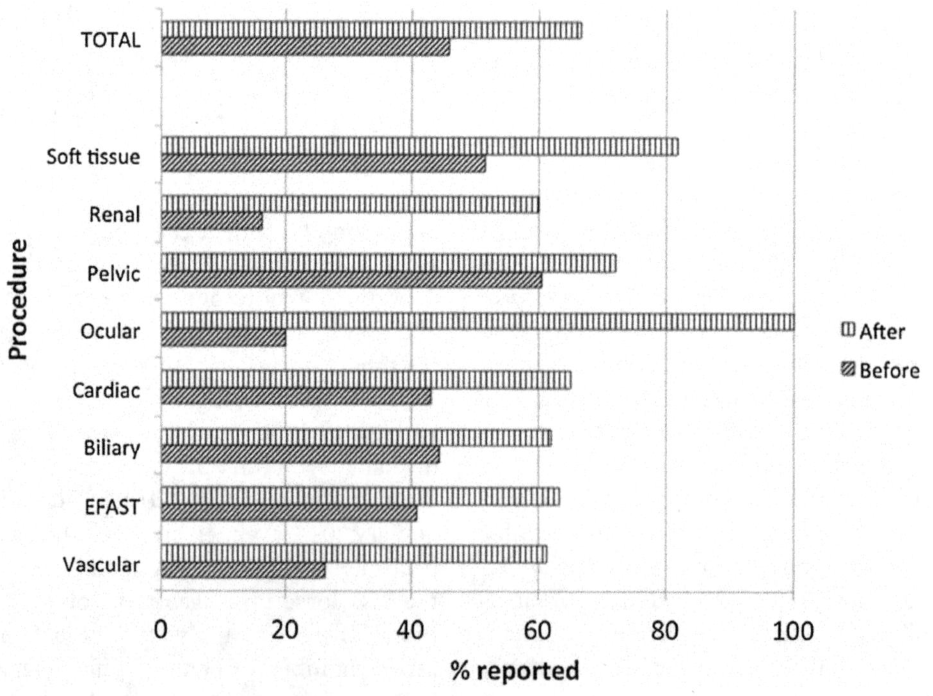

Fig. 1 The percentage of scans reported to the medical coders in the pre- and post-intervention periods. *X-axis* represents the percentage of POC u/s scans documented and reported for coding (*slanted dark hashed bar* pre-intervention data; *vertical hashed bar* post-intervention data). *Y-axis* identifies the number of application specific and number of total POC u/s examinations

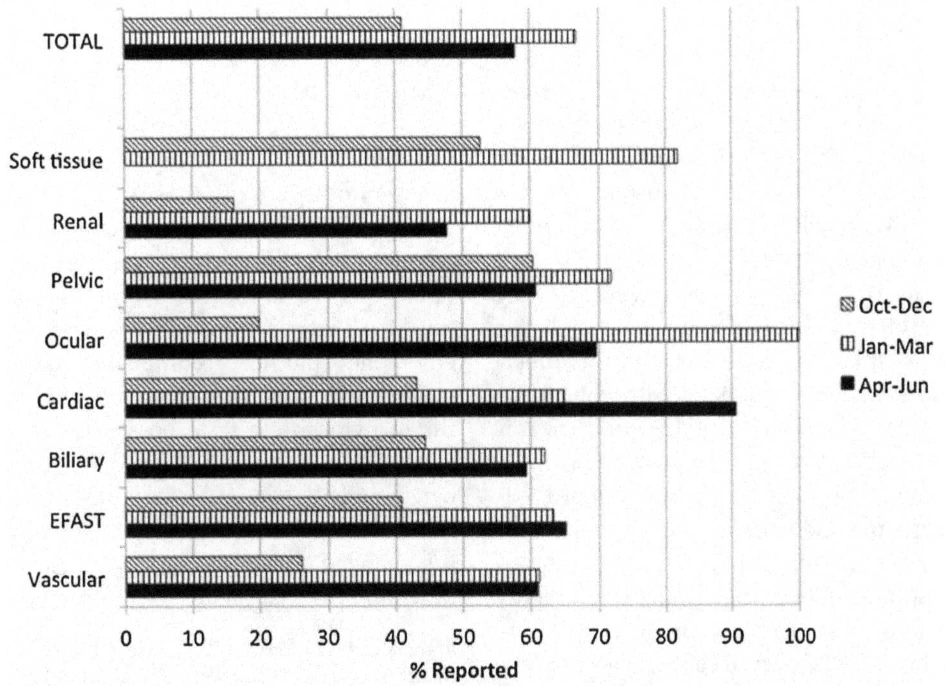

Fig. 2 The percentage of scans reported to the medical coders in the pre- and two 3-month post-intervention periods. *X-axis* represents the percentage of POC u/s scans documented and reported for coding (*dark slanted hashed bar* pre-intervention data; *vertical hashed bar* first post-intervention data; *solid dark bar* second post-intervention period). *Y-axis* identifies the number of application specific and number of total POC u/s examinations

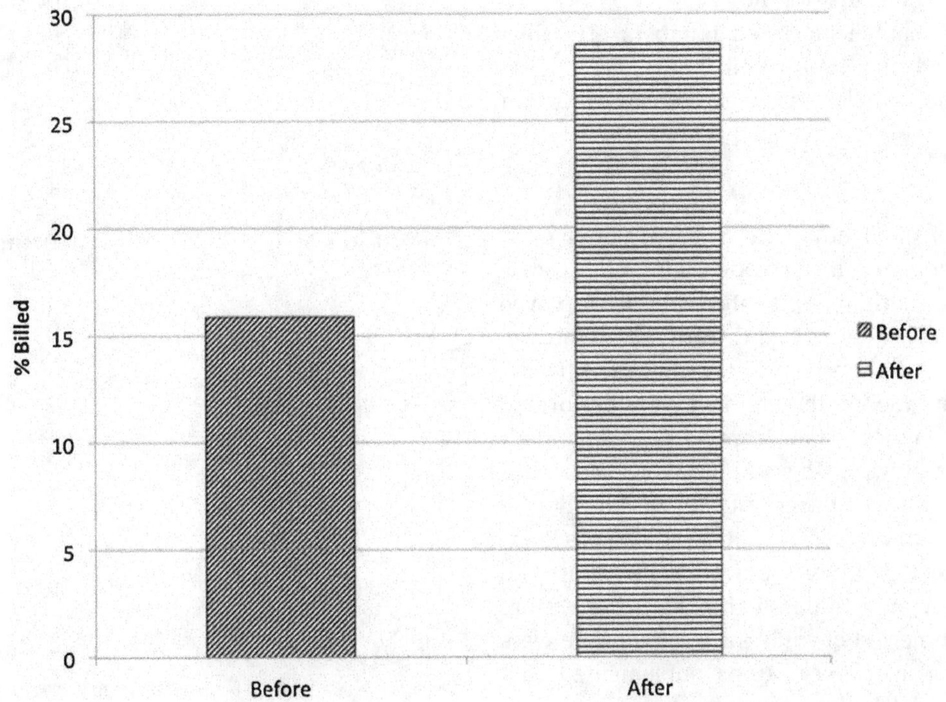

Fig. 3 The change in the percentage of scans billed after being reported to the medical coders by the department pre- and post-task force intervention. *X-axis* illustrates pre- and post-intervention periods (*dark slanted hashed bar* pre-intervention data; *horizontal hashed bar* post-intervention data). *Y-axis* represents the percentage of examinations billed

as possible. For example, we had the auto logout time increased significantly to allow the physicians to remain logged into the database longer thus reducing the time required to document studies during their shifts. Interestingly, feedback from several physicians focused on medico-legal concerns as they were now placing a report of their US findings in the medical record prior to review by our ultrasound division. This concern was somewhat surprising to the department leadership as faculty had been credentialed to use US for clinical decision making for several years and they were already responsible for their interpretations. Through discussion at faculty meetings as well as individual conversations with concerned faculty members, we were able to allay this concern. It is likely that the intervention that is most effective once the workflow concerns were resolved was daily email feedback by our chairman to individuals who had not completed the workflow for billable studies. Faculty reported that while bothersome initially, the emails were highly effective in increasing compliance. We instituted systemic changes to improve the overall ease and acceptance of new compliance standards in ultrasound. We found that in the 3- and 6-month periods after the task force initiative, the mean number of POC u/s examinations documented and transferred for billing and coding significantly increased. This intervention is one that could potentially be replicated at other academic institutions with an organized POC u/s workflow.

While we have shown increased numbers of studies being documented and transferred in the short term, we cannot predict the long-term sustainability of our interventions.

Limitations

One limitation of our study is the relatively brief post-intervention period. We may see deterioration in compliance over time. With multiple interventions employed at the same time, it is difficult to discern which form of feedback was most responsible for the change in behavior. A second limitation is the provider, who performed a "quick look" study for patient care without documentation or image archiving. This would not be accounted for in the denominator of the calculation. A third limitation is the Hawthorne or observer effect. Providers knew that the department chair was following the progress and completion of documentation so they have been more compliant for the period of study. In general, there were various time-intensive interventions implemented that changed practice in the short term; however, we do not know the long-term changes these will create. The interventions may not be feasible on a long-term basis. Finally, the study was performed at a single academic institution with an ultrasound division and fellowship. Some of the barriers and solutions may be specific to the institution and environment. A multi-centered study would be needed to analyze the specific effects in other practice environments.

Conclusion

We are not aware of other studies looking at the formation of a workflow solution task force with the analysis of resultant behavioral changes in the successful documentation of POC u/s ultrasound examinations. The formation of a workflow solution task force positively affected emergency physician compliance with POC u/s documentation in the EHR for coding and billing. Ultimately, the formation of a task force may prove to be an efficacious method for providing feedback and incentive for behavioral change. A future study should seek to provide not only how the frequency of documentation of POC u/s changed, but also quantify the costs of the intervention and how that relates to the enhanced yields.

Authors' contributions

REL, JC, AS, NA, NLK, JR, TS, SDS, DW participated in task force meetings and brain storming communications. REL, JC, AS, NA, NLK, JR, TS, SDS, DW participated in the project design, coordination, and drafting of the manuscript. REL, JC, NA, TS, provided final edits. All authors read and approved the final manuscript.

Author details

[1] Department of emergency medicine, Department of Radiology, University of Colorado Hospital, Aurora, CO, USA. [2] Department of emergency medicine, Yale-New Haven Hospital, New Haven, CT, USA. [3] Department of emergency medicine, Mount Sinai St. Luke's Mount Sinai West, New York, NY, USA. [4] Department of emergency medicine, St. Barnabas Hospital, Bronx, NY, USA. [5] Department of emergency medicine, Mount Sinai Beth Israel Hospital , New York, NY, USA. [6] Bronx-Lebanon Hospital Center, Bronx, NY, USA.

Acknowledgements

Sharda Budhan, head coder, for preparation of coded studies and billing reports. Emilia Bagiella, Ph.D. for her statistical support.

Meetings ACEP 2014 Scientific Assembly Oral Presentation, Chicago, Il.

Grants None.

References

1. Ortiz E, Clancy CM, AHRQ (2003) Use of information technology to improve the quality of health care in the United States. Health Serv Res 38(2):11–22
2. Milling TJ, Rose J, Briggs WM, Birkhahn R, Gaeta TJ, Bove JJ et al (2005) Randomized, controlled clinical trial of point-of-care limited ultrasonography assistance of central venous cannulation: the Third Sonography Outcomes Assessment Program (SOAP-3) Trial. Crit Care Med 33(8):1764–1769
3. Melniker LA, Leibner E, McKenney MG, Lopez P, Briggs WM, Mancuso CA (2006) Randomized controlled clinical trial of point-of-care, limited ultrasonography for trauma in the emergency department: the first sonography outcomes assessment program trial. Ann Emerg Med 48(3):227–235
4. Moore CL, Copel JA (2011) Point-of-care ultrasonography. N Engl J Med 364(8):749–757
5. Resnick J, Hoffenberg S, Tayal V, Dickman E. Ultrasound coding and reimbursement document 2009. ACEP
6. Adhikari S, Amini R, Stolz L, O'Brien K, Gross A, Jones T et al (2014) Implementation of a novel point-of-care ultrasound billing and reimbursement program: fiscal impact. Am J Emerg Med 32(6):592–595
7. Grimshaw JM, Shirran L, Thomas R, Mowatt G, Fraser C, Bero L et al (2001) Changing provider behavior: an overview of systematic reviews of interventions. Med Care 39(8 Suppl 2):II2–II45

6

Serial lung and IVC ultrasound in the assessment of congestive heart failure

Rachel Spevack[1*], Mohamed Al Shukairi[2], Dev Jayaraman[3], Jerrald Dankoff[4], Lawrence Rudski[5,6] and Jed Lipes[7]

Abstract

Background: Management of congestive heart failure (CHF) is dependent on clinical assessments of volume status, which are subjective and imprecise. Point-of-care ultrasound (POCUS) is useful in the diagnosis of CHF, but how POCUS findings correlate with therapy remains unknown. This study aimed to determine whether the changes in clinical evaluation of CHF with treatment are mirrored with changes in the number of B lines on lung ultrasound (LUS) and inferior vena cava (IVC) size. In this prospective observational study, investigators performed serial clinical and ultrasound assessments within 24 h of admission (T1), day 1 in hospital (T2) and within 24 h of discharge (T3). Clinical assessments included an evaluation of the jugular venous distension (JVD), hepatojugular reflux (HJR), pulmonary rales and a clinical congestion score was calculated. Ultrasound assessment included the IVC size and collapsibility, and the number of B lines in an 8-point scan.

Results: Fifty consecutive patients were recruited with a mean age of 71.2 years (SD 12.7). Mean clinical congestion score on admission was 5.6 (SD 1.4) and declined significantly over time to 1.3 (0.91), as did the JVP, HJR and pulmonary rales. No significant changes were found in the IVC size between T1 [1.9 (0.65)] and T3 [2.0 (0.50)] or in the IVC collapsibility index [T1 0.3 (0.19) versus T3 0.25 (0.16)]. The mean number of B lines decreased from 11 (6.1) at T1 to 8.3 (5.5) at T3, although this decrease did not reach statistical significance. Spearman correlation between JVP and HJR versus IVC collapsibility and total B lines did not yield significant results.

Conclusions: Clinical exam findings correlate over time during the management of CHF, whereas LUS and IVC results did not. The number of B lines did decrease with therapy, but did not reach statistical significance likely because the sampled population was small and had only mild heart failure. Further studies are warranted to further explore the use of lung ultrasound in this patient population.

Keywords: Vascular ultrasound, Lung ultrasound, Inferior vena cava, B lines, Heart failure

Background

Cardiovascular disease is the leading cause of mortality, representing 29% of all deaths, and costs the healthcare system 20.9 billion dollars annually in North America [1]. Congestive heart failure (CHF) is a complex clinical syndrome characterized by recurrent episodes of acute decompensation, requiring frequent hospitalizations and readmissions [2]. The diagnosis and management of CHF remain a clinical challenge; decisions are based on clinical assessments of volume status, which are used to estimate cardiac filling pressures [3]. Chest X-ray (CXR) has traditionally been used to suggest pulmonary congestion, but assessments can be subjective [4] and lack sensitivity and specificity [5]. Recently, serial assessments of brain natriuretic peptide (BNP) have been shown to correlate with the degree of hemodynamic congestion [6] and may be a reliable tool to guide management in heart failure patients [7].

The gold standard for determining cardiac congestion is cardiac catheterization with determination of right atrial and left atrial pressures, as estimated by the

*Correspondence: rachel.la.spevack@gmail.com
[1] Internal Medicine Training Program, Department of Medicine, Jewish General Hospital, McGill University, 3755 Chemin de la Cote St Catherine, Montreal H3T 1E2, Canada
Full list of author information is available at the end of the article

pulmonary capillary wedge pressures. These tests are invasive, time consuming and carry risk, and are not typically performed in patients admitted with decompensated heart failure [8]. As a result, physicians rely on clinical assessments to diagnose elevated cardiac filling pressures. Clinical evaluation, however, correlates poorly with invasive hemodynamics [9] and the physical exam lacks sensitivity and specificity for the diagnosis of heart failure, limiting its clinical utility [10].

Point of care ultrasound (POCUS) has been developed as an easy-to-learn, rapid, portable, and non-invasive adjunct to physical examination. Previous studies have shown that inferior vena cava size correlates with right atrial pressure and pulmonary capillary wedge pressure with good sensitivity and specificity [11, 12], and outperforms the physical exam in the detection of an elevated jugular venous pressure [13]. However, IVC as a surrogate for volume status has been increasingly questioned, as the correlation to CVP has been variable [14]. However, the American Society of Echo guidelines still recommend its use as a non-invasive measurement of CVP [15].

Similarly, lung ultrasound and B lines, an artifact representing extravascular lung water, similarly correlate significantly with pulmonary artery systolic pressure [16] and outperform classical signs and symptoms of congestion [17]. Both lung [18, 19] and vascular ultrasound [20–22] have been shown to be helpful in the assessment of undifferentiated dyspnea and in the diagnosis of heart failure. It is not clear how POCUS findings change with treatment.

Methods

The primary objective of the current study is to compare serial lung and vascular ultrasound exam with clinical findings upon CHF treatment. The secondary objective was to explore the relationship between the severity of ultrasound-measured degree of congestion and length of hospital stay, hospital readmission and mortality.

The current study recruited consecutive patients with a clinical diagnosis of left-sided congestive heart failure who require admission to the cardiology service, the admitting cardiology team having made the diagnosis. All hospitalized, spontaneously breathing adult patients, between the ages of 18 and 90, with an admitting diagnosis of either systolic or diastolic left-sided heart failure as per the admitting cardiologist were included. Exclusion criteria were as follows: patients undergoing invasive ventilation, patients with a primary diagnosis of right-sided heart failure, patients with active lung cancer, pulmonary fibrosis, interstitial lung disease, or pneumonia, patients who we are unable to have an ultrasound within the first 24 h of admission and patients who are not competent to sign the consent form. Patients underwent serial clinical and ultrasound assessments at three time points: within 24 h of admission (T1), day 1 of hospitalization (T2), and within 24 h prior to discharge (T3), for a total of three separate clinical and ultrasound exams (Fig. 1). The clinical assessments including the physical exam were performed by a senior resident in internal medicine and a senior critical care fellow. The assessors were aware of the time point of assessment.

Baseline patient demographics, including age, weight, sex, medical comorbidities, and etiology of heart failure were recorded from chart review. Laboratory values including hemoglobin, renal function and troponin values on admission were recorded from a chart review. Left ventricular ejection fraction (LVEF), diastolic function and valvulopathy were obtained from the most recent echocardiogram or during the current hospitalization. Chest X-ray (CXR) on admission was reviewed and graded by resident authors after they performed the clinical and ultrasound assessment as having interstitial edema or alveolar edema, where alveolar edema indicates more significant pulmonary congestion. Three months following discharge, a chart review was performed to assess for length of hospital stay, hospital readmissions and 90-day mortality. The hospital ethics committee approved the current study.

Clinical assessment

The Killip and clinical congestion score (CCS) were calculated for each patient at across the three time points. The Killip score (0–4) [23] was calculated to grade the severity of heart failure, with 0 indicating no heart failure and 4 indicating cardiogenic shock. Although this score has been designed specifically in the setting of acute myocardial infarction, it was used in this study as it is a widely known descriptor of the severity of heart failure.

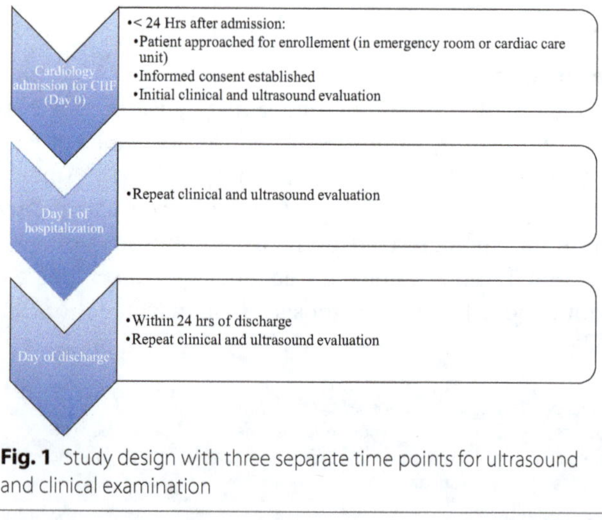

Fig. 1 Study design with three separate time points for ultrasound and clinical examination

The clinical congestion score (CCS) [24] was calculated based on pulmonary rales (scored 0–4), central venous pressure elevation (scored 0–4), S3 (presence 1, absence 0) and orthopnea (scored 0–4). The CCS has a maximum score of 13, where higher scores indicate more severe heart failure. The CCS was validated on an outpatient population with stable heart failure, and has been shown to correlate with echocardiographic findings of increased filling pressures [19].

Specifically, the following symptoms and physical exam findings were graded for the above scores as follows: the presence of dyspnea and PND was graded as present (1) or absent (0). Orthopnea was graded between 0 and 4, with a score of 0 indicating the need of one pillow during sleep, and 4 indicating at least one night spent sleeping in a sitting position. Central venous pressure elevation was graded as 0 if the crests of neither the internal nor the external jugular vein are visible above the clavicle, and 4 if the crests are visible at the earlobe with the patient assessed at 30–45°. The hepatojugular reflux was recorded as present (1) or absent (0). Rales/crackles were graded as being absent (0), present in less than 50% of the lung field (1), or more than 50% of the lung field (2). Peripheral edema was graded between 0 and 4 according to the depth of indentation at the ankle.

Ultrasound assessment

The POCUS ultrasound assessment was performed with the Zonare zone system (Zonare Medical Systems Inc, Mountain View, Ca, USA). Two authors (RS and MS) collected the ultrasound data after a 3-h training session and 10 supervised scans with an intensive care specialist with advanced cardiac echo and formal training in lung ultrasound prior to enrollment of patients. Brennan et al. [25] have shown that internal medicine residents with minimal training, including 4 h of formal didactic ultrasound teaching, and 20 sonographer supervised acquisitions were able to obtain adequate images of the IVC in 90% of patients. Each patient underwent serial scans at the time of the clinical assessments. Two authors (MS and JL) blinded to clinical information analyzed the stored images. A priori it was established that findings on vascular and LUS were not disclosed to the treating team unless they found a significant unexpected life-threatening diagnoses, such as venous thrombus, complex pleural effusion suggestive of empyema, pneumothorax or cardiac tamponade. As a result, no treatment decisions regarding the patient's heart failure were made based on the ultrasound findings.

The IVC was analyzed in the long axis via the subcostal window using a 4-MHz phased-array ultrasound transducer. The diameter of the intra-hepatic IVC within 1–2 cm of the right atrium and the response of the IVC to an inspiratory maneuvre was measured and recorded. The size of the IVC on expiration was recorded, and the IVC collapsibility index was calculated as (IVC size on expiration − IVC size on inspiration)/IVC size on expiration.

All lung ultrasounds were performed using a 6-MHz curved array probe and a 3-s clip was recorded in each quadrant. A bilateral 8-point LUS examination was performed to assess for B lines following the International consensus guidelines [8]. An oblique intercostal view was obtained to maximize the number of B lines, and the actual count was made at the moment the most B lines were visualized.

Data analysis

Clinical and ultrasound variables were analyzed using a paired *t* test. Pearson correlations were used to compare clinical and ultrasound variables. The impact of ultrasound and clinical assessments on hospital LOS and 90-day mortality was evaluated using univariate and multivariate analyses.

Results

Fifty patients were recruited in the study. Five patients were excluded because they had a primary diagnosis of pneumonia complicated by pulmonary edema, and one patient was excluded because CHF was not the final diagnosis. Mean age was 77 (SD 12.7); 52% were males. The mean LVEF was 47.8%, and mean highly sensitive troponin T (Roche) value on admission was 293 ng/L (SD 824). The etiology of CHF was ischemic (33%), followed by valvular (26%) and hypertensive (6%), whereas 22% had a new diagnosis of CHF when they were recruited (Table 1). Median hospital length of stay was 7 days (IQR 5–13), 24% of patients were readmitted within 30 days of discharge and there was a 12% mortality rate at 90 days. Seventy-two percent of patients completed the three scans.

Table 1 Baseline clinical characteristics at time of recruitment

	Mean age	Sex (% male)	LVEF (%)	Diastolic dysfunction (%)	CKD (%)	Hs-Tnt (ng/L)	Interstitial edema CXR (%)	Pulmonary edema CXR (%)	Creatinine (μmol/L)
Mean or %	77.2	52.3%	47	32.6	41	293	66	48	150
SD	12.7	–	19	–	–	824	–	–	115

The mean clinical congestion score on admission was 5.6 (SD 1.4) and decreased significantly over time to 1.3 (0.91) at T3 (Fig. 2). Other markers of clinical congestion, including orthopnea, dyspnea, JVD, hepatojugular reflux and pulmonary rales, also showed similar significant changes between T1 and T3. The median Killip score was 2.

The mean IVC size on expiration showed no significant change between T1 (1.9: SD 0.65) and T3 (2: SD 0.50), nor did the IVC collapsibility index [T1 0.3 (0.19) versus T3 0.25 (0.16)] (Fig. 3). The mean number of B lines did decrease [T1 11 (6.1) versus T3 8.3 (5.5)], but this decrease did not reach statistical significance (Fig. 2). Analysis using non-parametric test for trends or ANOVA did not alter these conclusions.

Pearson correlations between JVP and HJR showed significant correlations at T1 (0.58, $p < 0.0001$) and T2 (0.55, $p = 0.0003$). However, correlations between JVP or HJR and IVC size or collapsibility did not reach significance.

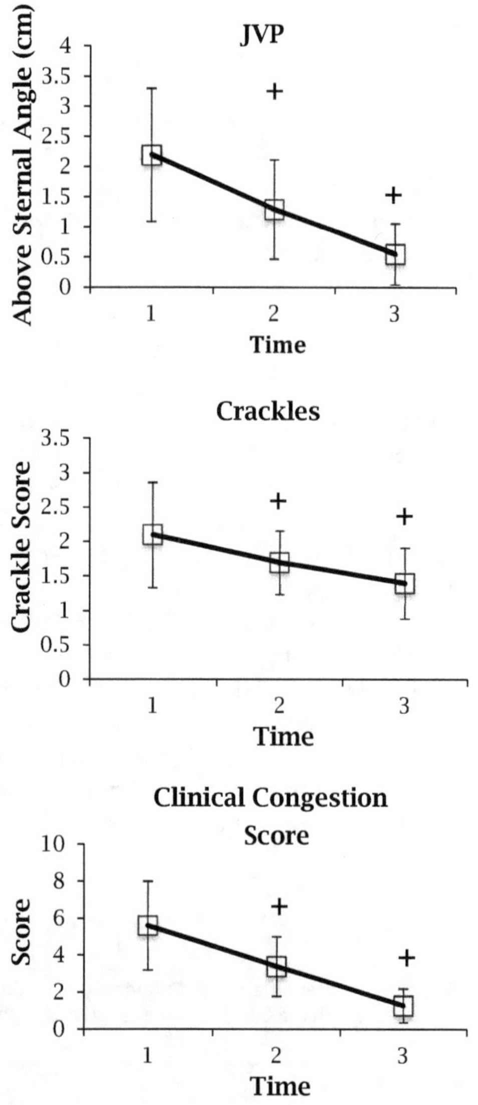

Fig. 2 Clinical exam findings at each time point

Similarly, pulmonary rales and number of B lines across all time points did not show significant correlations. Univariate and multivariate analysis did not show any clinical or ultrasound variables that correlate with hospital length of stay and 90-day mortality rate.

Ninety-eight percent of the IVC scans were interpretable and read; 1 out of 50 could not be read because of poor image quality. All LUS scans were interpretable and read offline. The quality of the scans was determined by expert opinion, an Intensive care specialist with advanced cardiac echo and formal training in lung ultrasound. There were no significant differences in the ultrasound variables between the two authors. Twenty-eight percent of patients did not complete all three time points.

Discussion

The present study showed no significant change in IVC size or collapsibility index despite significant improvement in clinical signs of congestion in patients treated for acute decompensated heart failure. The results did show a trend toward significance for number of B lines; there was a 38% decrease in the number of B lines with the treatment of heart failure.

There are several explanations for the current data. This study enrolled patients upon admission to the cardiac care unit, which occurred between hours and days after their presentation to the emergency department. Consequently, treatment for heart failure was already initiated in the emergency department prior to our first ultrasound assessment. Unfortunately, our hospital database does not track delay to admission for these patients in particular. With this delay, the degree of hemodynamic congestion was likely diminished, and any appreciable changes in IVC size and B lines subsequent to the initial findings were too small to detect. This may indicate that IVC size and B lines clear rapidly with treatment and the sensitivity of this technique to detect such changes is on the level of hours in the acute setting. Additionally, the patients in the current study had a median Killip score of 2, which indicates that this patient population had only mild heart failure.

In contrast to our results, Goonewardena et al. [26] demonstrated significant reduction in IVC size and increases in collapsibility index with heart failure treatment. This study found larger IVCs at admission (2.3 versus 1.9 cm in the current study). However, IVC size and collapsibility indices at discharge were identical between the two studies (2 cm in both studies). This may suggest that the greatest change in IVC size occurs early following initial therapy, and likely why the current study did not reach significance for this primary endpoint. However, IVC size as a surrogate for volume status has increasingly been questioned. Another explanation for

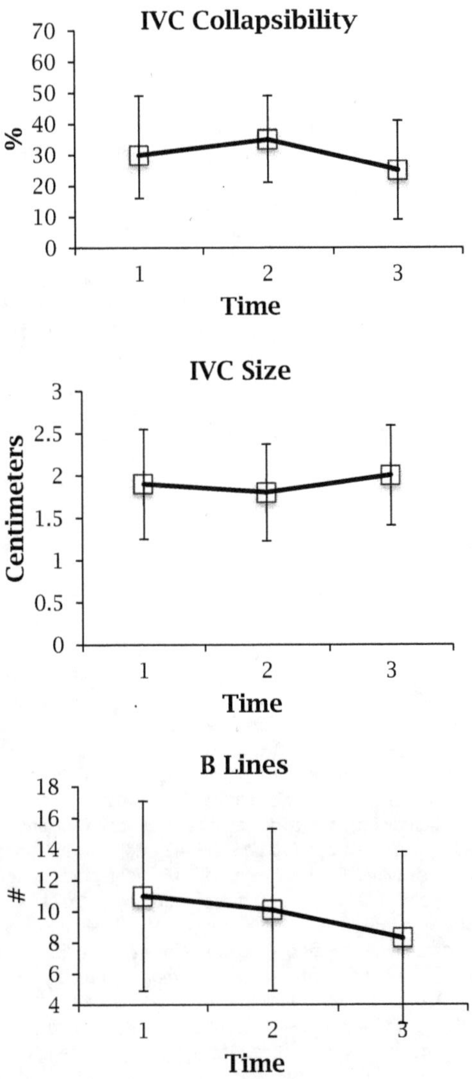

Fig. 3 Ultrasound findings at each time point

the current data is that IVC size may not accurately represent hypervolemic states, and thus may not be useful in the management of decompensated heart failure.

Volpicelli et al. [27] conducted a study where number of B lines was calculated at admission and discharge, and found significant clearing of B lines after treatment. However, this population had more severe heart failure than the current study. This study used an arbitrary clinical scale out of ten points to grade the clinical severity of heart failure which included the presence (1) or absence (0) of lower extremity edema, pulmonary rales and wheezing, jugular venous distension, orthopnea, high respiratory rates (>25 breaths/min) and low pulse oximeter saturation; median score was 8/10 on admission whereas in the current study, the mean CCS was 5.6 out of 13. In another study, Gargani et al. [27] showed a significant reduction in B lines with treatment from 48 on admission to 20 at discharge, compared to the current study which showed a non-significant reduction of B lines from 11 to 8.3. Both these studies found a larger number of B lines on admission and sampled patients with more severe heart failure. This may indicate that LUS is a useful indicator of improvement in pulmonary congestion in patients with severe heart failure, but may fail to identify significant changes in pulmonary congestion in patients with milder CHF.

Of note, Volpicelli [28] analyzed the B lines using a different method. Eleven regions were scanned, compared to eight regions in the current study. Additionally, a positive region was defined as number of B lines over 3, and they analyzed the data based on the number of positive regions as opposed to absolute number of B lines. However, we did not find a significant change even when our data were analyzed in a similar manner. There was no prospective strategy in the study protocol to quantify confluent B lines, and as a result, they were counted as a single B line. Although there is a suggested method to quantify confluent B lines by calculating the proportion of visualized pleural line/length of the confluent B lines [29], we felt that there is insufficient evidence to apply this technique at the current time. It is possible that we underestimated the overall quantity of B lines using this approach; however, this method was consistently used across all time points and should not affect the overall results.

There are several limitations in the current study. This was a small study with only 50 patients enrolled at a single center. We did not formally estimate sample size as there were no reliable data to estimate effect size in this population. However, based on our results, a sample size of approximately 150 would be required to detect a statistically significant difference (α 0.05 and β 0.20) for B lines and a sample size of approximately 1000 would be required for change in IVC diameter.

Additionally, there was a high dropout rate with 28% of patients not completing all three time points. The clinical assessments were not blinded; resident authors performing these assessments knew at which time point each patient was being assessed, which could have introduced bias.

As mentioned above, since treatment was initiated early upon presentation and prior to recruitment, the ability to detect a potential decrease in IVC size and number of B lines may have be reduced. The clinical score would be less influenced as resolution of peripheral edema and crackles would lag, and the clinical history of orthopnea and PND is retrospective.

Assessment of volume status is challenging and point of care ultrasound may provide greater sensitivity to detect subclinical congestion before overt clinical congestion occurs. While this may be true for patients with more severe heart failure, the current study suggests that lung and vascular ultrasound in patients with less severe heart failure may not be sensitive enough to detect such small changes in hemodynamic congestion. As a result, serial POCUS may perform less well in patients with mild versus more severe heart failure. Based on the current results, IVC size or collapsibility index is not an accurate marker of improvement in hemodynamic congestion. B lines may be a better marker of congestion as these did decrease with the treatment of heart failure as expected. The lack of statistical significance for the number of B lines may be a result of a small sample size, and a sampled population with less severe heart failure than previously published, and an initial small number of B lines. Another interpretation of our data is that given the significant correlation over time with clinical scores and not with ultrasound, it may suggest that clinical exam is more sensitive than ultrasound at detecting congestive symptoms, although this is hypothesis generating given the small sample size.

The current study is the only study to the authors' knowledge, which directly compared lung and IVC ultrasound in the dynamic clinical setting of heart failure management after hospital admission. Further studies are warranted to better understand the utility of bedside ultrasound in patients with mild heart failure, and which ultrasound modality provides the most accurate assessment of hemodynamic congestion for both diagnostic and prognostic purposes.

Conclusions

In conclusion, this study shows that vascular and lung ultrasound does not show significant changes with the management of heart failure in a hospitalized population with acute decompensated heart failure, although LUS shows a trend toward significance. This may indicate that vascular ultrasound parameters are less robust in patients with mild congestion and may show the greatest change during initial management.

Further larger scale studies are needed to explore how POCUS may be useful in the acute and sub-acute management of heart failure.

Abbreviations

CHF: congestive heart failure; POCUS: point-of-care ultrasound; LUS: lung ultrasound; IVC: inferior vena cava; JVP: jugular venous pressure; HJR: hepatojugular reflux; CCS: clinical congestion score.

Authors' contributions

Literature review, study design and implementation were performed by RS and JL. MAS and RS performed the clinical and ultrasound bedside assessments. MAS and JL performed the offline analysis of the ultrasound data. DJ performed all statistical analyses and assisted with the editing of the manuscript. JD and LR contributed to the study design and editing of the manuscript. All authors read and approved the final manuscript.

Author details

[1] Internal Medicine Training Program, Department of Medicine, Jewish General Hospital, McGill University, 3755 Chemin de la Cote St Catherine, Montreal H3T 1E2, Canada. [2] Critical Care Fellowship Training Program, McGill University, Montreal, Canada. [3] Division of General Internal Medicine, Department of Medicine, MUHC, McGill University & Adult Critical Care, Jewish General Hospital, McGill University, Montreal, Canada. [4] Department of Emergency Medicine, Jewish General Hospital, McGill University, Montreal, Canada. [5] Division of Cardiology, Department of Medicine, Jewish General Hospital, McGill University, Montreal, Canada. [6] Department of Adult Critical Care, Jewish General Hospital, McGill University, Montreal, Canada. [7] Division of General Internal Medicine, Department of Adult Critical Care, Jewish General Hospital, McGill University, Montreal, Canada.

Acknowledgements

None.

References

1. Writing Group Members, Lloyd-Jones D, Adams RJ et al (2010) Heart disease and stroke statistics—2010 update: a report from the American Heart Association. Circulation 121(7):e46–e215. doi:10.1161/CIRCULATIONAHA.109.192667
2. Jencks SF, Williams MV, Coleman EA (2009) Rehospitalizations among patients in the medicare fee-for-service program. N Engl J Med 360(14):1418–1428. doi:10.1056/NEJMsa0803563
3. Gheorghiade M, Follath F, Ponikowski P et al (2010) Assessing and grading congestion in acute heart failure: a scientific statement from the acute heart failure committee of the heart failure association of the European Society of Cardiology and endorsed by the European Society of Intensive Care Medicine. Eur J Heart Fail 12(5):423–433. doi:10.1093/eurjhf/hfq045
4. Mayhadoon H, Klein R, Eyler W et al (1989) Radiographic pulmonary congestion in end-stage congestive heart failure. Am J Cardiol 63:625–627
5. Mant J, Doust J, Roalfe A et al (2009) Systematic review and individual patient data meta-analysis of diagnosis of heart failure, with modelling of implications of different diagnostic strategies in primary care. Health Technol Assess 13(32):1–248. doi:10.3310/hta13320
6. Md SNG, Md JEAB, Md AM et al (2010) Use of hand carried ultrasound, B-type natriuretic peptide, and clinical assessment in identifying abnormal left ventricular filling pressures in patients referred for right heart catheterization. J Card Fail 16(1):69–75. doi:10.1016/j.cardfail.2009.08.004
7. Gackowski A, Isnard R, Golmard J et al (2004) Comparison of echocardiography and plasma B-type natriuretic peptide for monitoring the response to treatment in acute heart failure. Eur Heart J 25(20):1788–1796. doi:10.1016/j.ehj.2004.07.038
8. International Liaison Committee on Lung Ultrasound (ILC-LUS) for the International Consensus Conference on Lung Ultrasound (ICC-LUS), Volpicelli G, Elbarbary M et al (2012) International evidence-based recommendations for point-of-care lung ultrasound. Intensive Care Med 38(4):577–591. doi:10.1007/s00134-012-2513-4
9. Stevenson LW, Perloff JK (1989) The limited reliability of physical signs for estimating hemodynamics in chronic heart failure. JAMA 261:884–888
10. Cook DJ, Simel DL (1996) Does this patient have abnormal central venous pressure? JAMA 275(8):630–634. doi:10.1001/jama.1996.03530320054034
11. Brennan JM, Blair JE, Goonewardena S et al (2007) Reappraisal of the use of inferior vena cava for estimating right atrial pressure. J Am Soc Echocardiogr 20(7):857–861. doi:10.1016/j.echo.2007.01.005
12. Blair JE, Brennan JM, Goonewardena SN, Shah D, Vasaiwala S, Spencer KT (2009) Usefulness of hand-carried ultrasound to predict elevated left ventricular filling pressure. Am J Cardiol 103(2):246–247. doi:10.1016/j.amjcard.2008.08.061
13. Goonewardena SN, Spencer KT (2010) Handcarried echocardiography to assess hemodynamics in acute decompensated heart failure. Curr Heart Fail Rep 7(4):219–227. doi:10.1007/s11897-010-0030-8
14. Alavi-Moghaddam M, Kabir A, Shojaee M et al (2016) Ultrasonography of inferior vena cava to determine central venous pressure: a meta analysis and meta regression. Acta Radiol 18:1–5

15. Rudski LG, Wyman WL, Afilalo J et al (2010) Guidelines for the echocardiographic assessment of the right heart in adults: a report from the American Society of Echocardiography, a registered branch of the European Society of Cardiology, and the Canadian Society of Echocardiography. J Am Soc Echocardiogr 23:685–713
16. Platz E, Lattanzi A, Agbo C et al (2012) Utility of lung ultrasound in predicting pulmonary and cardiac pressures. Eur J Heart Fail 14(11):1276–1284. doi:10.1093/eurjhf/hfs144
17. Anderson KLI, Jenq KY, Panebianco NL, Dean AJ (2013) Diagnosing heart failure among acutely dyspneic patients with cardiac, inferior vena cava and lung ultrasonography. Am J Emerg Med 31(8):1208–1214
18. Vitturi N, Soattin M, Allemand E, Simoni F, Realdi G (2011) Thoracic ultrasonography: a new method for the work-up of patients with dyspnea. J Ultrasound 14(3):147–151. doi:10.1016/j.jus.2011.06.009
19. Miglioranza MH, Gargani L, Sant'Anna RT et al (2013) Lung ultrasound for the evaluation of pulmonary congestion in outpatients. JACC Cardiovasc Imaging 6(11):1141–1151. doi:10.1016/j.jcmg.2013.08.004
20. Miller JB, Sen A, Strote SR et al (2012) Inferior vena cava assessment in the bedside diagnosis of acute heart failure. Am J Emerg Med 30(5):778–783. doi:10.1016/j.ajem.2011.04.008
21. Pellicori P, Carubelli V, Zhang J et al (2013) IVC diameter in patients with chronic heart failure. JACC Cardiovasc Imaging 6(1):16–28. doi:10.1016/j.jcmg.2012.08.012
22. Md DJB, Md ED, Md RG (2009) Identification of congestive heart failure via respiratory variation of inferior vena cava diameter. Am J Emerg Med 27(1):71–75. doi:10.1016/j.ajem.2008.01.002
23. Killip T, Kimball JT (1967) Treatment of myocardial infarction in a coronary care unit: a 2 year experience with 250 patients. Am J Cardiol 20(4):457–464
24. Rhode LE, da-Silva Beck L, Goldraich L, Grazziotin TC, Palombini DV, Polanczyk CA, Claussell N (2004) Reliability and prognostic value of traditional signs and symptoms in outpatients with congestive heart failure. Can J Cardiol 20(7):697–702
25. Brennan JM, Blair JE, Goonewardena S, Ronan A, Shah D, Vasaiwala S et al (2007) A comparison by medicine residents of physical examination versus hand-carried ultrasound for estimation of right atrial pressure. Am J Cardiol 99(11):1614–1616. doi:10.1016/j.amjcard.2007.01.037
26. Goonewardena SN, Gemignani A, Ronan A et al (2008) Comparison of hand-carried ultrasound assessment of the inferior vena cava and N-terminal pro-brain natriuretic peptide for predicting readmission after hospitalization for acute decompensated heart failure. JACC Cardiovasc Imaging 1(5):595–601. doi:10.1016/j.jcmg.2008.06.005
27. Gargani L, Pang PS, Frassi F et al (2015) Persistent pulmonary congestion before discharge predicts rehospitalization in heart failure: a lung ultrasound study. Cardiovasc Ultrasound 13:1–9. doi:10.1186/s12947-015-0033-4
28. Volpicelli G, Caramello V, Cardinale L, Mussa A, Bar F, Frascisco MF (2008) Bedside ultrasound of the lung for the monitoring of acute decompensated heart failure. Am J Emerg Med 26(5):585–591. doi:10.1016/j.ajem.2007.09.014
29. Anderson KL, Fields JM, Panebianco NL, Jenq KY, Marin J, Dean AJJ (2013) Inter-rater reliability of quantifying pleural B-lines using multiple counting methods. Ultrasound Med 32(1):115–120

7

Ultrasonography in trauma: a nation-wide cross-sectional investigation

Jesper Weile[1,2*], Klaus Nielsen[3], Stine C. Primdahl[4], Christian A. Frederiksen[5], Christian B. Laursen[6], Erik Sloth[7] and Hans Kirkegaard[8]

Abstract

Background: The Focused Assessment with Sonography in Trauma (FAST) protocol is considered beneficial in emergent evaluation of trauma patients with blunt or penetrating injury and has become integrated into the Advanced Trauma Life Support (ATLS) protocol. No guidelines exist as to the use of ultrasonography in trauma in Denmark. We aimed to determine the current use of ultrasonography for assessing trauma patients in Denmark.

Methods: We conducted a nation-wide cross-sectional investigation of ultrasonography usage in trauma care. The first phase consisted of an Internet-based investigation of existing guidelines, and the second phase was a series of structured interviews of orthopedic surgeons, anesthesiologists, and radiologists on call in all hospitals receiving traumatized patients in Denmark.

Results: Guidelines were obtained from all 22 hospitals receiving traumatized patients in Denmark. Twenty-one (95.5%) of the guidelines included and recommended FAST as part of trauma assessment. The recommended person to perform the examination was the radiologist in $n = 11$ (50.0%), the surgeon in $n = 6$ (27.3%), the anesthesiologist in $n = 1$ (4.5%), and unspecified in $n = 3$ (13.6%) facilities. FAST indications varied between circulatory instability $n = 8$ (36.4%), team leader's discretion $n = 6$ (27.3%), abdominal trauma $n = 3$ (13.6%), and not specified $n = 6$ (27.3%). Telephone interviews revealed that exams were always $n = 8$ (36.4%) or often $n = 4$ (18.2%) registered in the patients' charts. The remaining $n = 10$ (45.5%) facilities either never registered $n = 2$ (9.1%), it was not possible to register $n = 1$ (4.5%), or unknown by the trauma leaders $n = 7$ (31.8%). Images were often stored in $n = 1$ (4.5%), never stored in $n = 10$ (45.5%), not possible to store in $n = 2$ (9.1%), and unknown in $n = 9$ (40.9%) facilities.

Conclusion: Ultrasonography was used in a non-uniform fashion by multiple specialties in Danish trauma facilities. Very few images from FAST examinations were stored and documentation was scanty. National guidelines on application and documentation of ultrasonography in trauma are called for.

Keywords: Trauma, Ultrasonography, Focused Assessment with Sonography in Trauma, FAST, Emergency Medicine

Background

The Focused Assessment with Sonography in Trauma (FAST) protocol is considered beneficial in emergent evaluation of trauma patients with blunt or penetrating injury [1]. FAST is a focused abdominal and cardiac ultrasound examination designed for assessment of free fluid in the peritoneum and the pericardium. The examination was initially introduced in the early 1990's and has spread throughout the world [2]. The protocol includes three views of the abdomen and one view of the heart, as shown in Fig. 1. The abdominal views are right upper quadrant, left upper quadrant, and pelvis for assessment of hemorrhage into the peritoneal cavity. The subcostal view of the heart is used for detecting blood in the pericardium. The parasternal long axis view can be used as an alternative if the subcostal view cannot be obtained [3]. Previous studies of sensitivity and specificity of FAST have found these to be 63–100% and 95–100%, respectively [4]. The likelihood ratio of positive test has been found to be >7.9 [5]. The FAST exam has been shown

*Correspondence: jesper.weile@clin.au.dk
[2] Research Center for Emergency Medicine, Aarhus University Hospital, Nørrebrogade 44, Building 1B, 8000 Aarhus C, Denmark
Full list of author information is available at the end of the article

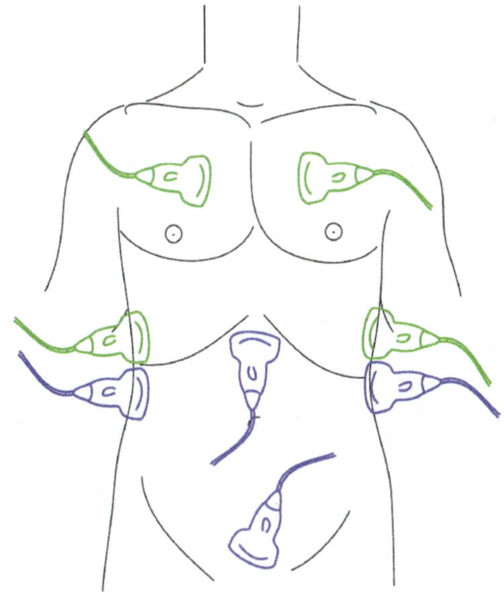

Fig. 1 The FAST and eFAST exam. The *blue* probes illustrate the scanning positions of the FAST exam. The green probes illustrate the scanning positions of the extended FAST exam assessing for pneumothorax and hemothorax

to decrease time to intervention, complication rate, and hospital length of stay [6]. The FAST protocol is reproducible and not correlated to adverse effects from radiation[6].

In 2004, Kirkpatrick et al. presented an extension adding anterior and dorsolateral thoracic images of the pleura to the FAST exam [7]. See Fig. 1. The intention of the Extended Focused Assessment with Sonography in Trauma (eFAST) was to add detection of pneumothorax or hemothorax to the basic FAST. Ultrasonography has a higher sensitivity detecting pneumothorax than does antero-posterior chest X-ray in the supine position (88–98.1% vs. 50–75.5%) and can detect very small amounts of intrathoracic fluid [6–16].

In Denmark, there are no strict recommendations for trauma facilities to implement FAST, eFAST, or other ultrasound examinations as standard of care for traumatized patients. According to the Advanced Trauma Life Support (ATLS) protocol, FAST scanning should be performed as an extension to the primary survey [17], and the American College of Emergency Physicians (ACEP) recommends ultrasonography as initial diagnostic modality for blunt and penetrating abdominal trauma in hemodynamic unstable patients[18]. A previous Danish national study found that anesthesiologists or surgeons, present as consultants in the emergency department, perform ultrasonography in 43 and 18% of the cases, respectively [19]. It is unknown whether these are FAST examinations performed on trauma patients or other point-of-care examinations. Application and development of ultrasonography in trauma care are difficult if little is known about the existing usage of ultrasonography in the trauma facilities.

This study aims to clarify the current use of ultrasonography in existing trauma facilities, including examination indication, ultrasound protocol choice, examiner characteristics, and examination documentation.

Methods

Inclusion criteria

All 22 hospitals in Denmark receiving acutely injured patients via ambulance services (air, ship, or ground) with a predefined multidisciplinary trauma team, were included in this study. We defined the trauma patient as a patient activating the trauma call where a multidisciplinary trauma team cares for the patient in the trauma room.

We conducted a cross-sectional observational study performed in two phases.

Phase 1

a. We gathered all local guidelines for trauma patient care from these 22 hospitals. This was done by searching publicly available resources on the Internet. If guidelines could not be accessed online, the Emergency Department was contacted by e-mail, and it sent the guideline.
b. The guidelines from trauma facilities were investigated for use of ultrasonography in trauma. All mentions of "ultrasonography," "ultrasound," or "FAST" were recorded.

Phase 2

a. The anesthesiologist, the orthopedic surgeon, and the radiologist on call in every trauma facility were interviewed via telephone by use of a structured questionnaire regarding the use of ultrasonography during treatment of traumatized patients. The questionnaire can be found in the Additional file 1: Appendix.
b. All phone calls were conducted during weekdays between 09:00 am to 08:00 pm. A phone call was repeated seven times if not answered. After the 7th missed call, an e-mail containing the same questionnaire as the structured telephone interview was sent to the department. The department was asked to forward the questionnaire to a doctor frequently involved in trauma care. A second reminder e-mail was sent, and if the department did not respond, it was designated as "not responding."

Endpoints

Our primary endpoint was to establish the proportion of trauma facilities recommending ultrasonography in local trauma care manuals. Secondary endpoints were to establish the specialty of the physician conducting the FAST examination, the indication(s) for performing FAST, and whether other ultrasonography examinations were recommended in trauma care. Lastly, we examined the proportion of facilities documenting examinations in the patient records and the frequency of trauma facilities storing images from sonography.

Statistics

Descriptive statistics was used to present actual numbers and percentages unless otherwise indicated in the text. We calculated Cohen's weighted kappa for multiple observers on interview answers as to who was performing the examinations. When interpreting Cohen's kappa, we used Landis and Koch's guidelines from 1977 [20]. The interobserver agreement was also expressed in percentage of agreement. Calculations were performed using Stata 13 (Statacorp, USA).

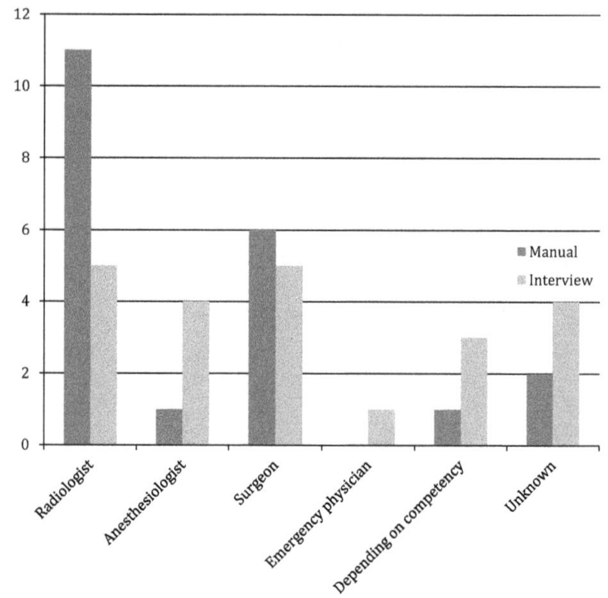

Fig. 2 Specialties performing FAST. Specialties performing FAST examinations in trauma according to trauma care manuals and interviews with trauma leaders

Results

Data were collected from August 2016 to December 2016. Trauma care manuals were obtained from all 22 facilities receiving traumatized patients in Denmark. A total of 64 (97.0%) out of 66 possible interviews were performed. Anesthesiologists, radiologists, and orthopedic surgeons on call on 22 hospitals were eligible for inclusion via telephone interviews. Anesthesiologists from all 22 hospitals participated in the study, while one eligible orthopedic department and one department of radiology failed to participate.

The FAST protocol was mentioned in 21 (95.5%) manuals for traumatized patients. One (4.5%) manual did not mention ultrasonography of any kind for trauma care.

The specialty of the performing physicians and the distribution of specialties are shown in Fig. 2. The results are from the 21 facilities mentioning ultrasonography in the trauma care manual, and from the interviews with trauma leaders from the 22 facilities. We interviewed orthopedic surgeons, anesthesiologists, and radiologists on call on the subject; Fig. 2 expresses the answer from the trauma leader. The numbers on the y axis are the number of hospitals. "Depending on competency" meant that the doctor present from either radiology, anesthesiology, or surgery with the highest level of competency performed the examination. In 8 (36.4%), all three interviewed physicians agreed on the person performing the FAST examination. In 6 (27.3%), two agreed, and in the remaining 8 (36.4%) there was total disagreement. Cohen's kappa on interrater agreement among radiologists, anesthesiologists, and orthopedic surgeons was $K = 0.35$, $p < 0.0001$ and interpreted as fair.

Indications for ultrasonography were either not mentioned, at the discretion of the trauma leader, abdominal trauma, or circulatory instability. The distribution is shown in Fig. 3. Because two trauma manuals stated indications as being abdominal trauma or circulatory instability, the total number of FAST indications ($n = 23$) was higher than the number of guidelines mentioning FAST ($n = 21$). The remaining facilities each stated a single indication as shown. One facility stated the indication as all circulatory unstable patients with suspected abdominal trauma; it was included as "circulatory instability" in the figure. In one manual, FAST exam was mentioned as a useful modality for "Trauma in Children." As this indication was unspecific, it was not included in the figure. It was the only manual mentioning ultrasonography specifically for children. In 16 (72.7%) manuals, the FAST exam was part of the primary survey, and in 2 (9.1%), it was part of the secondary survey. The remaining 3 (13.6%) trauma facilities did not specify when the examination was to be performed.

The use of the eFAST protocol for ruling out pneumothorax and hemothorax was mentioned in 6 (27.3%) facilities. Additional uses for ultrasound examinations were mentioned in 7 (31.8%) trauma manuals, categorized as follows. Ultrasonography of arterial flow in extremities was mentioned in 5 (22.7%) manuals, but none of the manuals specify which specialty should perform the examination. Ultrasonography of scrotal trauma performed by radiologist was mentioned in two (9.1%) manuals, and ultrasonography of internal organs by radiologist was mentioned in two (9.1%) manuals. One (4.5%)

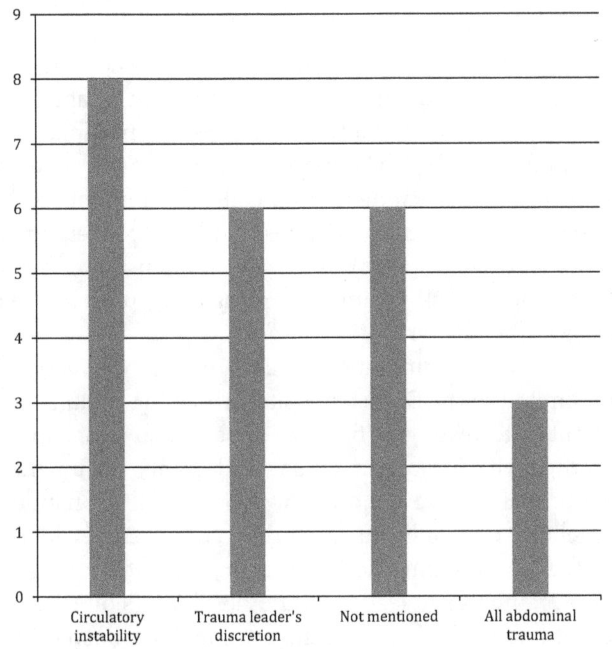

Fig. 3 Indications (total $n = 23$) for performing FAST. Indications for performing FAST examination mentioned in the trauma manuals and number of hospitals

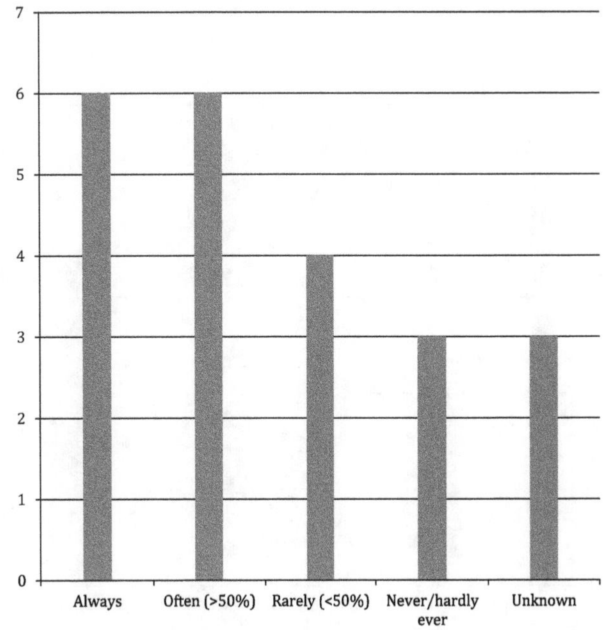

Fig. 4 Ultrasonography usage according to trauma leaders. Usage according to trauma leaders when asked how frequently ultrasonography is used in trauma care in their facility and number of hospitals

manual mentioned focused cardiac ultrasonography in the primary survey, but it did not mention indication or who was to perform the examination. Lastly, one (4.5%) manual mentioned unspecified thoracic ultrasonography for penetrating trauma.

Trauma leaders were questioned in regards to the frequency of use of ultrasonography in trauma care. Answers are shown in Fig. 4.

Lastly, trauma leaders were questioned about the frequency of storing images and entering descriptions of the ultrasound examinations into medical charts. Results are shown in Fig. 5.

Discussion

The FAST exam was recommended in 21 out of 22 local guidelines. In addition, our study revealed three main findings. First, different specialties seem to perform ultrasound examinations in different trauma facilities. Second, we found various indications for performing FAST, ranging from all "abdominal trauma" to "trauma leader's discretion." Third, we found that documentation of ultrasonography examinations and storing of images was sparse.

An e-mail survey from 2008 in the U.S. showed that 85% of hospitals reported using the FAST examination for trauma care [2]. Our investigation showed a recommendation of FAST in 95.5% of all facilities receiving traumatized patients in Denmark. The higher percentage in our study probably reflects the growing interest in ultrasonography over time. Repetition of the American study might reveal a higher percentage today, which is why we consider the difference as a reflection of general development in the area.

Our study revealed differing local recommendations regarding which specialties should perform the ultrasound examinations. We have not come across evidence in the literature that one specialty should outperform others. We found that fewer surgeons and radiologists, and more anesthesiologists, perform FAST examination according to interviews than according to the local trauma care guidelines. Earlier work has shown that the vast majority of physicians performing ultrasonography in the Emergency Department are anesthesiologists [19]. Our study suggests that in trauma it will more often be the person with the greatest skill who performs the FAST examination rather than the person recommended in the guidelines. These findings might reflect that anesthesiology often is the specialty present with the most experience, while radiologists may be on call but not present in the trauma room.

The FAST exam is user dependent, and the specificity and sensitivity are related to the experience of the provider. The examination has low sensitivity for organ injury without hemoperitoneum and low sensitivity for retroperitoneal bleeding [6]. To reach an overall sensitivity of 67% and specificity of 100%, extensive experience

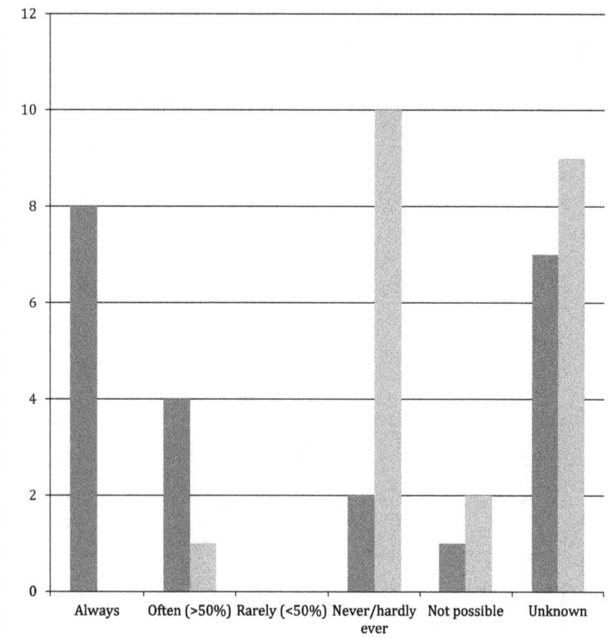

Fig. 5 Documentation. Documentation in patient charts and storage of ultrasonography images when ultrasonography is performed. Results from interviews with trauma leaders in all facilities. The *graph* shows the distribution of answers to two questions. *Dark gray*: "Are the results of the ultrasonography examination documented in the patient chart?" *Light gray*: "Are the images stored?"

of more than 100 FAST examinations is necessary [21]. A reliable and validated assessment tool for assessment of competency in point-of-care ultrasonography exists [22]. This evidence calls for a specification in the existing guidelines recommending the most experienced person to perform the examination. Preferably, the experience should be quantified, and an expected minimum of experience or a minimum required competency level should be outlined.

The indications for performing FAST differ between facilities, and, including extended FAST, views of the thorax are also heterogenic. Some facilities recommend other use of sonography beyond FAST, such as sonography of the scrotum. The addition of extended FAST views appears helpful in the literature as life-threatening injuries such as tension pneumothorax or massive hemothorax can be diagnosed at the bedside [11, 23]. Cardiac evaluation alone in penetrating trauma to the chest has been shown to decrease mortality [24]. Although the eFAST exam for trauma has not been shown to reduce mortality, it still has several advantages. Knowledge of thoracic injury with pneumothorax, hemothorax, or pericardial effusion at the time of arrival can be used to guide initial treatment even before a CT scan is performed. Future trials should seek to illuminate the clinical strength of the full eFAST over the FAST alone.

To our knowledge, the frequency of ultrasonography images being stored and documented has not previously been investigated in the trauma setting. Recommendations have been published on how to store images and document examinations [25], but these are not followed. Our findings, which show a surprisingly low frequency of storage and documentation, call for attention to the problem in the local guidelines. Without proper documentation, developing the field is immensely difficult. Furthermore, lack of image storing may present legal issues in the future.

Our study has limitations. First, the study is national and limited to the Danish hospitals receiving traumatized patients. However, our findings of particular problems in heterogeneity between facilities and scanty documentation undoubtfully exist abroad, and our call for national guidelines can only inspire other countries to do the same. A second limitation is ascribing value to interviews of the trauma team leaders and other doctors on call. We do not know whether the results would have been different if the phone call had been made on a different day or whether the answers were influenced by recollection bias.

Conclusion

Ultrasonography is applied in a heterogeneous manner by multiple specialties on multiple indications in trauma care in Denmark. Storage and documentation of examinations is sparse and desultory. Multispecialty national evidence-based guidelines, as well as unified implementation of existing guidelines, are called for.

Additional file

Additional file 1. Appendix 1

Abbreviations

ATLS: Advanced Trauma Life Support; eFAST: extended Focused Assessment with Sonography in Trauma; FAST: Focused Assessment with Sonography in Trauma.

Authors' contributions

JW, KN, ES, HK, CAF, and CBL contributed to conception and design the study. JW, SCP, and KN performed the telephone interviews. JW collected all trauma care manuals and drafted the manuscript. All authors critically revised drafts for important intellectual content and approved the final manuscript submitted. All authors read and approved the final manuscript.

Author details

[1] Emergency Department, Regional Hospital Herning, Herning, Denmark. [2] Research Center for Emergency Medicine, Aarhus University Hospital, Nørrebrogade 44, Building 1B, 8000 Aarhus C, Denmark. [3] Department of Medicine, Section of Respiratory Medicine, University Hospital Hvidovre, Hvidovre, Denmark. [4] Aarhus University, Aarhus, Denmark. [5] Department of Cardiology, Aarhus University Hospital, Aarhus, Denmark. [6] Department of Respiratory Medicine, Odense University Hospital, Odense, Denmark. [7] Department of Anesthesiology and Intensive Care, Aarhus University Hospital, Aarhus, Denmark. [8] Research Center for Emergency Medicine, Aarhus University Hospital, Aarhus, Denmark.

Acknowledgements
The authors would like to thank all departments and physicians participating in the interviews. Without this great help, this study could not have been performed. The authors especially wish to thank medical student Stig Holm Jensen for contributing to the data collection.

References

1. Melniker LA, Leibner E, McKenney MG, Lopez P, Briggs WM, Mancuso CA (2006) Randomized controlled clinical trial of point-of-care, limited ultrasonography for trauma in the emergency department: the first sonography outcomes assessment program trial. Ann Emerg Med 48:227–235
2. Scaife ER, Fenton SJ, Hansen KW, Metzger RR (2009) Use of focused abdominal sonography for trauma at pediatric and adult trauma centers: a survey. J Pediatr Surg 44:1746–1749
3. American Institute of Ultrasound in (2014) M, American College of Emergency P. AIUM practice guideline for the performance of the focused assessment with sonography for trauma (FAST) examination. J Ultrasound Med 33:2047–2056
4. Smith ZA, Wood D (2014) Emergency focussed assessment with sonography in trauma (FAST) and haemodynamic stability. Emerg Med J. 31:273–277
5. Quinn AC, Sinert R (2011) What is the utility of the Focused Assessment with Sonography in Trauma (FAST) exam in penetrating torso trauma? Injury 42:482–487
6. Ollerton JE, Sugrue M, Balogh Z, D'Amours SK, Giles A, Wyllie P (2006) Prospective study to evaluate the influence of FAST on trauma patient management. J Trauma 60:785–791
7. Kirkpatrick AW, Sirois M, Laupland KB, Liu D, Rowan K, Ball CG et al (2004) Hand-held thoracic sonography for detecting post-traumatic pneumothoraces: the Extended Focused Assessment with Sonography for Trauma (EFAST). J Trauma 57:288–295
8. Knudtson JL, Dort JM, Helmer SD, Smith RS (2004) Surgeon-performed ultrasound for pneumothorax in the trauma suite. J Trauma 56:527–530
9. Lichtenstein D, Meziere G, Biderman P, Gepner A (2000) The, "lung point": an ultrasound sign specific to pneumothorax. Intensive Care Med 26:1434–1440
10. Rowan KR, Kirkpatrick AW, Liu D, Forkheim KE, Mayo JR, Nicolaou S (2002) Traumatic pneumothorax detection with thoracic US: correlation with chest radiography and CT—initial experience. Radiology 225:210–214
11. Blaivas M, Lyon M, Duggal S (2005) A prospective comparison of supine chest radiography and bedside ultrasound for the diagnosis of traumatic pneumothorax. Acad Emerg Med 12:844–849
12. Whitson MR, Mayo PH (2016) Ultrasonography in the emergency department. Crit Care 20:227
13. Abu-Zidan F (1997) The role of ultrasonography and ultrasound-guided aspiration in blunt abdominal trauma. Ann Saudi Med 17:569–570
14. Rozycki GS, Feliciano DV, Davis TP (1998) Ultrasound as used in thoracoabdominal trauma. Surg Clin North Am 78:295–310
15. Ding W, Shen Y, Yang J, He X, Zhang M (2011) Diagnosis of pneumothorax by radiography and ultrasonography: a meta-analysis. Chest 140:859–866
16. Alrajhi K, Woo MY, Vaillancourt C (2012) Test characteristics of ultrasonography for the detection of pneumothorax: a systematic review and meta-analysis. Chest 141:703–708
17. Subcommittee A, American College of Surgeons' Committee on T, International Awg (2013) Advanced trauma life support (ATLS(R)): the ninth edition. J Trauma Acute Care Surg 74:1363–1366.
18. American College of Emergency P (2009) Emergency ultrasound guidelines. Ann Emerg Med 53:550–570
19. Nielsen K, Lauridsen JR, Laursen CB, Brabrand M (2015) Physicians using ultrasound in Danish emergency departments are mostly summoned specialists. Scand J Trauma Resusc Emerg Med 23:51
20. Landis JR, Koch GG (1977) An application of hierarchical kappa-type statistics in the assessment of majority agreement among multiple observers. Biometrics 33:363–374
21. Gracias VH, Frankel HL, Gupta R, Malcynski J, Gandhi R, Collazzo L et al (2001) Defining the learning curve for the Focused Abdominal Sonogram for Trauma (FAST) examination: implications for credentialing. Am Surg 67:364–368
22. Todsen T, Tolsgaard MG, Olsen BH, Henriksen BM, Hillingso JG, Konge L et al (2015) Reliable and valid assessment of point-of-care ultrasonography. Ann Surg 261:309–315
23. Lee C, Revell M, Porter K, Steyn R (2007) Faculty of Pre-hospital Care RCoSoE. The prehospital management of chest injuries: a consensus statement. Faculty of Pre-hospital Care, Royal College of Surgeons of Edinburgh. Emerg Med J 24:220–224
24. Arntfield RT, Millington SJ (2012) Point of care cardiac ultrasound applications in the emergency department and intensive care unit—a review. Curr Cardiol Rev 8:98–108
25. Laursen CB, Nielsen K, Riishede M, Tiwald G, Mollekaer A, Aagaard R et al (2014) A framework for implementation, education, research and clinical use of ultrasound in emergency departments by the Danish Society for Emergency Medicine. Scand J Trauma Resusc Emerg Med 22:25

8

Acute fissuration of a giant splenic artery aneurysm detected by point-of-care ultrasound

Philippe Le Conte[1*], David Trewick[1], Philippe Pes[1], Eric Frampas[2], Eric Batard[1] and Winfocus-France Group

Abstract

Background: Epigastric pain is frequent in Emergency Medicine and remains a challenging situation. Besides benign etiologies such as gastritis or uncomplicated cholelithiasis, it could reveal myocardial infarction or vascular disease. Point-of-care ultrasound (POCUS) could be performed in such situation.

Case presentation: A healthy 66-year-old man with no previous medical history was admitted to the Emergency Department for a rapid onset epigastric pain. He reported taking non-steroidal anti-inflammatories for 1 week prior to admission. His pain had rapidly subsided and the physical examination was inconclusive. ECG and blood samples were normal. POCUS revealed a vascular mass located between the spleen and the left kidney measuring 80 * 74 mm associated with small amounts of free peritoneal fluid. Computed tomography diagnosed a fissurated giant aneurysm of the splenic artery. The aneurysm was managed emergently by endovascular exclusion by selective splenic artery embolization. The post-intervention course was uneventful and the patient was discharged home 3 days later. The patient has remained free from any complications of the embolization 6 months after the procedure.

Conclusion: Spontaneously regressive epigastric pain with a normal physical and biology/ECG should not necessarily reassure the physician, in particular if patients have cardiovascular risk factors. A POCUS should be considered for these patients.

Background

Epigastric pain is a frequent and often challenging situation in the Emergency Department (ED) [1]. Besides benign etiologies such as gastritis or uncomplicated cholelithiasis, it could reveal myocardial infarction, aortic, or vascular diseases. The risk is neglecting vascular dissection or rupture leading to a possible fatal hemorrhagic shock [2]. Splenic artery aneurysms (SAA) are rare, often asymptomatic, and usually discovered incidentally [3] but remain potentially life threatening lesions [4]. SAA were reported in 0.78% of 3600 non-selective angiograms [4]; the incidence increases with female gender, in older patients and portal hypertension [5]. The ED incidence was reported as 0.011% in a retrospective study [6].

*Correspondence: philippe.leconte@chu-nantes.fr
[1] Service des Urgences, CHU de Nantes, 44093 Nantes, France
Full list of author information is available at the end of the article

We report a case of a patient consulting in the ED for epigastric pain in whom point-of-care ultrasound (POCUS) revealed an acute fissuration of a giant splenic aneurysm.

Case report

A healthy 66-year-old man with no previous medical history was admitted to the ED for a first episode of rapid onset severe epigastric pain. It appeared at rest without associated symptoms such as dyspnea or vomiting. He reported taking non-steroidal anti-inflammatories for 1 week prior to admission for an epicondylitis. On admission, his pain had rapidly subsided and the physical examination was inconclusive: blood pressure, temperature, heart rate, and capillary filling were normal. Thoracic auscultation and abdominal palpation revealed only slight epigastric pain. ECG and troponin assay were normal as was hemoglobin, bilirubin, liver enzymes, and lipase levels. As a part of our department's policy, a POCUS was performed essentially to rule out cholelithiasis. It was performed using a Philips CX50 with a 3.5–5 MHz abdominal probe. There were no gallstones; however, POCUS revealed a mass located between the spleen and the left kidney (Fig. 1 and Additional file 1: Video 1) measuring 80 * 74 mm. The mass was vascular with a strong color Doppler signal (Fig. 2 and Additional file 2: Video 2) and an intraluminal thrombus which explains why the Doppler signal does not fill all the lumen. The maximum velocity in the aneurysm was only 18 cm/s because of the large diameter. The aorta was explored from diaphragm to bifurcation. No other aneurysm was found. Small amounts of free peritoneal fluid were detected around the spleen.

Urgent computed tomography diagnosed a fissurated giant aneurysm of the splenic artery (Figs. 3, 4, 5). A selective angiography (Fig. 6) was then performed under general anesthesia; a complete exclusion of the aneurysm was obtained with glue/lipiodol embolization. The post-intervention course was uneventful and the patient was discharged home 3 days later. The patient has remained free from any complications of the embolization 6 months after the procedure.

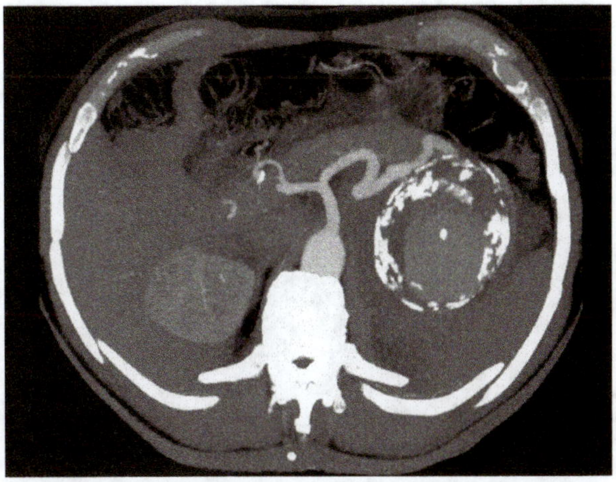

Fig. 3 Axial arterial phase contrast-enhanced MDCT. Maximal Intensity Projection view: Giant calcified aneurysm of the splenic artery

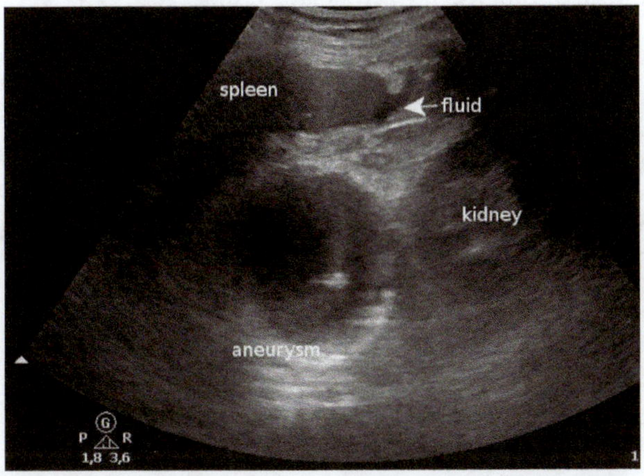

Fig. 1 POCUS scan of the left upper quadrant of a patient presenting with epigastric pain. See the vascular mass located between spleen and kidney

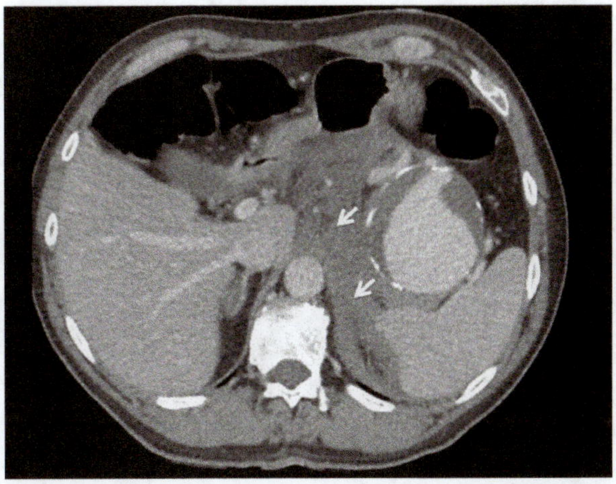

Fig. 4 Axial portal venous phase contrast-enhanced MDCT. Hemoretroperitoneum (white arrows)

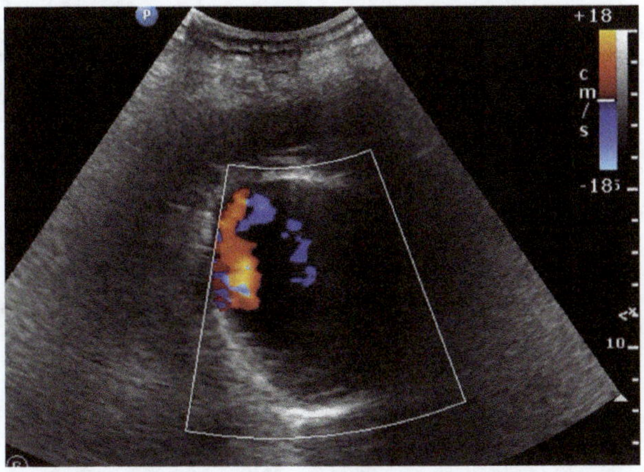

Fig. 2 POCUS color Doppler scan of left upper quadrant in a patient presenting an epigastric pain. See the strong Doppler signal

Discussion

We report the case of a patient presenting an acute fissuration of a previously asymptomatic giant splenic artery aneurysm detected by POCUS. Thanks to early detection, the aneurysm was embolized before full rupture and the patient was discharged home without complication. The occurrence of fissuration allowed an effective

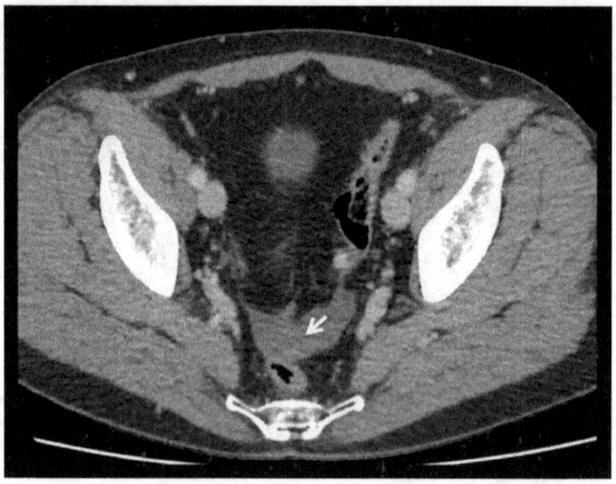

Fig. 5 Axial portal venous phase contrast-enhanced MDCT. Pelvic hemoperitoneum (white arrow)

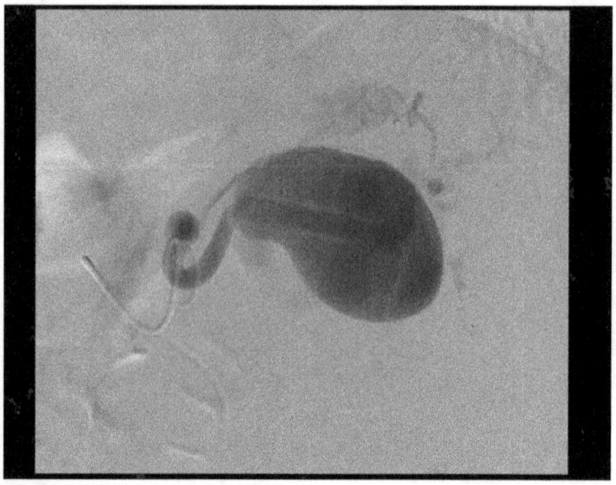

Fig. 6 Splenic angiography. Morphological aspect of the aneurysm

treatment before a catastrophic hemorrhagic shock. Although POCUS was used in other similar cases with SAA, the ultrasound was not conclusive and the diagnosis was made by CT-scan [2, 7]. To our knowledge, detection by POCUS of a fissuration episode has not been published. The "detection" of the SAA was done by POCUS in the case of Lo and Mok published in this journal [2], but the suspicion was of abdominal aortic aneurysm, so even if they detected it by POCUS, the correct and final diagnosis was made by CT-scan. There are many other similar cases [8] described in the literature, where POCUS showed an anechoic mass that sometimes was confused with a pancreatic cyst and others with an aortic aneurysm, and CT-scan was needed to reach the correct diagnosis [7, 9]. Rupture occurs in approximately 10% of SAA, especially when diameter exceeds 2 cm [10], with a mortality rate of 10–25% [2]. Even if incidence and rupture rates are particularly increased in the third trimester of pregnancy [10], the risk is higher from the first trimester [11]. In all patients, endovascular embolization should be considered as the first-line treatment [3, 12] rather than surgery, but strong evidence is still lacking.

Abdominal pain accounted for 8 million ED visits in USA in 2006 [1]. Epigastric pain remains a challenging situation in particular in older patients. A pragmatic pathway could include a thorough physical exam, an ECG, appropriate biological workup, and POCUS.

Conclusion

Point-of-care ultrasound performances allow the trained Emergency Physician to rule in/out pericardial effusion [13], aortic aneurysms [14], and gallstones [15]. It is thus an invaluable tool and is recommended by the American College of Emergency Physicians [16].

Additional files

Additional file 1: Video 1. POCUS scan of the left upper quadrant of a patient presenting with epigastric pain. See the vascular mass located between spleen and kidney.

Additional file 2: Video 2. POCUS color Doppler scan of left upper quadrant in a patient presenting an epigastric pain. See the strong Doppler signal.

Authors' contributions

PLC realized POCUS, EF CT, and embolization; DT, PP and EB helped in case-report redaction. All authors read and approved the final manuscript.

Author details

[1] Service des Urgences, CHU de Nantes, 44093 Nantes, France. [2] Radiologie centrale, CHU de Nantes, Nantes, France.

Acknowledgements

None.

References

1. Pitts SR, Niska RW, Xu J, Burt CW (2008) National hospital ambulatory medical care survey: 2006 emergency department summary. Natl Health Stat Rep 7:1–38
2. Lo WL, Mok KL (2015) Ruptured splenic artery aneurysm detected by emergency ultrasound—a case report. Crit Ultrasound J 7:9. https://doi.org/10.1186/s13089-015-0026-4
3. Akbulut S, Otan E (2015) Management of giant splenic artery aneurysm. Medicine (Baltimore) 94:e1016. https://doi.org/10.1097/MD.0000000000001016
4. Stanley JC, Fry WJ (1974) Pathogenesis and clinical significance of splenic artery aneurysms. Surgery 76:898–909
5. Al-Habbal Y, Christophi C, Muralidharan V (2010) Aneurysms of the splenic artery—a review. Surgeon 8:223–231
6. Liu C-F, Kung C-T, Liu B-M et al (2007) Splenic artery aneurysms encountered in the ED: 10 years' experience. Am J Emerg Med 25:430–436. https://doi.org/10.1016/j.ajem.2006.08.017
7. Iyanaga M, Watts S, Kasai T (2010) A patient with splenic artery aneurysm rupture and the importance of rapid sonography in the ED. Emerg Med Int. https://doi.org/10.1155/2010/893606

8. Davis T, Minardi J, Knight J et al (2015) Ruptured splenic artery aneurysm: rare cause of shock diagnosed with bedside ultrasound. West J Emerg Med 16:762–765. https://doi.org/10.5811/westjem.2015.7.25934
9. Abdulrahman A, Shabkah A, Hassanain M, Aljiffry M (2014) Ruptured spontaneous splenic artery aneurysm: a case report and review of the literature. Int J Surg Case Rep 5:754–757. https://doi.org/10.1016/j.ijscr.2014.08.021
10. Sadat U, Dar O, Walsh S, Varty K (2008) Splenic artery aneurysms in pregnancy—a systematic review. Int J Surg 6:261–265. https://doi.org/10.1016/j.ijsu.2007.08.002
11. Groussolles M, Merveille M, Alacoque X et al (2011) Rupture of a splenic artery aneurysm in the first trimester of pregnancy. J Emerg Med 41:e13–e16. https://doi.org/10.1016/j.jemermed.2010.04.023
12. Yamamoto S, Hirota S, Maeda H et al (2008) Transcatheter coil embolization of splenic artery aneurysm. Cardiovasc Interv Radiol 31:527–534. https://doi.org/10.1007/s00270-007-9237-9
13. Labovitz AJ, Noble VE, Bierig M et al (2010) Focused cardiac ultrasound in the emergent setting: a consensus statement of the American Society of Echocardiography and American College of Emergency Physicians. J Am Soc Echocardiogr 23:1225–1230. https://doi.org/10.1016/j.echo.2010.10.005
14. Kuhn M, Bonnin RLL, Davey MJ et al (2000) Emergency department ultrasound scanning for abdominal aortic aneurysm: accessible, accurate, and advantageous. Ann Emerg Med 36:219–223. https://doi.org/10.1067/mem.2000.108616
15. Kendall JL, Shimp RJ (2001) Performance and interpretation of focused right upper quadrant ultrasound by emergency physicians. J Emerg Med 21:7–13. https://doi.org/10.1016/S0736-4679(01)00329-8
16. ACEP (2016) Ultrasound guidelines: emergency, point-of-care, and clinical ultrasound guidelines in medicine. https://www.acep.org/Clinical---Practice-Management/Ultrasound/. Accessed 23 Jan 2018

9

Minimal training sufficient to diagnose pediatric wrist fractures with ultrasound

Henrik Hedelin[1,3*], Christian Tingström[1], Hanna Hebelka[2] and Jon Karlsson[1]

Abstract

Background: In children, non-fractured wrists generally need no treatment and those that are fractured may only require a 3-week cast without any clinical follow-up. The ability to perform a point-of-care triage decision if radiographs are needed could improve patient flow and decrease unnecessary radiographs. The aim of this study was to evaluate the role of ultrasound (US) as a point-of-care triage tool for pediatric wrist injuries with limited training.

Methods: Physicians with no previous US experience attended a 1.5 h course in the use of US to diagnose distal radius fractures at the Emergency Department (ED). The physicians firstly used US to diagnose a potential fracture and, if the patient had a fracture, grouped the patient according to how they wanted him/her to be treated based on US. The physician then interpreted the subsequent radiographs and decided on a treatment based on this information. Consultant traumatologists and a senior radiologist established a gold standard for correct treatment and radiological diagnosis, respectively.

Results: One hundred and sixteen injuries in 115 patients were included. The ED physician identified 75 fractures on radiographs. With the exception of a minimal buckle fracture, all were identified on US. US had a tendency to interpret complete fractures on radiographs as incomplete ($n = 7$) leading to incorrect treatment decisions.

Conclusions: In the hands of an US novice, US examination is comparable with radiographs as a point-of-care tool to distinguish a fractured wrist from a non-fractured one. US is not, however, as good as radiographs for placing fractured wrists into the correct treatment group.

Level of Evidence: Level III. Diagnostic study of non-consecutive patients.

Keywords: Ultrasound, Pediatric, Fracture, Emergency, Wrist

Background

At Emergency Departments (ED) children with wrist trauma constitute a large proportion of the admitted patients in all age groups. Approximately 30% of all fractures in children are located in the forearm [1, 2] and the majority of those fractures are in the distal radius. Radiographs are the standard diagnostic tool for pediatric patients with trauma to the wrist. Treatment and acceptable angulations vary greatly depending on the age of the child and the fracture type. Exact guidelines for treatment also vary between individual physicians, hospitals, and countries.

*Correspondence: henrik.hedelin@vgregion.se
[3] Barnortopeden Östra sjukhuset, Sahlgrenska Universitetssjukhuset, Smörslottsgatan 1, 416 78 Gothenburg, Sweden
Full list of author information is available at the end of the article

The general use of ultrasound (US) by non-radiologists has increased over the last decade and in many cases focus has shifted toward using US in the ED and in the pre-hospital setting to exclude a specific injury rather than to visualize an entire organ system [3, 4]. In the orthopedic field, the diagnosis of many fracture types have been evaluated [5–10] in this setting and results have been shown to be promising. US as a triage tool for ankle fractures in adults has been shown to greatly decrease the need for radiographs with only minimal training of the involved physicians [11]. A recent systematic review and meta-analysis of the use of US in the diagnosis of distal forearm fractures in children including 1204 patients showed a high accuracy of US as a diagnostic tool with a sensitivity and specificity of 97 and 95%, respectively [12]. The authors conclude that US can safely be used to establish the diagnosis of distal forearm fractures in children. In a sub-group of the meta-analysis, there was no difference in sensitivity based on the experience of the examining physician. However, there is no standardized method to quantify experience. The use of US as a primary screening tool is still under debate.

Ultrasound as a point-of-care triage tool to select the children with wrist trauma who need radiographs could decrease the need for unnecessary radiographs. This would reduce radiation and possibly save resources for the hospital and the average time a patient needs to spend at the ED.

The primary aim of the study was to add information to the current debate by investigating if US can be used as a point-of-care triage tool in the hands of non-radiologists with standardized minimal training to differentiate between a fracture and no fracture. The secondary aim was to evaluate if US can differentiate between complete fractures (usually needing follow-up) and buckle fractures (that can often be treated without a follow-up at the hospital).

Methods

The Queen Silvia Children's Hospital (DSBUS) is the only regional hospital for pediatric trauma in the western region of Sweden. On a normal day the orthopedist on call takes care of between 10 and 40 patients. All follow-ups were made at the same hospital's orthopedic outpatient department.

Six physicians ranging from junior doctors to consultants participated in the inclusion of patients, all without previous experience of US diagnostics.

They attended a 1.5 h intensive course designed by a pediatric radiologist and an orthopedic surgeon (both authors). The course focused only on the diagnosis of suspected wrist fractures in children. The study physicians performed one examination each on a patient with a fracture to verify that they were acquainted with the method. A fracture was diagnosed only if a cortical gap, torus formation, or displacement was seen (Figs. 1, 2). Indirect signs like subperiosteal hematoma was not used since these signs are deemed more subtle and difficult to learn and interpret for an US novice.

When present at the ED during the study period between February and September 2015, study physicians included all patients eligible. The US equipment used was only available for this time period and was only used for the purpose of this study. Inclusion criteria were all patients between 3 and 16 years with wrist pain after recent (last 3 days) trauma. Patients were excluded if there was an uncertain clinical finding (i.e., pain from proximal forearm or hand), an open fracture, or if the parents did not have the language skills to understand the information material.

Distal radial fractures in children can be categorized in a variety of ways such as buckle (or torus) fractures, greenstick fractures, complete fractures, and fractures involving the physis (classified according to the Salter–Harris classification [13]). For the purpose of this study the exact radiological classification was of less importance since the focus was on the effects of the treatment.

At our department the vast majorities of cases are treated with only a splint or closed reduction followed by a splint [2]. The treatment guidelines for the ED doctors

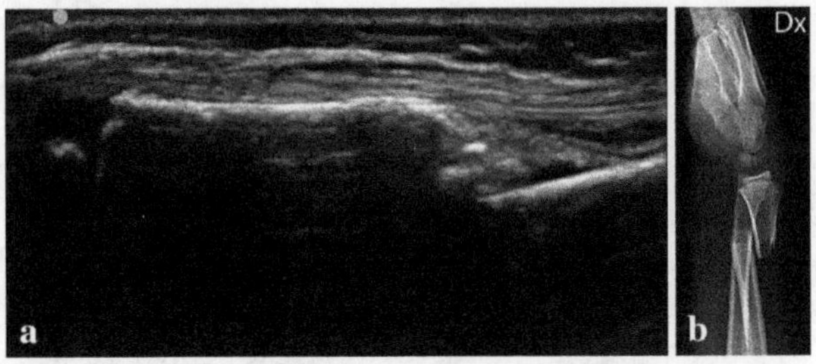

Fig. 1 **a** Displaced complete fracture of the distal radius. US dorsal longitudinal view. **b** (Same case as image **a**) Radiograph lateral view. Displaced complete fracture of the distal radius

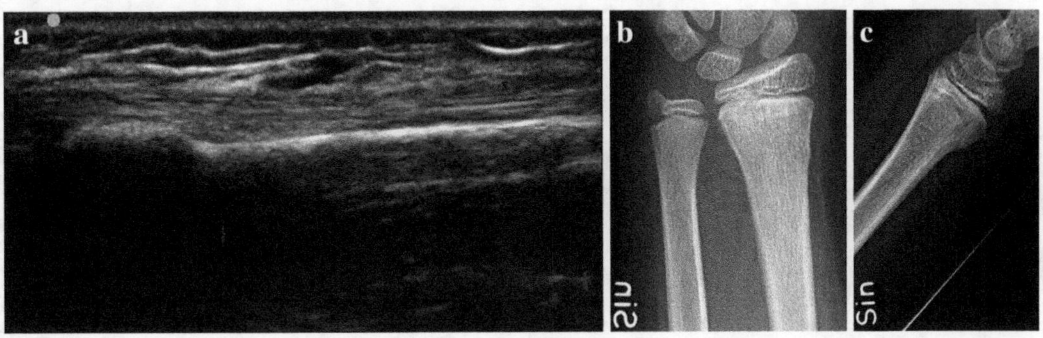

Fig. 2 **a** Infraction/torus fracture of the distal radius, US dorsal longitudinal view. **b, c** (Same case as **a**) Infraction/torus fracture of the distal radius on lateral and AP radiographs

at the hospital can, in a simplified manner, be divided into four groups:

1. No fracture.
   Advised treatment: No splint or immobilization.
2. A buckle or greenstick fracture with acceptable angulation.
   Advised treatment: A dorsal forearm plaster of Paris splint for 3 weeks that is removed by the parents. No follow-up is needed.
3. A buckle or greenstick fracture with borderline angulation or complete fracture with minor angulation or displacement.
   Advised treatment: A dorsal forearm splint for 3–4 weeks with a radiographic control of the fracture position after 5–7 days.
4. A buckle or greenstick fracture with unacceptable angulation or complete fractures with little angulation or displacement.

   Advised treatment: Closed reduction with or without surgical intervention.

The term "acceptable angulation" is relative since, as noted above, indications for intervention or follow-up depends on the age of the child and other factors. It is therefore up to the ED physician to make a qualified decision with all factors taken into account.

A radiographic follow-up is thus, according to the guidelines for ED doctors, needed if (a) the angulation or displacement is such that any further angulation is unacceptable or (b) the fracture is potentially unstable. The latter is the case for many complete fractures with even minor displacement (Fig. 3). Rare fractures involving the actual joint (Salter–Harris type 3 or 4) generally require a follow-up radiograph or surgery. No such fractures were found in the present study.

Each patient had a physical examination of the wrist and US of the wrist was performed with a Fujifilm SonoSite, Inc. Edge® using a linear 15–6 MHz probe. The US examination took 5–10 min to perform and consisted of longitudinal images in the sagittal plane of the distal 10 cm of the radius with special focus on painful areas. Dorsal, radial, and volar aspects of the distal radius were visualized. Imaging of the radial portion of the wrist in the sagittal plane on US visualized the same plane as a lateral view on radiographs. The decision of the study physician was stored in a coded closed envelope in order to blind the result from the results of the radiograph. The patient was asked if he or she found the examination painful.

The possible outcomes of the US examination correspond to the treatment groups 1–4 described above. The study physician first grouped each patient based only on the US interpretation. The alternative "uncertain finding" was used when the study physician was not able make a decision based on the US findings alone or could not achieve adequate images.

After the US examination standard radiographs of the wrist, using AP and lateral views, were performed in all patients. The same four outcomes were used. The study physician interpreted the images and stored the results in a second envelope.

To validate the accuracy of the radiographic readings by the study physicians the radiographs were also, at a later time, inspected by an independent senior radiologists blinded to the US and radiograph interpretation of the study physician. The radiologist did not sort the fractures according to the four groups used by the study physicians, since the radiologist were not involved in the decision making of the treatment, and the interpretation was used only to analyze the specific fractures where the two diagnostic modalities did not agree. The senior radiologist did no interpret the US images.

To obtain a gold standard for treatment, two senior consultants in pediatric orthopedic surgery, specialized in fractures, analyzed all the radiographs and decided on the most appropriate treatment. This second look was

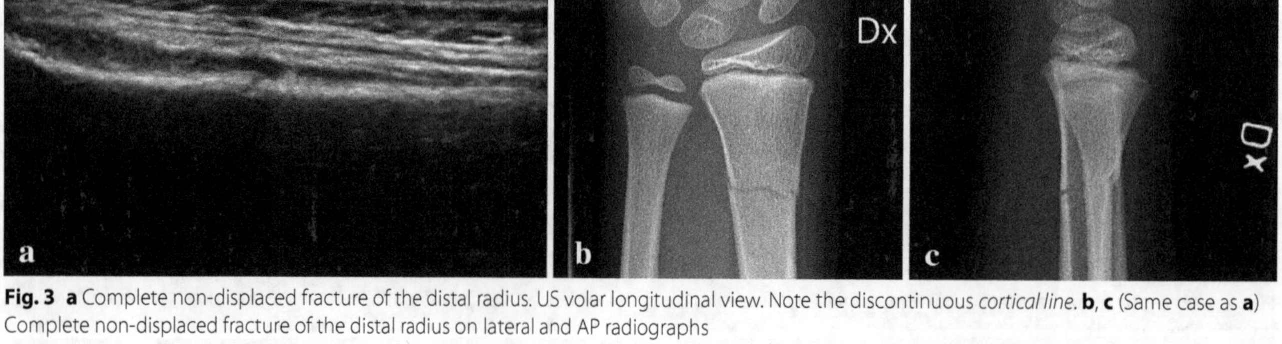

Fig. 3 **a** Complete non-displaced fracture of the distal radius. US volar longitudinal view. Note the discontinuous *cortical line*. **b, c** (Same case as **a**) Complete non-displaced fracture of the distal radius on lateral and AP radiographs

blinded to all other results and interpretations. The consultants were asked "what is the optimal treatment for a patient of this age with this injury based on the radiograph" with the treatment groups corresponding to numbers 1–4 presented above. The consultants established a joint consensus and there were no cases of dispute. This method was used in order to evaluate the clinical relevance of the results and not limit the study to if the US and radiological findings correlated perfectly.

Ethics, consent, and permissions

Participation was voluntary but all patients who met the inclusion criteria approved of participation and subsequent publishing of obtained material. Ethical approval was obtained from the Human Ethics Committee at the Medical Faculty, Gothenburg University (DNR 956-14).

Statistics

To reach the desired level of evidence based on pre-study power analysis, a study group of 130 patients was desirable. The sample size was depending on 80% power and $p < 0.05$ together with normal distribution, estimating that using US 75% of the fractures would be detected. The very conservative 75% sensitivity estimate was chosen based on the lowest sensitivity that was found in relevant studies [14]. However, only 117 cases were included due to the limited time the ultrasound equipment was available. As mentioned in the result section the sensitivity was shown to be clearly higher than the conservative estimate used to estimate power.

Results

Examinations of 117 injuries in 116 patients were included between February and August 2015. One patient was excluded due to loss of data and therefore 116 injuries in 115 patients (62 female/53 male) were analyzed. The median age was 11 years (range 3–16). The patients were fairly evenly distributed among the study physicians (range 10–43, median 16). None of the patients described the procedure as more than mildly painful.

Ultrasound by study physician vs radiograph interpretation by study physician (shown in Table 1)

The results of US and radiographic examination are reported in Table 1. Out of 75 fractures seen on radiographs by the study physician, one was interpreted as a non-fractured wrist on US. This misdiagnosed case was interpreted as a minimal dorsal buckle fracture by the radiologists on the radiographs.

Seven out of 21 complete fractures were interpreted as a "greenstick or a buckle fracture" on the US examination. All of the fractures in question were, incorrectly, assumed to be greenstick fractures by the study physician. Misinterpreted fractures were evenly distributed among the study physicians.

Radiographic interpretation by study physician vs radiograph interpretation by radiologist

The senior radiologist identified a total of 79 fractures which illustrates that the radiographic interpretation by the study physician was not completely accurate. Three cases that the ED physicians considered "uncertain findings" on radiographs proved to be fractures. The one fracture that was overlooked on the radiograph by the ED physician was an undisplaced distal tip ulna fracture that was stable but was treated with splint for pain relief. This fracture was also missed on US. The study physician identified all complete or displaced fractures on radiographs but three did not need the follow-up suggested by the study physician. Out of 54 fractures judged by the study physician to be buckle fractures or greenstick fractures, not needing follow-up, five were considered complete fractures by the radiologist. Only three of these needed a follow-up according to the senior traumatologists.

Table 1 The examination outcomes of the US and radiographs as interpreted by the study physician

		Radiographic assessment by study physician				Total
		No fracture	Buckle fracture/ greenstick fracture	Complete fracture or unacceptable angulation	Uncertain finding	
US assessment by study physician	No fracture	27	1	0	2	30
	Buckle fracture/ greenstick fracture	4	51	7	2	64
	Complete fracture or unacceptable angulation	0	1	14	0	15
	Uncertain finding	4	1	0	2	7
Total		35	54	21	6	116

The radiologist's interpretation is not shown here

Radiographic interpretation by study physician vs correct treatment based on radiographs according to senior traumatologists (shown in Table 2)

Two patients that needed a follow-up were missed using radiographs as the tool to inform treatment decision by the study physician. One patient who was judged not to need any treatment needed a cast for 3 weeks according to senior traumatologists.

Ultrasound by study physician vs correct treatment based on radiographs according to senior traumatologists (shown in Table 3)

Two patients judged to have no fracture needed a cast for 3 weeks. Five patients believed to have a buckle or greenstick fracture (with acceptable angulation) turned out to need a follow-up (they were complete). One patient with a greenstick fracture needed repositioning according to senior traumatologists despite being grouped as an acceptable angulation by the study physician. Thus a total of eight fractures would not have received necessary treatment using only US as a triage tool to decide treatment. There was also, a tendency to over-treat benign fractures or non-fractured wrists.

Sensitivity and specificity

Compared with the radiologist's gold standard the study physicians ability to distinguish a fracture from a non-fracture using US has a sensitivity of 97.4% (95% CI 90.9–99.7%) and a specificity of 84% (95% CI 67.2–94.7%), assuming normal distribution and omitting uncertain findings (Table 4). Since US was evaluated as a triage tool to see if the patient needed a radiograph "uncertain findings" could be included as true positive for the calculation since these cases would have been triaged to need a radiograph. Omitting these cases for the above calculations produces a more conservative estimate of the sensitivity. The isolated stable ulna fissure was not included as a fracture since the distal ulna was not examined using US. Apart from the calculations of sensitivity and specificity above regarding the ability of US to identify the non-fractured wrist, the results regarding the correct treatment of identified fractures are presented only as descriptive statistics.

Table 2 The study physician's interpretation of the radiographs at the ED cross-tabulated with the gold standard treatment decided by senior traumatologists based on radiographs

		Appropriate treatment based on radiographs				Total
		No treatment	Cast for 3 weeks without follow-up	Cast with radiographic follow-up	Reposition or operation needed	
Radiograph assessment by study physician	No fracture	34	1	0	0	35
	Buckle fracture/ greenstick fracture	0	52	2	0	54
	Complete fracture or unacceptable angulation	0	3	14	4	21
	Uncertain finding	4	2	0	0	6
Total		38	58	16	4	116

The radiologist's interpretation is not shown here

Table 3 The study physician's interpretation of the US examination at the ED cross-tabulated with the gold standard treatment decided by senior traumatologists based on radiographs

		Appropriate treatment based on radiographs				Total
		No treatment	Cast for 3 weeks without follow-up	Cast with radiographic follow-up	Reposition or operation needed	
US assessment by study physician	No fracture	28	2	0	0	30
	Buckle fracture/ greenstick fracture	5	53	5	1	64
	Complete fracture or unacceptable angulation	0	2	10	3	15
	Uncertain finding	5	2	0	0	7
Total		38	59	15	4	116

Table 4 Sensitivity and specificity for US to detect any fracture type

	US examination positive	US examination negative	Total
Fracture present	75	2	77 (2 uncertain)
Fracture absent	5	27	32 (5 uncertain)
Total	80	29	116 (77 + 32 + 2 + 5)
	Sensitivity: 97.4% (95% CI 90.9–99.7%)	Specificity: 84% (95% CI 67.2–94.7%)	

Discussion

The main finding of the current study is that physicians with limited but standardized training can use point-of-care US examination to distinguish distal radius fracture from non-fracture trauma in an age mixed pediatric patient group.

A number of studies on the use of US for forearm fractures in children report approximately 95% sensitivity and specificity for fracture detection, which are in accordance with the results of the present study [10, 12, 14–18]. Some previous studies have included all forearm fractures, leading to lower sensitivity and specificity [14, 19, 20].

With few exceptions previous studies have included experienced ultrasonographers (or do not present the experience of the examiner). US is considered user-dependent and therefore this constitutes a weakness in most studies. What an expert can find is very different from what can be expected to be found by a novice and the ED is generally staffed by physicians with limited US experience. We regard limited training as training that can take place in a few hours requiring only a few sample cases. The studies limited to physicians without any prior experience in US and examining only wrist fractures showed results comparable to the present study. [16, 21]. A recent meta-analysis did, however, not see any significant differences between trained and untrained personnel, supporting the idea that limited training can prove sufficient for this task [12]. All the above-mentioned studies have also used radiographs as a gold standard despite the fact that ED doctors may need to interpret radiographs without the support of a radiologist.

In the present study the aim was to address the above-mentioned limitations. The results also showed that US can be used to distinguish between different types of fractures and subsequently treat them accordingly. The purpose would be to limit the use of radiographs to the cases that may need repositioning or surgery. US was in this study not as good as radiographs for this purpose as seen in the results above. No specific statistical analysis was made for this group as it was obvious from the results presented in the tables.

A more detailed analyses of the misdiagnosed cases shows that the 4/21 complete fractures that should have received a radiographic follow-up (three were considered stable) were all stable without any dislocation at the 1-week radiographic follow-up.

In the present study the sensitivity of the US examination to distinguish fractures needing follow-up from fractures that do not need it is not completely satisfactory if one adheres to the follow-up indications used at the hospital of the study. It is also, however, evident that radiographs are not perfect for this purpose if ED doctors need to interpret the radiographs without the support of a radiologist. Most errors in both groups did, however, result in over-treatment with an unnecessary follow-up rather than under-treatment. The results also serve as a reminder to always properly visualize the distal parts of ulna when examining the wrist.

Since this study evaluates the reliability of US as a triage method to decide which patients needed radiographs, false positives ($n = 4/116$) are of less concern since this group would only need an "unnecessary" radiograph. The same reasoning is valid for the group of uncertain US results ($n = 7/116$).

Point-of-care US in the hands of non-radiologists is a method that has gained scientific support over the last decade and it appears like its use will continue to expand in the ED environment [4, 22–26]. From a global perspective, the World Health Organization has recommended the use of US imaging in developing countries and established minimum specifications for a "general purpose scanner" [27]. In situations like these, the ability to exclude a fracture can be even more valuable and US could also be used to predict the correct treatment, accepting the slightly lower sensitivity compared to radiographs.

Limitations

The relatively low number of patients included in our study is a limitation as we did not reach the original numbers needed in the pre-study power analysis. Due to the higher than expected accuracy of the US the study group must, however, be considered to be of adequate size to make a valid interpretation. Future studies should further elucidate the field and show the possibilities and limitations of point-of-care ultrasound triage for fractures at the ED.

Conclusion

Emergency physicians with relevant but limited training can use US to safely rule out a suspected wrist fracture in children and it can significantly decrease the need for radiographs if used as a point-of-care triage tool. US can also be used as a more advanced tool to decide if a suspected fracture warrants a radiograph to decide on further treatment. In the latter case, US examination appears to be less accurate than radiographs as a diagnostic aid for the ED physician.

Additional file

Additional file 1. Ultrasound wrist study.

Authors' contributions

All authors have contributed to both the collection of data and the writing of the article. All authors read and approved the final manuscript.

Author details

[1] Department of Orthopedics, Sahlgrenska University Hospital, Instititute of Clinical Sciences, Sahlgrenska Academy, University of Gothenburg, Gothenburg, Sweden. [2] Department of Radiology, Institute of Clinical Sciences, Sahlgrenska Academy, University of Gothenburg, Gothenburg, Sweden. [3] Barnortopeden Östra sjukhuset, Sahlgrenska Universitetssjukhuset, Smörslottsgatan 1, 416 78 Gothenburg, Sweden.

Acknowledgements

None.

References

1. Hart ES, Albright MB, Rebello GN, Grottkau BE (2006) Broken bones: common pediatric fractures–part I. Orthop Nurs 25(4):251–256
2. Pretell Mazzini J, Rodriguez Martin J (2010) Paediatric forearm and distal radius fractures: risk factors and re-displacement—role of casting indices. Int Orthop 34(3):407–412. doi:10.1007/s00264-009-0904-0
3. Heegaard W, Hildebrandt D, Spear D, Chason K, Nelson B, Ho J (2010) Prehospital ultrasound by paramedics: results of field trial. Acad Emerg Med 17(6):624–630. doi:10.1111/j.1553-2712.2010.00755.x
4. Tirado A, Wu T, Noble VE, Huang C, Lewiss RE, Martin JA, Murphy MC, Sivitz A (2013) Ultrasound-guided procedures in the emergency department-diagnostic and therapeutic asset. Emerg Med Clin North Am 31(1):117–149. doi:10.1016/j.emc.2012.09.009
5. Hunter JD, Mann CJ, Hughes PM (1998) Fibular fracture: detection with high resolution diagnostic ultrasound. J Accid Emerg Med 15(2):118
6. Wang CL, Shieh JY, Wang TG, Hsieh FJ (1999) Sonographic detection of occult fractures in the foot and ankle. J Clin Ultrasound 27(8):421–425
7. Marshburn TH, Legome E, Sargsyan A, Li SM, Noble VA, Dulchavsky SA, Sims C, Robinson D (2004) Goal-directed ultrasound in the detection of long-bone fractures. J Trauma 57(2):329–332
8. Rutten MJ, Jager GJ, de Waal Malefijt MC, Blickman JG (2007) Double line sign: a helpful sonographic sign to detect occult fractures of the proximal humerus. Eur Radiol 17(3):762–767. doi:10.1007/s00330-006-0331-1
9. Taggart I, Voskoboynik N, Shah S, Liebmann O (2012) ED point-of-care ultrasound in the diagnosis of ankle fractures in children. Am J Emerg Med 30(7):1321–1323. doi:10.1016/j.ajem.2011.06.037
10. Joshi N, Lira A, Mehta N, Paladino L, Sinert R (2013) Diagnostic accuracy of history, physical examination, and bedside ultrasound for diagnosis of extremity fractures in the emergency department: a systematic review. Acad Emerg Med 20(1):1–15
11. Hedelin H, Goksor LA, Karlsson J, Stjernstrom S (2013) Ultrasound-assisted triage of ankle trauma can decrease the need for radiographic imaging. Am J Emerg Med 31(12):1686–1689. doi:10.1016/j.ajem.2013.09.005
12. Douma-den Hamer D, Blanker MH, Edens MA, Buijteweg LN, Boomsma MF, van Helden SH, Mauritz G-J (2016) Ultrasound for distal forearm fracture: a systematic review and diagnostic meta-analysis. PLoS ONE 11(5):e0155659. doi:10.1371/journal.pone.0155659
13. Cepela DJ, Tartaglione JP, Dooley TP, Patel PN (2016) Classifications In brief: salter-harris classification of pediatric physeal fractures. Clin Orthop Relat Res 474(11):2531–2537. doi:10.1007/s11999-016-4891-3
14. Weinberg ER, Tunik MG, Tsung JW (2010) Accuracy of clinician-performed point-of-care ultrasound for the diagnosis of fractures in children and young adults. Injury 41(8):862–868. doi:10.1016/j.injury.2010.04.020
15. Chen L, Kim Y, Moore CL (2007) Diagnosis and guided reduction of forearm fractures in children using bedside ultrasound. Pediatr Emerg Care 23(8):528–531. doi:10.1097/PEC.0b013e318128f85d
16. Patel DD, Blumberg SM, Crain EF (2009) The utility of bedside ultrasonography in identifying fractures and guiding fracture reduction in children. Pediatr Emerg Care 25(4):221–225
17. Chaar-Alvarez FM, Warkentine F, Cross K, Herr S, Paul RI (2011) Bedside ultrasound diagnosis of nonangulated distal forearm fractures in the pediatric emergency department. Pediatr Emerg Care 27(11):1027–1032. doi:10.1097/PEC.0b013e318235e228
18. Eckert K, Ackermann O, Schweiger B, Radeloff E, Liedgens P (2012) Sonographic diagnosis of metaphyseal forearm fractures in children: a safe and applicable alternative to standard x-rays. Pediatr Emerg Care 28(9):851–854. doi:10.1097/PEC.0b013e318267a73d
19. Waterbrook AL, Adhikari S, Stolz U, Adrion C (2013) The accuracy of point-of-care ultrasound to diagnose long bone fractures in the ED. Am J Emerg Med 31(9):1352–1356. doi:10.1016/j.ajem.2013.06.006
20. Hubner U, Schlicht W, Outzen S, Barthel M, Halsband H (2000) Ultrasound in the diagnosis of fractures in children. J Bone Joint Surg Ser B 82(8):1170–1173
21. Rowlands R, Rippey J, Tie S, Flynn J (2017) Bedside ultrasound vs X-ray for the diagnosis of forearm fractures in children. J Emerg Med 52(2):208–215. doi:10.1016/j.jemermed.2016.10.013
22. Chan SS (2009) Emergency bedside ultrasound for the diagnosis of rib fractures. Am J Emerg Med 27(5):617–620. doi:10.1016/j.ajem.2008.04.013
23. Budhram GR, Schmunk JC (2014) Bedside ultrasound AIDS identification and removal of cutaneous foreign bodies: a case series. J Emerg Med 47(2):e43–e48. doi:10.1016/j.jemermed.2014.01.033
24. Rippey JC, Royse AG (2009) Ultrasound in trauma. Best Pract Res Clin Anaesthesiol 23(3):343–362
25. Pare JR, Liu R, Moore CL, Sherban T, Kelleher MS Jr, Thomas S, Taylor RA (2015) Emergency physician focused cardiac ultrasound improves diagnosis of ascending aortic dissection. Am J Emerg Med. doi:10.1016/j.ajem.2015.12.005
26. Mantuani D, Frazee BW, Fahimi J, Nagdev A (2016) Point-of-care multi-organ ultrasound improves diagnostic accuracy in adults presenting to the emergency department with acute dyspnea. West J Emerg Med 17(1):46–53. doi:10.5811/westjem.2015.11.28525
27. Lutz HBE (2011) Manual of diagnostic ultrasound, 2nd edn. World Health Organization, Geneva

10

Teaching the internist to see: effectiveness of a 1-day workshop in bedside ultrasound for internal medicine residents

Ryan D. Clay[1,3], Elizabeth C. Lee[1], Marc F. Kurtzman[1] and Renee K. Dversdal[2*]

Abstract

Background: A growing body of evidence supports the use of bedside ultrasound for core Internal Medicine procedures and increasingly as augmentation of the physical exam. The literature also supports that trainees, both medical students and residents, can acquire these skills. However, there is no consensus on training approach.

Aim: To implement and study the effectiveness of a high-yield and expedited curriculum to train internal medicine interns to use bedside ultrasound for physical examination and procedures.

Setting: The study was conducted at a metropolitan, academic medical center and included 33 Internal Medicine interns.

Program description: This was a prospective cohort study of a new educational intervention consisting of a single-day intensive bedside ultrasound workshop followed by two optional hour-long workshops later in the year. The investigation was conducted at Oregon Health & Science University in Portland, Oregon. The intensive day consisted of alternating didactic sessions with small group hands-on ultrasound practice sessions and ultrasound simulations. A 30-question assessment was used to assess ultrasound interpretation knowledge prior to, immediately post, and 6 months post intervention.

Results: Thirty-three interns served as their own historical controls. Assessment performance significantly increased after the intervention from a mean pre-test score of 18.3 (60.9 % correct) to a mean post-test score 25.5 (85.0 % correct), *P* value of <0.0001. This performance remained significantly better at 6 months with a mean score of 23.8 (79.3 % correct), *P* value <0.0001. There was significant knowledge attrition compared to the immediate post-assessment, *P* value 0.0099.

Conclusions: A single-day ultrasound training session followed by two optional noon conference sessions yielded significantly improved ultrasound interpretation skills in internal medicine interns.

Keywords: Bedside ultrasound, Physical examination, Point-of-care ultrasound, Graduate medical education, Ultrasound education, Internal Medicine education

Background

The twenty-first century has witnessed a dramatic and rapid expansion of the availability and use of technology in patient care. Improvement of pre-existing technologies, such as the miniaturization of ultrasound devices, has significantly expanded the range of use for these devices. Trauma Surgery pioneered the use of point-of-care ultrasound. Emergency Medicine followed by Critical Care then embraced and popularized bedside, provider-performed ultrasound, beginning in the 1970s. Many bedside ultrasound applications have been validated, and several specialties have ACGME training requirements for training in ultrasound. The Internal Medicine community has been slower to incorporate

*Correspondence: dversdar@ohsu.edu
[2] Division of Hospital Medicine, Department of Medicine, Oregon Health & Science University, 3181 SW Sam Jackson Park Road, OP-30, Portland, OR 97239, USA
Full list of author information is available at the end of the article

bedside ultrasound into daily practice. However, the literature examining the use of bedside ultrasound by generalists and hospitalists for diagnostic and procedural purposes is now growing.

Now that the value of ultrasound use is increasingly recognized by Internal Medicine providers, focus has also expanded to ultrasound education in residency training. In 2012, approximately 25 % of Internal Medicine residency programs had some form of ultrasound training with another 25 % planning on incorporating ultrasound training in the next year [1]. Additionally, there is an increasing body of literature describing the efficacy of curricular modules to teach ultrasound skills to Internal Medicine residents [2]. Programs using both cadaver models and standardized patients have demonstrated improvement in resident ultrasound examination skills after a hands-on training module [3, 4]. Other approaches include a 30-h ultrasound course covering many applications held during intern orientation, and an integrated three-year curriculum focused on the cardiovascular limited ultrasound examination (CLUE) [2, 5]. When these ultrasonography skills are applied to clinical care, patients may receive a more accurate or nuanced diagnosis, expediting their appropriate workup and treatment [6].

In addition, residents also gain confidence from formal training in using ultrasound for invasive procedures [7]. Studies demonstrate that ultrasound-guidance improves the safety of central line placement and thoracentesis [8, 9]. There is evidence that the patients of residents trained in bedside ultrasound-guided paracentesis not only received less post-procedural blood product transfusions compared to patients that underwent paracentesis by Interventional Radiology, but also benefitted from an average total cost reduction of over $500 per procedure for bedside ultrasound-guided paracentesis [10]. This is potentially related to Interventional Radiology versus American Association for the Study of Liver Diseases consensus guidelines regarding ideal INR and platelet count before paracentesis, and is an important consideration in the ever-important concept of High Value Care.

In order to foster career-long proficiency with ultrasound technology, it was deemed important to introduce skills training early in Internal Medicine residency. However, the optimal timing and intervention to fit high-yield ultrasound training into a crowded curriculum with limited resources is not clear. The Oregon Health and Sciences University Internal Medicine residency program is located at a metropolitan academic medical center in Portland, Oregon, and includes 33 interns. This intervention focused on a single-day bedside ultrasound training followed by two optional 1-h-long workshops later in the year. It was hypothesized that after 1 day of intensive ultrasound training interns would demonstrate significantly improved ultrasound interpretation skills, along with significant retention at 6 months.

Methods

This was a prospective cohort study with 33 interns serving as their own historical controls. A 1-day bedside ultrasound workshop was developed as one component of a comprehensive 5-day intern "boot-camp" designed to improve interns' cognitive, affective and psychomotor skills using active learning techniques including simulation, standardized patients and communication workshops. The "boot-camp" was purposefully placed 3 months into the academic year so that these key concepts did not get lost during the intern's busy orientation time.

The bedside ultrasound training day consisted of alternating didactics with small group hands-on sessions. Six topics pertinent to Internal Medicine patient management were covered including ultrasound basics (physics, knobology, artifacts), cardiac limited ultrasound exam (CLUE) [5], basic pulmonary exam, abdominal exam, basic vascular anatomy of the aorta, and neck anatomy. The abdominal exam was a modified FAST exam adapted for internal medicine, assessing for free intraperitoneal fluid, inferior vena cava collapse as an assessment of intravascular volume status [11], and ruling out hydronephrosis. Each topic was introduced with a 15- to 20-min didactic. Following the brief didactic session, interns worked within 12 pre-assigned groups of 2–3 learners for 40-min hands-on sessions. Each session was divided into 20 min for completing modules demonstrating pathology on SonoSim® machines and 20 min for facilitator-led hands-on practice with a SonoSite Edge® machine and volunteer models. Volunteers were solicited from the pre-health student list serve of a local university. Facilitators included two clinical trainers from SonoSite® in addition to emergency medicine residents, fellows and faculty, cardiology fellows, and Internal Medicine faculty. All facilitators had experience and training in bedside ultrasound. The teaching during the intensive intervention was re-enforced by two additional 1-h ultrasound training sessions within the first 6 months. However, these were held during noon conference sessions with untracked attendance.

To assess image acquisition, optimization, interpretation and application within the clinical context, study investigators designed a 30-question assessment covering ultrasound basics, neck anatomy, abdomen, limited cardiac, volume assessment, and basic vascular ultrasound. Subject areas were determined by group consensus and based on existing literature supporting the use of bedside ultrasound in the practice of internal medicine.

Questions were vetted by the four co-investigators with final edits by the PI. Seventeen questions tested image interpretation, 7 tested concepts of image acquisition/optimization and 6 tested clinical application. A copy of the assessment can be obtained by emailing the corresponding author. See Fig. 1 for an example, test question.

Interns completed the ultrasound knowledge assessment in a proctored room directly before and after the bedside ultrasound training day. They subsequently completed the ultrasound knowledge assessment approximately 6 months after the bedside ultrasound training day on their own time in an unproctored setting. Each individual testing session randomized the question order and did not provide feedback regarding test performance to minimize subjects' ability to "learn the test".

Qualitative feedback on the entire training week and each session was collected from learners at the completion of the week via survey.

This study was approved by the Oregon Health & Science University Institutional Review Board. All participants in the intern intensive week gave informed consent to be studied as part of this educational initiative; however, the IRB did waive documentation of consent and interns were notified that the research portion was optional. Each intern selected a unique identifier that test results could be traced to at the onset of the study. Intern identifiers were not known to the data assessors, and all participants were assured that their scores were used only for research purposes rather than summative feedback.

Statistical analysis was calculated using Stata v. 11 using Student's t test for mean comparison.

Results

After assessing for proper matching of the pre- and post-test data sets, as well as verifying individual respondents based upon their unique identifiers, 33 interns completed

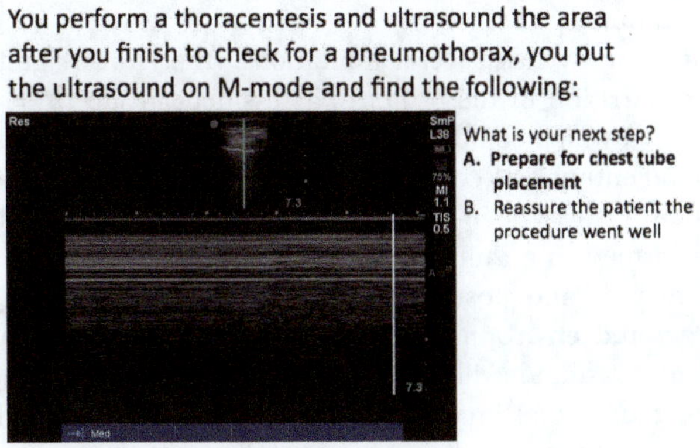

Fig. 1 Sample test question of clinical application of bedside ultrasound

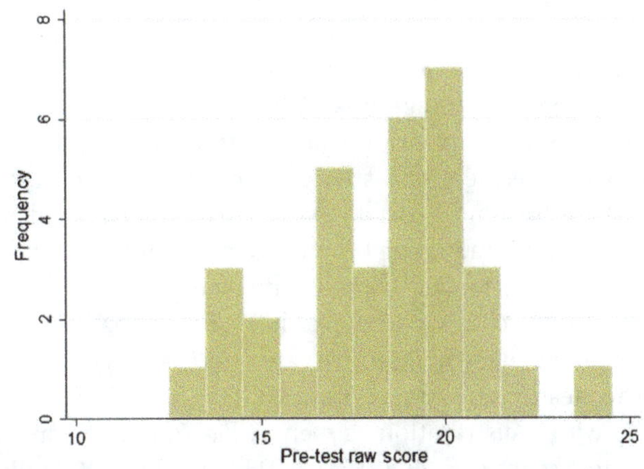

Fig. 2 Distribution of pre-test raw scores (of a possible 30 points), $n = 33$

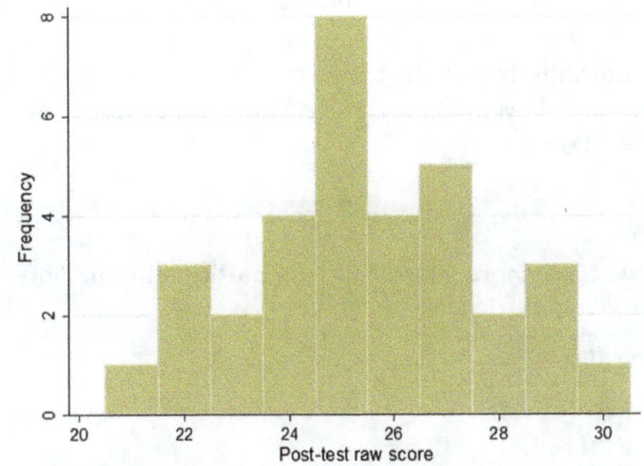

Fig. 3 Distribution of immediate post-test raw scores (of a possible 30 points), $n = 33$

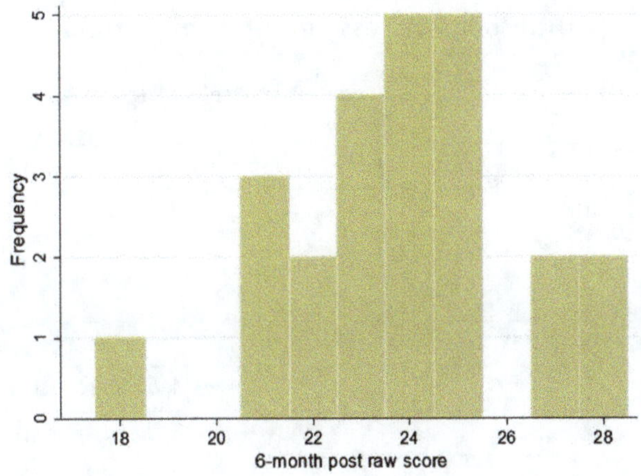

Fig. 4 Distribution of 6-month post-test raw scores (of a possible 30 points), $n = 24$

both the pre and post-assessment. The 6-month post-assessment was completed by 24 of the original respondents. This gave a follow-up response rate of 72.7 %. The average intern age was 28.3 years old; only 29.4 % reported significant prior exposure to ultrasound teaching before residency. A strong majority (88.2 %) anticipated performing procedures as part of their medical practice after graduating from residency (Table 1). Nearly all of the interns had some inpatient experience by the time of the workshop and over half of them had rotated through the medical intensive care unit (Table 1).

The mean pre-test score was 18.3 (60.9 %, 95 % CI 17.4–19.2) with a distribution as seen in Fig. 2, and the mean post-test score was 25.5 (85.0 %, 95 % CI 24.7–26.3) distrubution demonstrated in Fig. 3. A two-sample paired t test demonstrated that the post-test scores were significantly higher with a P value of <0.0001. Interns then completed the assessment 6 months after their initial training session. The mean 6-month post-test score was 23.8 (79.3 %), 95 % confidence interval 22.8–24.8, with distrubution demonstrated in Fig. 4. This remained statistically significantly higher than the pre-test score ($P < 0.0001$), but was lower than the immediate post-assessment ($P = 0.0099$).

Table 1 Demographics of interns participating in "intensive week" curriculum

Interns ($n = 33$)	
Average age (years)	28.3
Percent female	66.7
Percent with prior ultrasound training	29.4
Anticipates performing procedures in post residency career? (% yes)	88.2

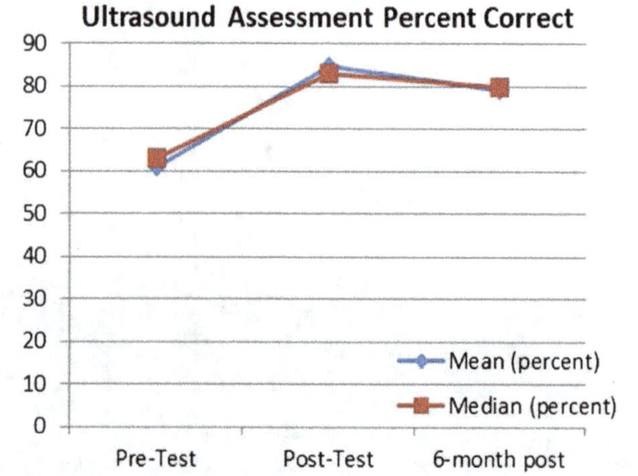

Fig. 5 Assessment percent correct—mean and median

Mean and median test scores were closely associated as demonstrated by Fig. 5, and the mean fell within the standard deviation for all assessment periods. Additionally, the histograms reflect a change in the distribution of scores after the teaching intervention and this change was partially maintained 6 months out from the initial intervention.

The study also included a qualitative assessment of the ultrasound intervention based upon intern feedback where each session of the intern boot-camp was ranked on a 1–5 Likert scale. The ultrasound course was rated a mean of 4.4, fitting with an overwhelmingly positive response from the interns. One intern acknowledged that ultrasound is "such a common bedside tool." Another noted that bedside sonography "is an ongoing skill, but something that will definitely be a part of my future practice." Participants expressed a desire for more hands-on practice and less didactic time. Learner opinion of ultrasound simulators compared to volunteer subjects was not specifically quantified; however, 2 of the 33 subjects commented on desiring more time scanning the live models as opposed to practice scenarios on the simulator.

Discussion

These results show that an innovative 1-day bedside ultrasound curriculum timed early in the academic year supplemented by two 1-h workshops results in significant improvement in point-of-care ultrasound knowledge pertaining to image acquisition, optimization, interpretation and clinical application. This knowledge was retained to a statistically significant degree 6 months later, though with some knowledge decay. Additionally, the intervention was very positively received by learners who felt that these skills would serve them well in their future Internal Medicine careers. Timing this intervention as a distinct entity, separate from intern orientation, may have allowed for better focus on ultrasound-specific educational goals.

This study has several limitations. There was significant attrition in the 6-month assessment group ($n = 7$, 27.3 %), which could leave a self-selecting group of ultrasound enthusiasts completing the knowledge assessment. Additionally, the 6-month knowledge assessment was performed in an unsupervised setting, while the immediate pre- and post assessments were conducted in a proctored environment. Finally, this assessment evaluated ultrasound skills and use by multiple-choice testing, and thus actual image acquisition at the bedside could not be tested. However, we carefully crafted questions that referred to image aquisition such as probe selection for a specific exam, optimization techniques such as depth adjustment, and clinical interpretation such as appropriate next step in an attempt to assess more than simple ultrasound interpretation skills.

Strengths of this study include the condensed time frame with minimal time investment in an already overcrowded curriculum, demonstration of knowledge retention that persisted after the immediate post-training assessment, and relative lack of expense to recreate with the use of volunteer faculty instructors and volunteer ultrasound scanning models.

It is clear that a landmark-based approach to procedures is less safe than ultrasound-guided approach for procedures in Internal Medicine. Furthermore bedside sonography adds to the physical exam to offer the opportunity to better understand complex patients early in the course of their illness [12–14]. The majority of intern participants anticipate performing procedures as part of their practice after residency. However, less than 1/3 of the entering class had prior ultrasound teaching, despite bedside ultrasound's essential role in bedside procedures. As an internal medicine residency training tomorrow's general internist, we feel it is our duty to include high-quality training in ultrasound for our trainees. But as noted, funding and time constraints raise a considerable challenge to adding new curricula.

Including a module with just 80 min of hands-on practice significantly increased internal medicine residents' comfort in interpreting and acquiring images [7]. However, the optimal training duration is still unclear, as another program's experience with a 3-h stand-alone training session did not demonstrate improved diagnostic accuracy [15]. This study shows that a 1-day workshop with two 1-h sessions within the next 6-month results in sustained knowledge of image acquisition theory and image interpretation as well as improved attitudes towards the use of bedside ultrasound. At a time when Medicare funding for post-graduate medical education stagnates, it is ever more important to implement cost-effective educational interventions while expanding the breath of Internal Medicine curricula to embrace technologic advances in patient care.

Conclusion

While there are many ways to introduce and teach ultrasound skills to learners, timing and funding constraints may pose a barrier to adopting new curricula. In this study, a focused one-day intensive curriculum with two supplemental 1-h workshops yielded improved ultrasound interpretation, troubleshooting and clinical application knowledge immediately afterwards and at 6-month post-training. Future studies are needed to formally assess ultrasound image acquisition skills, and clinical outcomes related to the addition of bedside ultrasound to the standard clinical assessment by Internal Medicine physicians.

Abbreviations

ACGME: Accrediting Committee of Graduate Medical Education; CLUE: Cardiovascular limited ultrasound examination; FAST: Focused assessment with sonography in Trauma.

Authors' contributions

RC—literature review, original writing, figure design. EL—literature review, original writing. MK—original writing. RD—concept design, original writing, table generation. All authors participated in method design, manuscript editing and approval. All authors read and approved the final manuscript.

Author details

[1] Department of Medicine, Oregon Health & Science University, Portland, USA. [2] Division of Hospital Medicine, Department of Medicine, Oregon Health & Science University, 3181 SW Sam Jackson Park Road, OP-30, Portland, OR 97239, USA. [3] Present Address: Mayo Clinic Minnesota, 200 First Street SW, Rochester, MN, USA.

References

1. Schnobrich DJ, Gladding S, Olson APJ, Duran-Nelson A (2013) Point-of-care ultrasound in internal medicine: a National Survey of Educational Leadership. J Grad Med Educ 5(3):498–502. doi:10.4300/JGME-D-12-00215.1
2. Schnobrich DJ, Olson APJ, Broccard A, Duran-Nelson A (2013) Feasibility and acceptability of a structured curriculum in teaching procedural and basic diagnostic ultrasound skills to internal medicine residents. J Grad Med Educ 5(3):493–497. doi:10.4300/JGME-D-12-00214.1
3. Dulohery MM, Stoven S, Kurklinsky AK et al (2014) Ultrasound for internal medicine physicians: the future of the physical examination. J Ultrasound Med 33(6):1005–1011. doi:10.7863/ultra.33.6.1005
4. Skalski JH, Elrashidi M, Reed DA, McDonald FS, Bhagra A. Using standardized patients to teach point-of-care ultrasound-guided physical examination skills to internal medicine residents. 2015. http://www.jgme.org/doi/abs/10.4300/JGME-D-14-00178.1. Accessed 14 July 2015
5. Kimura BJ, Amundson SA, Phan JN, Agan DL, Shaw DJ (2012) Observations during development of an internal medicine residency training program in cardiovascular limited ultrasound examination. J Hosp Med 7(7):537–542. doi:10.1002/jhm.1944
6. Andersen GN, Graven T, Skjetne K et al (2015) Diagnostic influence of routine point-of-care pocket-size ultrasound examinations performed by medical residents. J Ultrasound Med 34(4):627–636. doi:10.7863/ultra.34.4.627
7. Keddis MT, Cullen MW, Reed DA et al (2011) Effectiveness of an ultrasound training module for internal medicine residents. BMC Med Educ 11:75. doi:10.1186/1472-6920-11-75
8. Randolph AG, Cook DJ, Gonzales CA, Pribble CG (1996) Ultrasound guidance for placement of central venous catheters: a meta-analysis of the literature. Crit Care Med 24(12):2053–2058. http://www.ncbi.nlm.nih.gov/pubmed/8968276. Accessed 14 July 2015
9. Barnes TW, Morgenthaler TI, Olson EJ, Hesley GK, Decker PA, Ryu JH (2005) Sonographically guided thoracentesis and rate of pneumothorax. J Clin Ultrasound 33(9):442–446. doi:10.1002/jcu.20163
10. Barsuk JH, Cohen ER, Feinglass J et al (2014) Cost savings of performing paracentesis procedures at the bedside after simulation-based education. Simul Healthc 9(5):312–318. doi:10.1097/SIH.0000000000000040
11. Kircher BJ, Himelman RB, Schiller NB (1990) Noninvasive estimation of right atrial pressure from the inspiratory collapse of the inferior vena cava. Am J Cardiol 66(4):493–496. http://www.ncbi.nlm.nih.gov/pubmed/2386120. Accessed 16 July 2015
12. Riegert-Johnson DL, Bruce CJ, Montori VM, Cook RJ, Spittell PC (2005) Residents can be trained to detect abdominal aortic aneurysms using personal ultrasound imagers: a pilot study. J Am Soc Echocardiogr 18(5):394–397. doi:10.1016/j.echo.2004.12.019

13. Jacoby J, Cesta M, Axelband J, Melanson S, Heller M, Reed J (2007) Can emergency medicine residents detect acute deep venous thrombosis with a limited, two-site ultrasound examination? J Emerg Med 32(2):197–200. doi:10.1016/j.jemermed.2006.06.008
14. Martin LD, Howell EE, Ziegelstein RC et al (2009) Hand-carried ultrasound performed by hospitalists: does it improve the cardiac physical examination? Am J Med 122(1):35–41. doi:10.1016/j.amjmed.2008.07.022
15. Ojeda JC, Colbert JA, Lin X et al (2015) Pocket-sized ultrasound as an aid to physical diagnosis for internal medicine residents: a randomized trial. J Gen Intern Med 30(2):199–206. doi:10.1007/s11606-014-3086-4

11

Postural lung recruitment assessed by lung ultrasound in mechanically ventilated children

Gerardo Tusman[1*], Cecilia M. Acosta[1], Stephan H. Böhm[2], Andreas D. Waldmann[3], Carlos Ferrando[4], Manuel Perez Marquez[5] and Fernando Suarez Sipmann[6,7,8]

Abstract

Background: Atelectasis is a common finding in mechanically ventilated children with healthy lungs. This lung collapse cannot be overcome using standard levels of positive end-expiratory pressure (PEEP) and thus for only individualized lung recruitment maneuvers lead to satisfactory therapeutic results. In this short communication, we demonstrate by lung ultrasound images (LUS) the effect of a postural recruitment maneuver (P-RM, i.e., a ventilatory strategy aimed at reaerating atelectasis by changing body position under constant ventilation).

Results: Data was collected in the operating room of the Hospital Privado de Comunidad, Mar del Plata, Argentina. Three anesthetized children undergoing mechanical ventilation at constant settings were sequentially subjected to the following two maneuvers: (1) *PEEP trial* in the supine position PEEP was increased to 10 cmH_2O for 3 min and then decreased to back to baseline. (2) *P-RM* patient position was changed from supine to the left and then to the right lateral position for 90 s each before returning to supine. The total P-RM procedure took approximately 3 min. LUS in the supine position showed similar atelectasis before and after the PEEP trial. Contrarily, atelectasis disappeared in the non-dependent lung when patients were placed in the lateral positions. Both lungs remained atelectasis free even after returning to the supine position.

Conclusions: We provide LUS images that illustrate the concept and effects of postural recruitment in children. This maneuver has the advantage of achieving recruitment effects without the need to elevate airways pressures.

Keywords: Children, Airways, Outcome, Respiration, Lung ultrasound, PEEP, Anesthesia-induced atelectasis, Lung recruitment, Mechanical ventilation

Background

The incidence of atelectasis in mechanically ventilated children with healthy lungs is as high as 68–100% [1–4]. Anesthesia-induced atelectasis has been well described by different imaging techniques such as CT, MRI and lung ultrasound (LUS) [1–5]. The main mechanism leading to atelectasis formation during anesthesia is a decrease in functional residual capacity due to lung compression through the dysfunctional diaphragm by abdominal content [6, 7]. During such conditions, the trans-pulmonary pressure (Ptp = airways − pleural pressure) is no longer sufficient to offset these compressive forces on the most gravity-dependent parts of the lungs, where Ptp is naturally the lowest. *Compression atelectasis* has clearly been demonstrated in anesthetized children and adults [3, 7–10].

Rationale of postural lung recruitment

Lung recruitment maneuvers are ventilator strategies that elevate airway pressures for a few breaths to reaerate atelectasis [11, 12]. Such maneuvers are safe and easily to conduct in mechanically ventilated children [3, 13]. However, potential hemodynamic side effects of high intrathoracic pressures necessitate close hemodynamic

*Correspondence: gtusman@hotmail.com
[1] Department of Anesthesiology, Hospital Privado de Comunidad, 7600 Mar del Plata, Buenos Aires, Argentina
Full list of author information is available at the end of the article

monitoring and that such maneuvers are performed in normovolemic patients, only [12].

In this short communication, we explain the rationale of a new type of lung recruitment maneuver—the postural recruitment (P-RM). It can be defined as an active reaeration of atelectatic lung tissue by intentional changes of a patient's body position under constant ventilatory conditions. This concept makes use of the influence that gravity has on respiratory physiology, more precisely on Ptp. The superimposed pressure within the thorax caused by the lung's own weight decreases Ptp by approximately 0.25 cmH_2O for every 1 cm of ventral-to-dorsal thoracic diameter. Therefore, in supine mechanically ventilated patients Ptp decreases along the gravitational axis causing the lungs to collapse in their most dorsal parts (lowest Ptp) while keeping the ventral zones (highest Ptp) aerated and thus "open" during the entire respiratory cycle [12]. No matter in which body position the patient is placed, dorsal lung zones will always be prone to atelectasis and airways closure [6, 7, 10].

Considering this gravity-dependent physiology, the additive effect of the two following principles can be used therapeutically to recruit lungs by intentionally changing the body position of ventilated patients:

- The *first principle* refers to the relationship between Ptp and body position. It postulates that collapsed tissue in dependent lung zones can be recruited by placing the patient in the opposite position (i.e., from supine to prone or from the left to the right lateral decubitus position). This way, previously collapse lung tissue is now located in the non-dependent position where it is being subjected to the expanding forces of higher Ptps.
- The *second principle* refers to the stabilizing effect of positive end-expiratory pressure (PEEP) on airways and alveoli. It postulates that—provided sufficient PEEP is applied—well ventilated and fully aerated non-dependent lung areas will remain "open" even when becoming dependent again after returning the body to its initial position.

Based on the above principles, we propose a postural recruitment maneuver in which a supine patient is first turned onto his left, then onto his right side and finally to his original supine position (Fig. 1). Thus, we speculate that lung recruitment can be achieved by postural changes without having to elevate airway pressures [11, 12].

Mechanically ventilated children are a sub-population that could especially benefit from this intervention for two reasons: (1) the respiratory physiology of pediatric patients makes them more susceptible to lung collapse after tracheal intubation than adults [8, 9], and (2) children are usually of light weight and can thus be easily turned by one single operator.

In this short communication, we present lung ultrasound (LUS) images which confirm the recruitment effect of intentional changes of body position in anesthetized children. LUS is a good non-invasive tool for

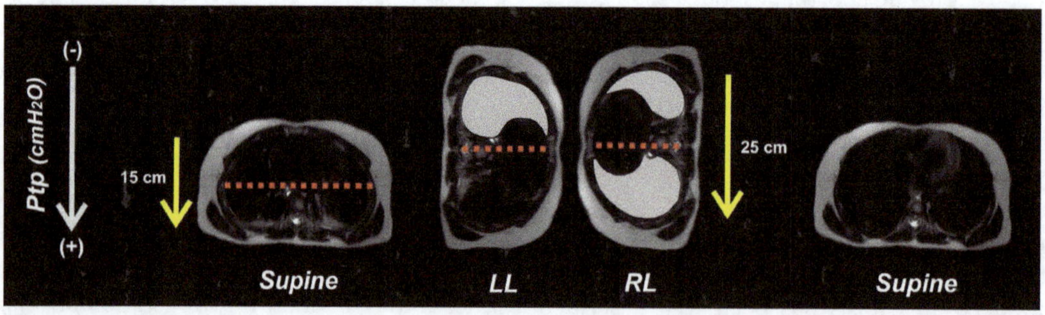

Fig. 1 Concept of postural lung recruitment. Theoretical explanations of the postural recruitment maneuver in an anesthetized child 6 years of age. The maneuver consists of sequential changes in body position from supine to both lateral positions and back to supine again, keeping ventilatory settings constant. The gradient of trans-pulmonary pressures (Ptp) differs between body positions due to the elliptical shape of the chest with the gravity-dependent thoracic dimension being larger in lateral than in the supine position (yellow arrows). Thus, the lower half of the lungs is predisposed to collapse while the upper half is usually aerated and "open" during the entire respiratory cycle (red dotted line). In the left lateral position (LL), the entire right upper lung has the chance to open up at a low plateau pressures even under standard ventilator settings (gray lung). Once open, this right lung can maintain its "open lung" condition when turned to the right lateral positioning (RL) provided sufficient PEEP is applied. Notice the larger vertical distance in the lateral position required a higher PEEP to counteract the potential decrease in Ptp in the dependent lung. Now, the left lung is being recruited as it is placed in the uppermost gravity non-dependent position. At the end of the postural recruitment maneuver both lungs are free from atelectasis although the patient has returned to the baseline supine position

monitoring lung aeration during and after lung recruitment maneuvers in real-time fashion [14–16].

Effects of postural lung recruitment

We analyzed three anesthetized children undergoing open inguinal hernia repair. Children aged 12, 24 and 34 months weighing 10, 12 and 18 kg, respectively. After approval by the local Ethical Committee and after obtaining Informed Consent from the parents, patients received general anesthesia under standard monitoring. Their lungs were ventilated in a pressure-controlled mode using an Aespire 7900 (Datex-Ohmeda, GE Healthcare, Helsinki, Finland) with the inspiratory pressure set to achieve a tidal volume of 7 mL/kg (approx. 12 cmH_2O) and a respiratory rate adjusted between 20 and 25 bpm to keep end-tidal of carbon dioxide between 35 and 40 mmHg. PEEP was 5 cmH_2O, I:E 1:1 and FIO_2 0.5.

Lung aeration was assessed by LUS using the linear 7–12 MHz transducer of the Esaote (MyLab Gamma, Genova, Italy). After anesthesia induction a standard bilateral LUS examination was performed in the supine position. Thereafter the echo probe was placed in an oblique direction between the ribs in the most dependent position as previously described [5]. All patients presented subpleural consolidations, air bronchograms and B-lines as signs of atelectasis (Figs. 2, 3).

Each patient was subjected to the following protocol sequence (Fig. 2):

- *Testing the reaerating effect of 10 cmH_2O of PEEP* After anesthesia induction in the supine position, PEEP was increased from 5 to 10 cmH_2O keeping ventilation constant for 3 min. Then, ventilation returned to baseline settings but keeping PEEP at 8 cmH_2O to maintain any potential recruitment that 10 cmH_2O of PEEP may have induced.
- *Testing the effect of postural recruitment* Before emergence from anesthesia, patients were placed in the left lateral decubitus position for 90 s at constant ventilation but raising PEEP to 10 cmH_2O. Thereafter, patients were turned on their right side for another 90 s. At the end of the 3rd min, patients were placed back in the supine position returning to baseline ventilation, however, at a PEEP of 8 cmH_2O to keep the lungs open.

Figure 2 depicts the results of the protocol in one patient (case 1–24 months). LUS images taken at 8 cmH_2O of PEEP show that 3 min of ventilation with 10 cmH_2O of PEEP in the supine position did not have any measurable recruitment effect. Atelectasis persisted during and after PEEP elevation in all patients. Figure 3 shows the effect of the P-RM in the other two patients (case 2–12 months and case 3–34 months). The Additional file 1: video S1, Additional file 2: video S2 and Additional file 3: video S3 show the corresponding results than Figs. 2 and 3.

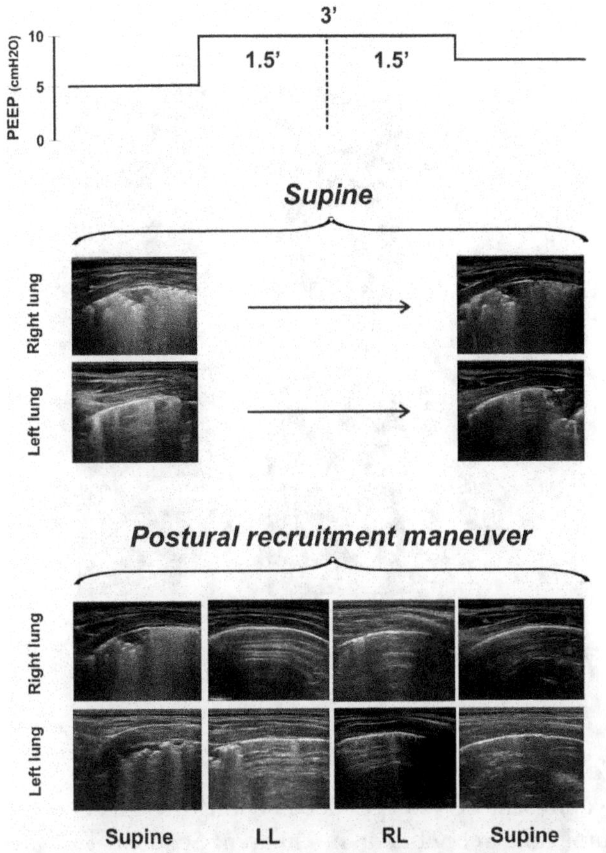

Fig. 2 Lung ultrasound images of postural recruitment. Example of the postural recruitment effect in one anesthetized child (case 1–24 months). This patient was subjected to 10 cmH_2O of positive end-expiratory pressure (PEEP) in the supine position and then during the postural recruitment maneuver. Bilateral atelectasis was diagnosed placing the ultrasound linear probe in the oblique position over the juxta-diaphragmatic lung areas. The same pulmonary areas were assessed in each body position. Note that atelectatic areas are reaerated only after the postural changes

By contrast, the changing body positions of the P-RM clearly restored lung aeration in the atelectatic areas at the same ventilator settings. Reaeration of previously collapsed dependent lung areas was always observed as soon as they became non-dependent in the uppermost position; first in the right lung with the patient lying in the left lateral position and then in the left one with the patient in the right lateral decubitus. After the P-RM, both lungs remained free from atelectasis in the final supine position (Figs. 2, 3; Additional file 1: video S1, Additional file 2: video S2 and Additional file 3: video S3). Hemodynamics maintained stable throughout the protocol.

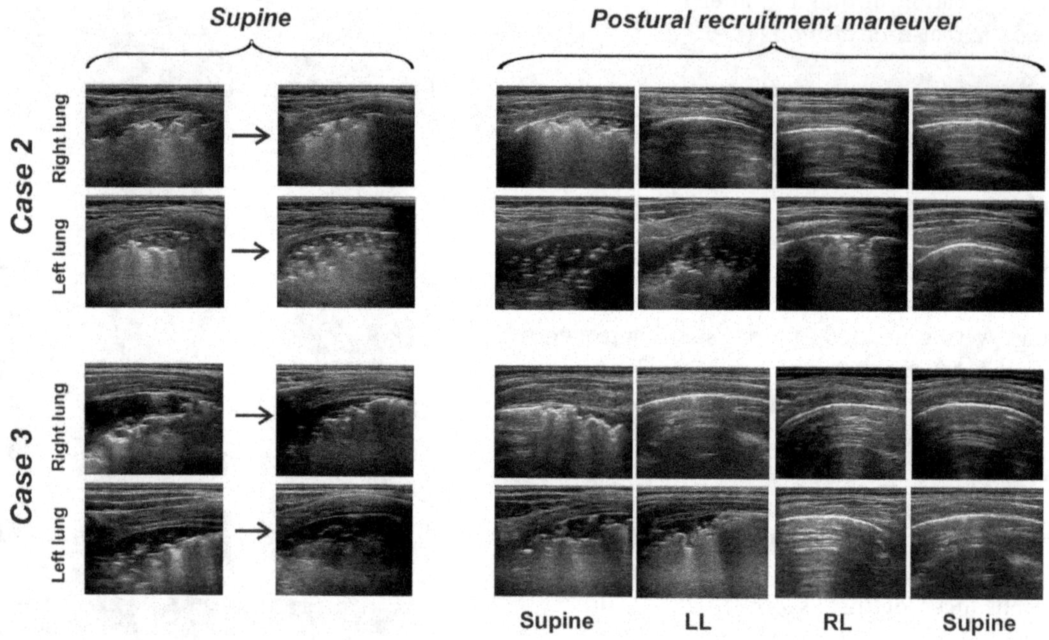

Fig. 3 Lung ultrasound images of postural recruitment in case 2 and 3

Commentary

We present LUS images documenting the effects of postural lung recruitment in children. Sequential changes in body position during constant ventilation at PEEP 10 cmH_2O decreased atelectasis even without applying the high airways pressures of classical recruitment maneuvers.

The therapeutic effect of P-RM seems to result from an increased Ptp caused by a gravity-dependent decrease in pleural pressure in the dorsal lungs and not by elevated airway pressures. As the right-to-left thoracic diameter is much larger than the anterior–posterior one, when a patient is placed in the lateral position, the resulting inspiratory Ptp within the uppermost lung will increase reaching the effective opening pressure of the collapsed lung tissue located in this region (Fig. 1). After the P-RM, a PEEP of 8 cmH_2O was enough to maintain an "open lung" condition in these three healthy patients [11].

The therapeutic implications of P-RM can be derived from the known negative consequence that atelectasis have on mechanically ventilated lungs. Perioperative respiratory complications such as hypoxemic events, bacterial translocation and pneumonia [17–21] adversely affect patient's outcomes while increasing health care cost in both, adults and pediatric patients [22, 23]. Lung recruitment maneuvers easily overcome atelectasis in children with healthy and sick lungs alike [3, 13]. They quickly abort hypoxemic events and could have some protective effect in atelectasis-mediated pneumonias [17, 24, 25].

However, the main objections against recruitment maneuvers are related to their potential hemodynamic side effects, especially in children. Reflexes triggered by high intrathoracic pressures cause bradycardia, compression of pulmonary capillaries and reduced venous return. Each of these either acting in isolation or combined are responsible for the hemodynamic impairment frequently encountered during recruitment maneuvers, predominantly in hypovolemic patients. In view of such undesirable consequences, the P-RM introduced in this paper presents an effective and efficient low risk alternative intervention for treating atelectasis in children. Turning the patients while applying 10 cmH_2O of PEEP for just 3 min seems to be uncritical in normovolemic children.

As far as we know, a postural lung recruitment maneuver has never before been described in children, although we found studies related to the effect of body positioning on respiratory function of mechanically ventilated patients. Some studies describe positive effects of lateral and prone positioning on respiratory function [26, 27] while others do not [28–30]. In these studies, body position was changed leaving ventilatory settings and PEEP constant. The lack of adequate PEEP adaptations—an essential therapeutic intervention of any recruitment strategy such as ours—may have led to these contradictory results. We reasoned that a slightly elevated PEEP should be applied for two reasons: (1) to obtain a plateau pressure high enough to reach the opening pressure of the uppermost lung areas and (2) to maintain the new recruited regions open when returning the patient to the supine position.

Conclusions

In this short communication, we present LUS images documenting the positive effects of postural recruitment in children. Changes in body position during constant ventilation at 10 cmH_2O of PEEP decreased atelectasis without the need to elevate airway pressures as in conventional recruitment maneuvers. Bedside imaging techniques such as LUS can help identify the best settings for a P-RM adapting them to the individual patient.

Additional files

Additional file 1: Video S1. Lung ultrasound images (LUS) of the isolated effect of 10 cmH_2O of PEEP and postural recruitment maneuver—case 1.

Additional file 2: Video S2. Lung ultrasound images (LUS) of the isolated effect of 10 cmH_2O of PEEP and postural recruitment maneuver—case 2.

Additional file 3: Video S3. Lung ultrasound images (LUS) of the isolated effect of 10 cmH_2O of PEEP and postural recruitment maneuver—case 3.

Authors' contributions

GT and CMA made the clinical cases. GT, CMA, SHB, ADW, CF, MPM and FSS worked on the interpretation of the findings and in the final edition of the manuscript. All authors read and approved the final manuscript.

Author details

[1] Department of Anesthesiology, Hospital Privado de Comunidad, 7600 Mar del Plata, Buenos Aires, Argentina. [2] Hepa Wash GmbH, Munich, Germany. [3] Swisstom AG, Landquart, Switzerland. [4] Department of Anesthesiology, University Hospital Valencia, Valencia, Spain. [5] Department of Intensive Care Medicine, Instituto de Investigación Sanitaria Fundación Jiménez Díaz, IIS-FJD, Madrid, Spain. [6] Hedenstierna Laboratory, Department of Surgical Sciences, Section of Anesthesia and Critical Care, Uppsala University Hospital, Uppsala, Sweden. [7] CIBERES, Madrid, Spain. [8] Department of Critical Care, Hospital La Fe, Valencia, Spain.

Acknowledgements

Not applicable.

References

1. Damgaard-Pedersen K, Qvist T (1980) Pediatric pulmonary CT-scanning: anesthesia-induced changes. Pediatr Radiol 9:145–148
2. Sargent MA, McEachern AM, Jamieson DH, Kahwaji R (1999) Atelectasis on pediatric chest CT: comparison of sedation techniques. Pediatr Radiol 29:509–513
3. Tusman G, Bohm SH, Tempra A, Melkun F, García E, Turchetto E, Mulder PG, Lachmann B (2003) Effects of recruitment maneuver on atelectasis in anesthetized children. Anesthesiology 98:14–22
4. Lutterbey G, Wattjes MP, Doerr D, Fischer NJ, Gieseke J, Schild HH (2007) Atelectasis in children undergoing either propofol infusion or positive pressure ventilation anesthesia for magnetic resonance imaging. Pediatr Anesth 17:121–125
5. Acosta CM, Maidana GA, Jacovitti D, Belaunzaran A, Cereceda S, Rae E, Molina A, Gonorazky S, Böhm SH, Tusman G (2014) Accuracy of transthoracic lung ultrasound for diagnosing anesthesia-induced atelectasis in children. Anesthesiology 120:1370–1379
6. Froese AB, Bryan AC (1974) Effects of anesthesia and paralysis on diaphragmatic mechanics in man. Anesthesiology 41:242–255
7. Brismar B, Hedenstierna G, Lundquist H, Strandberg Å, Svensson L, Tokics L (2002) Pulmonary densities during anaesthesia with muscular relation: a proposal of atelectasis. Anesthesiology 62:422–428
8. Motoyama EK, Finder JD (2010) Respiratory physiology in infants and children. Smith's Anesth Infants Child Expert Consult Prem 5(6):22
9. Taussig LM, Hanis TR, Lebowitz MD (1977) Lung function in infants and young children: functional residual capacity, tidal volume, respiratory rate. Am Rev Respir Dis 116:233–239
10. Hedenstierna G, Edmark L (2010) Mechanisms of atelectasis in the perioperative period. Best Pract Res Clin Anaesthesiol 24:157–169
11. Lachmann B (1992) Open up the lung and keep the lung open. Intensive Care Med 18:319–321
12. Tusman G, Böhm SH (2010) Prevention and reversal of lung collapse during the intra-operative period. Best Pract Res Clin Anaesthesiol 24:183–197
13. Duff JP, Rosychuk RJ, Joffe AR (2007) The safety and efficacy of sustained inflations as a lung recruitment maneuver in pediatric intensive care unit patients. Intensive Care Med 33:1778–1786
14. Bouhemad B, Brisson H, Le-Guen M, Arbelot C, Lu Q, Rouby JJ (2015) Bedside ultrasound assessment of positive end-expiratory pressure-induced lung recruitment. Am J Respir Crit Care Med 183:341–347
15. Song IK, Kim EH, Lee JH (2016) Effects of an alveolar recruitment manoeuvre guided by lung ultrasound on anaesthesia-induced atelectasis in infants: a randomised, controlled trial. Anaesthesia. doi:10.1111/anae.13713
16. Tusman G, Acosta CM, Costantini M (2016) Ultrasonography for the assessment of lung recruitment maneuvers. Crit Ultrasound J 8:8
17. Scohy TV, Bikker IG, Hofland J, De JONG, Peter L, Bogers AJ, Gommers D (2009) Alveolar recruitment strategy and PEEP improve oxygenation, dynamic compliance of respiratory system and end-expiratory lung volume in pediatric patients undergoing cardiac surgery for congenital heart disease. Pediatr Anesth 19:1207–1212
18. Tusman G, Böhm SH, Warner DO, Sprung J (2012) Atelectasis and perioperative pulmonary complications in high-risk patients. Curr Opin Anesthesiol 25:1–10
19. Van Kaam AH, Lachmann RA, Herting E, De Jaegere A, Van Iwaarden F, Noorduyn LA, Kok JH, Haitsma JJ, Lachmann B (2004) Reducing atelectasis attenuates bacterial growth and translocation in experimental pneumonia. Am J Respir Crit Care Med 169:1046–1053
20. Brooks-Brunn JA (1995) Postoperative atelectasis and pneumonia. Heart Lung 24:94–115
21. Elward AM, Warren DK, Fraser VJ (2002) Ventilator-associated pneumonia in pediatric intensive care unit patients: risk factors and outcomes. Pediatrics 109:758–764
22. Canet J, Mazo V (2010) Postoperative pulmonary complications. Minerva Anestesiol 76:138–143
23. Murat I, Constant I, Maud'Huy H (2004) Perioperative anaesthetic morbidity in children: a database of 24.165 anaesthetics over a 30-month period. Paediatr Anaesth 14:158–166
24. Lachmann RA, van Kaam AH, Haitsma JJ, Lachmann B (2007) High positive end-expiratory pressure levels promote bacterial translocation in experimental pneumonia. Intensive Care Med 33:1800–1804
25. Futier E, Constantin JM, Paugam-Burtz C, Pascal J, Eurin M, Neuschwander A, Allaouchiche B (2013) A trial of intraoperative low-tidal-volume ventilation in abdominal surgery. N Engl J Med 369:428–437
26. Remolina C, Khan A, Santiago T, Edelman NH (1981) Positional hypoxemia in unilateral lung disease. N Engl J Med 304:523–525
27. Chang SC, Chang HI, Shiao GM, Perng RP (1993) Effect of body position gas exchange in patients with unilateral central airway lesions: down with the good lung? Chest 103:787–791
28. Montgomery K, Choy NL, Steele M, Hough J (2014) The effectiveness of quarter turn from prone in maintaining respiratory function in premature infants. J Paediatr Child Health 50:972–977
29. Balaguer A, Escribano J, Roque M (2006) Infant position in neonates receiving mechanical ventilation. Cochrane Database Syst Rev 4:68
30. Numa AH, Hammer J, Newth CJL (1997) Effect of prone and supine positions on functional residual capacity, oxygenation, and respiratory mechanics in ventilated infants and children. Am J Respir Crit Care Med 156:1185–1189

12

Point-of-care lung ultrasound for diagnosis of *Pneumocystis jirovecii* pneumonia: notes from the field

Maria Teresa Giordani[1*], Francesca Tamarozzi[2], Daniel Kaminstein[3], Enrico Brunetti[4] and Tom Heller[5]

Abstract

Background: Thoracic ultrasound is helpful to evaluate lung pathology in patients with acute dyspnea. Several studies have demonstrated the efficacy of point-of-care ultrasound in patients with extrapulmonary TB and HIV co-infection. This retrospective, open-label case–control study explores the role of lung ultrasound in the diagnosis of *Pneumocystis jirovecii* pneumonia (PJP) in HIV-positive patients. In particular, it highlights the potential role of specific sonographic features that may be unique to this population.

Methods: The record of all HIV-positive patients admitted from 1.1.2013 to 31.6.2017 to the Department of Infectious Diseases and Tropical Medicine of san Bortolo Hospital, Vicenza, Italy, with a discharge diagnosis of acute lung injury (ALI) and who received point-of-care ultrasound of the chest for clinical purposes was included in the analysis. The patients were scanned according with the evidence-based recommendation.

Results: Of 273 HIV-positive patients whose records were reviewed, 81 (29.6%) were diagnosed with ALI. Complete documentation was available for 24 patients, of which 14 (58.3%) had microbiologically confirmed PJP (PJP+) and 10 (41.7%) had other conditions (PJP−). B-lines, subpleural consolidations, and cystic changes were significantly more frequent in patients with PJP (14/14 vs. 6/10, $p = 0.0198$; 14/14 vs. 4/10, $p = 0.0016$; 8/14 vs. 0/10, $p = 0.0019$, respectively). In particular, B-lines and subpleural consolidations were present in all PJP+ patients in our cohort giving a sensitivity of 100%, but their specificity was low (45 and 60%, respectively). On the contrary, the presence of consolidations with cystic changes had a very high specificity for PJP (100%), but low sensitivity (57%). Pleural effusions and consolidations with linear air bronchograms were not observed in PJP+ patients.

Conclusions: B-lines, subpleural consolidations, and cystic changes are suggestive of PJP. Lung consolidation with air bronchograms and pleural effusion should prompt suspicion of other etiologies. These findings have the potential to be useful in the daily management of HIV-positive patients in resource-limited settings where other diagnostic tools are rarely available.

Keywords: POC ultrasound, Lung, *Pneumocystis* pneumonia, AIDS, HIV, Pneumonia, Lung ultrasound

Background

The interpretation of artifacts created during ultrasound of the thoracic cavity was first described over 20 years ago [1]. Since then thoracic ultrasound has become a well-established imaging modality used by clinicians at the bedside of acutely dyspneic patient. The BLUE protocol [2] is a helpful approach to lung ultrasound as it outlines a step-by-step decision tree to differentiate between potential causes of dyspnea. In low-resource settings where even a basic chest X-ray (CXR) may not be available [3] ultrasound of the chest has profound implications. Point-of-care ultrasound (POCUS) has an established role as a diagnostic tool in HIV-positive patients with extrapulmonary tuberculosis (TB) [4], and has been shown to complement CXR [5]. Furthermore, it is a frequent POCUS application in settings with high TB and

*Correspondence: giordanimt@gmail.com
[1] Infectious and Tropical Diseases Unit, San Bortolo Hospital, Via Rodolfi 37, 36100 Vicenza, Italy
Full list of author information is available at the end of the article

HIV prevalence [6]. Recent case series describe sonographic lung finding seen in HIV-positive patients [7] and in patients with miliary TB [8].

Pneumocystis jirovecii pneumonia (PJP) is one of the most common opportunistic infections in HIV-positive patients [9] who are not receiving prophylaxis especially when CD4– counts fall below 200 cells/mm^3 [10]. Without timely diagnosis and treatment PJP carries a high mortality [11], though survival rates have increased in the era of antiretroviral therapy (ART) [12]. Diagnosis of PJP poses a significant challenge, due to its non-specific clinical presentation. Computed tomography (CT) of the chest remains the mainstay of diagnosis [13]. In cross-sectional CT imaging, PJP presents with bilateral geographic or patchy ground-glass opacities with septal thickening, lung consolidation, nodules, cysts, and pneumothorax, while pleural effusions are uncommon [14]. Microbiological confirmation relies on bronchoalveolar lavage (BAL) followed by microscopy or PCR. BAL is invasive, poorly tolerated by patients with respiratory distress and analysis requires a well-equipped laboratory with specific expertise.

In resource-limited settings, where the majority of HIV-positive patients live, the risk of PJP is high [15]; CT and bronchoscopy are generally not available. As POCUS has been found a promising tool for other diseases in these settings [16, 17], our study aimed to explore the diagnostic potential of sonographic lung features in the diagnosis of HIV-positive patients with PJP.

Methods

Study design and data collection

This retrospective unmatched case–control study of HIV-positive patients with and without microbiologically confirmed PJP was conducted in the Tropical Medicine and Infectious Diseases Department, San Bortolo Hospital, Vicenza, Italy, that cares for approximately 1000 HIV-positive individuals yearly.

The department operates a clinical ultrasound service including bedside POCUS. Chest POCUS is performed by an infectious disease specialist (MTG) using an Aplio XG Model SSA-790A with a 3.5-MHz convex and an 8-MHz linear probe (Toshiba, Tokyo, Japan). All patients included in this study were examined with both probes; the anterior, posterior, and lateral chest wall was bilaterally scanned in longitudinal (cranio-caudal orientation) and transverse (aligned with the intercostal space) orientation from apex to base with patients in supine, sitting or near-to-supine position, trying to achieve the maximum extension of the visible pleural line. No standard protocol was followed, although the International evidence-based recommendations for point-of-care lung ultrasound were taken into consideration [18].

All records of HIV-positive patients admitted from 1.1.2013 to 31.6.2017 were reviewed and patients with a discharge diagnosis of acute lung injury (ALI) according to Diagnosis-Related-Group (DRG) classification (http://www.salute.gov.it/imgs/C.pdf) were identified. Inclusion criteria were as follows: (1) HIV infection; (2) discharge diagnosis of ALI; (3) BAL followed by microbiological examination for *P. jirovecii* (microscopy or PCR); and (4) POCUS of the chest performed during the first week of admission blinded to CT scan findings. Extracted patient information included demographics, history of ART, CD4+ count, HIV viral load, microbiological, and imaging data. Stored static images and video files of all patients were reviewed for the study (Additional files 1, 2, 3).

Statistical methods

Patients included were classified as microbiologically confirmed PJP (PJP+) or control patients with ALI without microbiologically confirmed PJP (PJP−). Data are presented as medians, interquartile ranges (IQR), and counts with percentages, as appropriate. Differences in proportions were analyzed by Fisher's Exact test; continuous variables by Mann–Whitney-*U* test. All tests were two-sided; p-values < 0.05 were considered significant. Analyses were done using MedCalc version 17.8 (Ostend, Belgium).

Description of ultrasound findings

An ultrasound was considered normal when a normal lung surface, a pleural line with lung sliding, and A-lines were present and a maximum of two B-lines per single view was seen. Pathological ultrasound findings extracted for analysis were increased number of B-lines, pleural effusions, subpleural consolidation, lung consolidation with air bronchogram patterns or a cystic pattern, and presence of pneumothorax. Ultrasound findings are described in detail in Table 1.

Results

Patient characteristics

The records of 273 HIV-positive patients admitted during the study period were reviewed. 81 patients (29.6%) were diagnosed with ALI. Complete documentation was available for 24 patients, 18 males, and 6 females, of which 14 (58.3%) had microbiologically confirmed PJP (PJP+) and 10 (41.7%) were diagnosed with other conditions (PJP−). Clinical and demographic data are summarized in Table 2.

The frequency of lung ultrasound findings is summarized in Table 3. B-lines, subpleural consolidations, and cystic changes were more frequently seen in patients with PJP, and reached statistical significance. In particular,

Table 1 Clinical and demographic characteristics of the patients included in the study

	Total *n* = 24 (100%)	PJP+ *n* = 14 (58.33%)	PJP− *n* = 10 (41.66%)	*p*-value
Sex males/females (% males)	18/6 (75.00%)	13/1 (92.85%)	5/5 (50.00%)	0.0501
Median age in years (IQR)	44 (36–53)	43 (35–54)	44 (41–51)	0.8602
Ethnic origin (*n*)				
Caucasian	18	11	7	
African	3	1	2	
Latin-American	3	2	1	
Median CD4+T cells/μl on admission (IQR)	56.5 (18–172.25)	39.5 (16–73.5)	137.5 (59.75–325)	0.0608
Median viral load in copies/ml on admission (IQR)	345,000 (91,427–607,400)	262,450 (61,291–587,150)	391,200 (195,400–790,400)	0.8291
PJP as first AIDS-defining condition	n.a.	13/14 (92.85%)	n.a.	
Final diagnosis	-	PJP	See note[a]	

PJP, *Pneumocystis jirovecii* pneumonia; IQR, inter quartile range; n.a., not applicable

[a] Final diagnoses of PJP-patients: bacterial pneumonia (n = 3), TB (n = 3), disseminated Cytomegalovirus infection (n = 1) and *Mycobacterium avium* complex infection (n = 1) with lung involvement, non-Hodgkin's T cell lymphoma (n = 1) and adenocarcinoma (n = 1) of the lung

Table 2 Diagnostic performances of the lung ultrasound findings

Lung ultrasound sign	PJP+ *n* (%)	PJP− *n* (%)	*p*-value	Se (95% CI)	Sp (95% CI)	PPV (95% CI)	NPV (95% CI)	LR+ (95% CI)	LR− (95% CI)
B-lines (> 2 per view) no B-lines in the scan	14 (100%)	6 (60%)	0.0198	100% (76.84–100)	45.45% (16.75–76.62)	70% (57.64–80.01)	100% –	1.83 (1.07–3.14)	0.00 –
Pleural effusion	0 (0%)[a]	5 (50%)	0.0059	0.00% (0.00–23.16)	50.00% (18.71–81.29)	0.00% –	26.32% (16.12–39.90)	0.00 –	2.00 (1.08–3.27)
Pneumothorax	4 (28.5%)	1 (10%)	0.3577	40.00% (12.16–73.76)	90.00% (55.50–99.75)	80.00% (34.93–96.75)	60.00% (46.48–72.15)	4.00 (0.54–29.81)	0.67 (0.39–1.15)
Subpleural consolidation	14 (100%)	4 (40%)	0.0016	100% (76.84–100)	60.00% (16.24–87.84)	77.78% (62.10–88.20)	100% –	2.50 (1.17–5.34)	0.00 –
Lung consolidation, any lung consolidations with "cystic" changes at the pulmonary basis	8 (57.1%)	5 (50%)	1.0000	57.14% (28.86–82.34)	50.00% (18.71–81.29)	61.54% (42.60–77.52)	45.45% (25.95–66.46)	1.14 (0.53–2.46)	0.86 (0.36–2.04)
Lung consolidation with air bronchogram	0 (0%)	4 (40%)	0.0198	0.00% (0.00–23.16)	60.00% (26.24–87.84)	0.00% –	30.00% (20.53–41.55)	0.00 –	1.67 (1.00–2.76)
Lung consolidation with cystic pattern	8 (57.1%)	0 (0%)	0.0019	57.14% (28.86–82.34)	100% (69.15–100)	100% –	62.50 (47.65–75.32)	–	0.43 0.23–0.78

PJP, *Pneumocystis jirovecii* pneumonia; Se, sensitivity; Sp, specificity; PPV, positive predictive value; NPV, negative predictive value; LR+, positive likelihood ratio; LR−, negative likelihood ratio; CI, confidence interval

[a] One patient developed bilateral pleural effusion later during the stay in the Intensive Care Unit

B-lines and subpleural consolidations were present in all PJP+ patients in our cohort giving a sensitivity of 100%. The specificity of these two findings was low (45 and 60%, respectively). The presence of consolidations with cystic changes had a very high specificity for PJP. Pleural effusions and consolidations with linear air bronchograms were not seen in PJP+ patients.

As most HIV-positive patients admitted for acute lung disease underwent routine CXR and CT scan, we were able to compare the POCUS findings with radiologic findings from other modalities. Examples from three patients are shown in Table 4. We found a strong correlation between the imaging pattern seen on ultrasound and that of other imaging modalities. Of the six PJP+ patients without "cystic changes," three had CT scans demonstrating normal air-filled lung throughout the subpleural region, two had only intralobular opacities, and one patient had physical limitations to the scan (pectus excavatum).

Discussion

This is to our knowledge the first study systematically reporting POCUS findings of the lung in HIV-related PJP. Ultrasound patterns for several lung diseases in HIV-positive patients have been described in a recently published case series [7]; however, the diagnostic accuracy of

Table 3 Description of lung ultrasound findings

Findings	Image	Description	Interpretation
A-lines	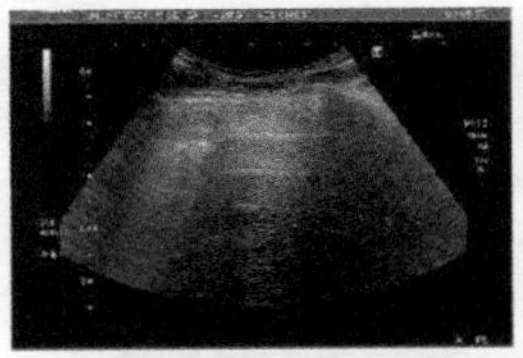	Horizontal lines separated from the pleural line by regular intervals that are equal to the distance between skin and pleural line Pleural line remains intact	Normal
B-lines	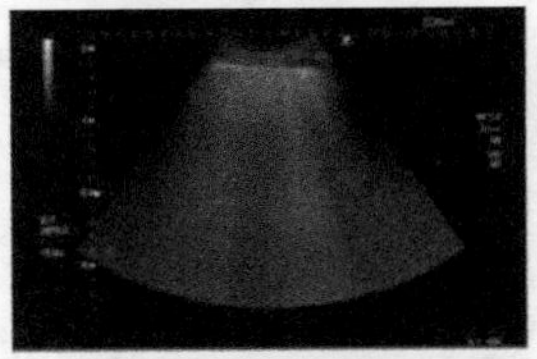	Vertical, hyperechoic reverberation artifacts originating from the pleural line and extending throughout the field of view Pleural line remains intact	Up to 2 B-lines per view are normal, otherwise fluid in the interstitial space is suspected
Pleural effusion	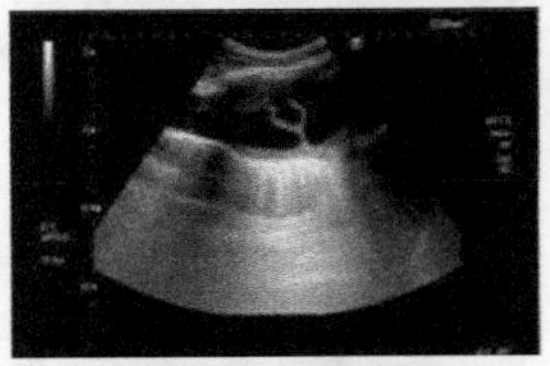	Anechoic areas that separate lung tissue from pleura and diaphragm, may be simple "black" fluid or contain complex septations Separation of visceral and parietal pleura by fluid	Collection of pleural transudate or exudate
Pneumothorax	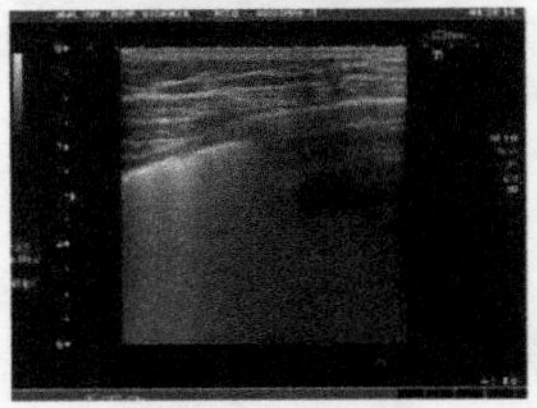	Absence of dynamic pleural sliding, a lung point represents the transition between loss of pleural sliding and the return of pleural sliding (the border of the pneumothorax) Separation of visceral and parietal pleura by air	Air in the pleural space
Subpleuric consolidation	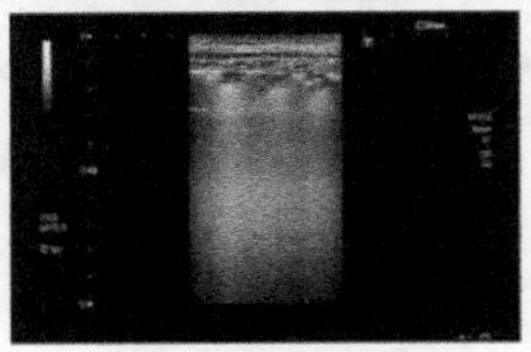	Small hypoechoic areas (< 2 cm) disrupt the visceral pleura Parietal pleura acquires a "ragged" or "shredded" appearance	Small consolidations are present on the visceral pleura itself

Table 3 continued

Findings	Image	Description	Interpretation
Consolidation with linear bronchogram	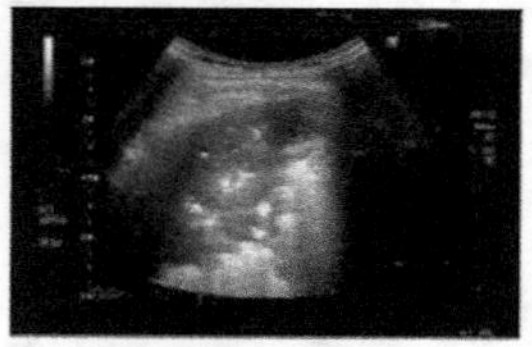	Larger irregular hypoechoic areas containing linear hyperechoic air bronchograms (bright areas with linear arrangement casting a vertical shadow artifact)	Alveolar parenchymal involvement, with air trapped in the obstructed airways
Consolidation with "cystic bronchogram"	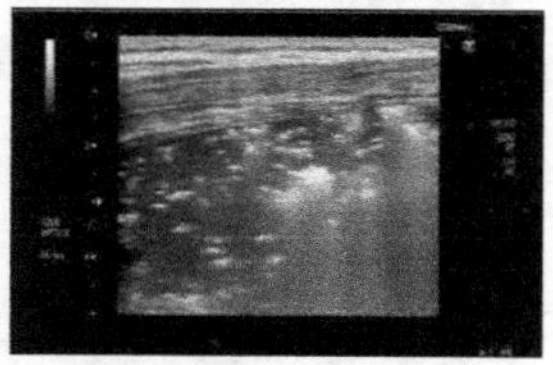	Larger irregular hypoechoic areas disrupting the visceral pleura with small disseminated hyperechoic areas within consolidated lung (without marked shadow artifacts)	Alveolar parenchymal involvement, possible cystic changes as explanation for the echogenic areas

Table 4 Comparison of findings on CT scan, CXR, and ultrasound of three patients with *Pneumocystis jirovecii* pneumonia PJP

	CT scan	CXR	Ultrasound
Patient 1	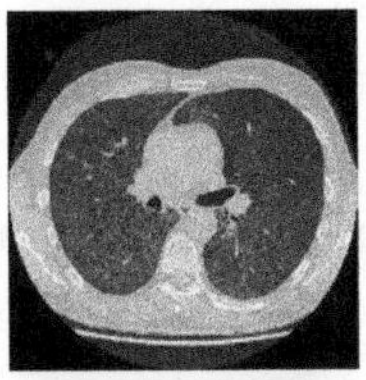	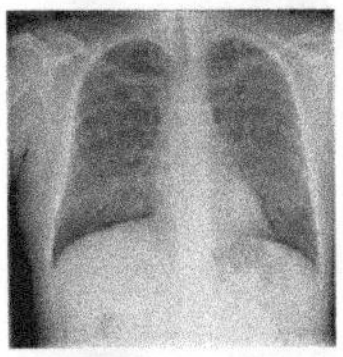	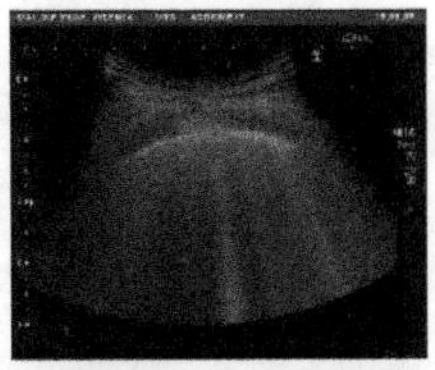
Patient 2	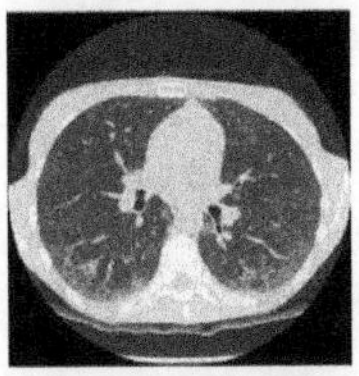	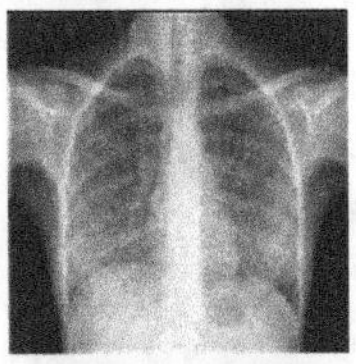	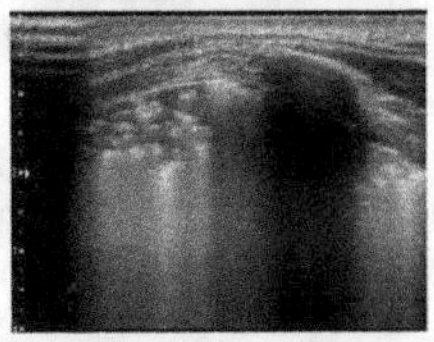
Patient 3	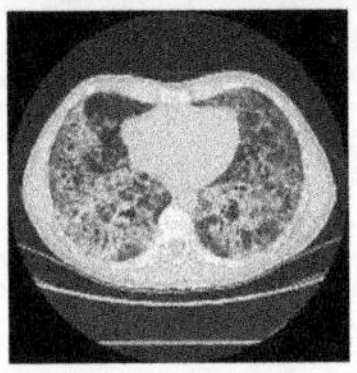	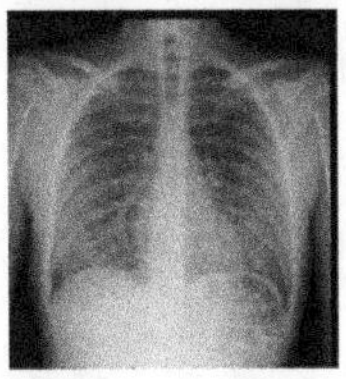	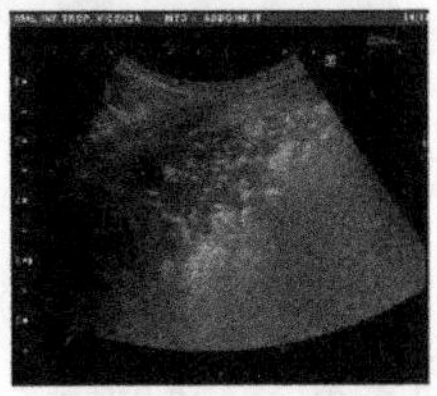

The infection spares the subpleural areas in patient 1, involves mainly the subpleural areas in patient 2, and involves wider lung parenchyma in patient 3

chest POCUS in this patient population has never been assessed. Our study suggests that there are thoracic ultrasound findings with significant predictive value for PJP in HIV-positive patients. B-lines, subpleural consolidations and cystic changes are suggestive of PJP. Lung consolidation with air bronchograms and pleural effusion should prompt suspicion of other etiologies.

In particular, the finding of "cystic changes" needs to be highlighted, as it was very specific in our cohort. The sign was characterized by a hypoechoic consolidation including widely scattered echogenic regions suggestive of air-containing cysts. The pattern was consistently present in serial scans of patients and seems to correlate with the type of lung consolidation seen on CT scan. The typical CT features include a "ground glass" pattern, septal thickening, and walled cysts next to the areas of ground-glass attenuation [14]. These may represent pathological changes of lung tissue with filling of the bronchioles and alveoli with foamy debris and macrophages as well as fungal cysts demonstrated in autopsies [18].

Our results should be considered preliminary, given the small numbers and the fact that a single operator performed the ultrasounds. The strength of this study is the use of a referral setting where all diagnostic methods considered to be the gold standard for diagnosing PJP (bronchoscopy, PCR, and CT scan) are routinely available. The discharge diagnosis in our population carries thus a high level of certainty.

Consolidation with "cystic changes," the most specific ultrasound finding, was only detected in 57% of PJP+ patients and thus has a suboptimal sensitivity. This may be in part due to the inherent limitations in scanning critically ill, dyspneic patients. Also the inhomogeneous spatial distribution of the inflammatory changes may add to this problem. Early stages of the infection seem to spare the subpleural areas [19]. Normal air-filled lung prevents ultrasound from detecting underlying areas of consolidation. Nevertheless, the presence of the pattern seems helpful to "rule-in" the diagnosis.

While no single finding yielded optimal sensitivity and specificity a combination of the described findings on thoracic ultrasound could be helpful in informing clinicians about the likelihood of various lung pathologies in HIV+ patients admitted with ALI.

Conclusion

POCUS is useful in diagnostic work-up of HIV-positive patients with acute lung disease and ultrasound patterns can help in diagnosing PJP. The use of lung POCUS poses an attractive option for HIV-patients as it combines affordability, non-invasiveness, and availability at patients' bedside regardless of clinical condition. This is even more relevant in resource-limited settings where the majority of patients reside. Our case series should encourage larger prospective studies to validate the described thoracic ultrasound findings in HIV-positive patients.

Additional files

Additional file 1: Clip SA. Subpleural consolidation: a hypoechoic area is visible in the superficial parts of the lung less than 2 cm below the pleural line.

Additional file 2: Clip SB. Lung consolidation with linear air bronchogram: large hypoechoic area (consolidation) visible containing hyperechoic bright areas casting a vertical shadow artifact. The bright areas are distributed in a linear pattern representing air trapped in the bronchi (sonographic air bronchogram).

Additional file 3: Clip SC. Lung consolidation with cystic changes: large hypoechoic area (consolidation) disrupting the visceral pleura with small, diffusely disseminated hyperechoic areas within the consolidated lung (without marked shadow artifacts). The spatial distribution of is not linear as in clip B.

Abbreviations

CXR: X-ray; POCUS: point-of-care ultrasound; TB: tuberculosis; PJP: *Pneumocystis jirovecii* pneumonia; CT: computed tomography; ART: antiretroviral therapy; BAL: bronchoalveolar lavage; ALI: acute lung injury.

Authors' contributions

MTG conceived the study, performed the ultrasound exams, and collected the data. FT analyzed the data. MTG, FT, DK, and TH drafted the manuscript. All authors critically discussed the results and approved the paper. All authors read and approved the final manuscript.

Authors' information

MTG is a full time clinician in Infectious Diseases and Tropical Medicine in San Bortolo Hospital, Vicenza, Italy. She started using ultrasound, POCUS and interventional US in the setting of Infectious and Tropical Diseases and HIV/TB patients in 1995 and exported her experience in remote settings with very constrained resources as Tibetan Plateau, Andes, and rural Africa.

FT graduated in medicine from Pavia University (Italy) in 2009, was granted her Ph.D. from the Liverpool School of Tropical Medicine (UK) in 2012 and her specialization in microbiology and virology from Milan University (Italy) in 2017. She is currently working in the Center for Tropical Diseases of Negrar hospital (Verona, Italy). Her broad professional research focus is the diagnosis of parasitic disease and, within this, the use of ultrasound for the diagnosis and epidemiology of parasitic infections.

DK is a full time practicing emergency medicine physician who holds dual fellowship degrees in Global Health and Ultrasound. He received a diploma in tropical medicine from the London School of Hygiene and Tropical Medicine. He is extensively involved in ultrasound training and research globally and serves as co-director of several ultrasound training courses in Africa and South America. His primary research interest is the application of ultrasound in the evaluation of tropical infectious diseases. He helps lead his university's ultrasound center and is passionate about advancing clinician ultrasound around the globe.

EB is an Infectious Disease clinician with over 30 years of experience in clinical ultrasound, working in a 900-bed teaching hospital in Pavia, Italy. He is a specialist in Internal Medicine and in Infectious Disease and an Associate Professor of Infectious Diseases at the University of Pavia. His research interests include the clinical management of a number of neglected tropical diseases and he has ongoing collaborations in this field with institutions in Europe, Asia, Africa, and the Americas. He directs the international Short Course on Ultrasound in Infectious Diseases and Tropical Medicine, held yearly at the University of Pavia.

TH graduated from medical school at the Technical University Munich, Germany in 1995. He specialized in general internal medicine, as well as in infectious diseases and worked in Germany, Saudi Arabia, and South Africa. He is currently working as a clinical advisor at Lighthouse Trust, operating three large HIV/TB clinic in Malawi. Throughout his career, his research interests were ultrasound applications in the resource-limited setting and sonographic diagnosis and treatment of infectious diseases. He has conducted ultrasound trainings in Germany, Italy, Zimbabwe, Ethiopia, South Africa, Ghana, Malawi, Kuwait, Saudi Arabia, Peru, and Laos.

Author details

[1] Infectious and Tropical Diseases Unit, San Bortolo Hospital, Via Rodolfi 37, 36100 Vicenza, Italy. [2] Center for Tropical Diseases, Sacro Cuore-Don Calabria Hospital, Negrar, Verona, Italy. [3] Department of Emergency Medicine and Hospitalist Service, Medical College of Georgia at Augusta University, Augusta, GA, USA. [4] Division of Infectious and Tropical Diseases, University of Pavia, IRCCS S. Matteo Hospital Foundation, Pavia, Italy. [5] Lighthouse Clinic, Lilongwe, Malawi.

Acknowledgements

We thank Sergio Savastano, MD, for reviewing CXR and CT scans. We thank the U.L.SS. 8 Berica Service Management Control Office for the support, and overall Colleagues and nurses of the San Bortolo Hospital, Vicenza, Italy, for having worked as a tight-knit team with these patients.

References

1. Lichtenstein D, Mézière G, Biderman P, Gepner A, Barré O (1997) The comet-tail artifact, an ultrasound sign of alveolar–interstitial syndrome. Am J Respir Crit Care Med 156:1640–1646
2. Lichtenstein DA, Mezière GA (2008) Relevance of lung ultrasound in the diagnosis of acute respiratory failure. Chest 134:117–125
3. Pedrazzoli D, Lalli M, Boccia D, Houben R, Kranzer K (2017) Can tuberculosis patients in resource-constrained settings afford chest radiography? Eur Respir J 49:1601877
4. Heller T, Wallrauch C, Goblirsch S, Brunetti E (2012) Focused assessment with sonography for HIV-associated tuberculosis (FASH)—a short protocol and a pictorial review. Crit Ultrasound J 4:21
5. Heller T, Goblirsch S, Bahlas S, Ahmed M, Giordani MT, Wallrauch C, Brunetti E (2013) Diagnostic value of FASH ultrasound and chest X-ray in HIV co-infected patients with abdominal TB. Int J Tuberc Lung Dis 17:342–344
6. van Hoving DJ, Lamprecht HH, Stander M, Vallabh K, Fredericks D, Louw P, Muller M, Malan JJ (2012) Adequacy of the emergency point-of-care ultrasound core curriculum for the local burden of disease in South Africa. Emerg Med J 30:312–315
7. Heuvelings CC, Bélard S, Janssen S, Wallrauch C, Grobusch MP, Brunetti E, Giordani MT, Heller T (2016) Chest ultrasonography in patients with HIV: a case series and review of the literature. Infection 44:1–10
8. Hunter L, Bélard S, Janssen S, van Hoving DJ, Heller T (2016) Miliary tuberculosis: sonographic pattern in chest ultrasound. Infection 44:243–246
9. Kaplan JE, Hanson D, Dworkin MS, Frederik T, Bertolli J, Lindegren ML, Holmberg S, Jones JL (2000) Epidemiology of human immunodeficiency virus-associated opportunistic infections in the United States in the era of highly active antiretroviral therapy. Clin Infect Dis 30(Suppl 1):S5–S14
10. Sepkowitz KA (2002) Opportunistic infections in patients with and patients without acquired immunodeficiency syndrome. Clin Infect Dis 34:1293
11. Wang HW, Lin CC, Kuo CF, Lee CM (2011) Mortality predictors of *Pneumocystis jirovecii* pneumonia in human immunodeficiency virus-infected patients at presentation: experience in a tertiary care hospital of northern Taiwan. J Microbiol Immunol Infect 44:274–281
12. Palella FJ Jr, Delaney KM, Moorman AC, Loveless MO, Fuhrer J, Satten GA, Aschman D, Holmberg SD (1998) Declining morbidity and mortality among patients with advanced human immunodeficiency virus infection. HIV Outpatient Study Investigators. N Engl J Med 338:853–860
13. Lichtenberger JP 3rd, Sharma A, Zachary KC, Krishnam MS, Greene RE, Shepard JA, Wu CC (2012) What a differential a virus makes: a practical approach to thoracic imaging findings in the context of HIV infection—part 1, pulmonary findings. Am J Roentgenol 198:1295–1304
14. Chou CW, Chao HS, Lin FC, Tsai HC, Yuan WH, Chang SC (2015) Clinical usefulness of HRCT in assessing the severity of *Pneumocystis jirovecii* pneumonia: a cross-sectional study. Medicine (Baltimore) 94:e768
15. Walzer PD, Eans HE, Copas AJ, Edwards SG, Grant AD, Miller RF (2008) Early predictors of mortality from *Pneumocystis jirovecii* pneumonia in HIV-infected patients: 1985–2006. Clin Infect Dis 46:625–633

16. Brunetti E, Heller T, Richter J, Kaminstein D, Youkee D, Giordani MT, Goblirsch S, Tamarozzi F (2016) Application of ultrasonography in the diagnosis of infectious diseases in resource-limited settings. Curr Infect Dis Rep 18:6
17. Bélard S, Tamarozzi F, Bustinduy AL, Wallrauch C, Grobusch MP, Kuhn W, Brunetti E, Joekes E, Heller T (2016) Point-of-care ultrasound assessment of tropical infectious diseases—a review of applications and perspectives. Am J Trop Med Hyg 94:8–21
18. Volpicelli G, Elbarbary M, Blaivas M, Lichtenstein DA, Mathis G, Kirkpatrick AW, Melniker L, Gargani L, Noble VE, Via G, Dean A, Tsung JW, Soldati G, Copetti R, Bouhemad B, Reissig A, Agricola E, Rouby JJ, Albelot C, Liteplo A, Sargsyan A, Silva F, Hoppmann R, Breitkreutz R, Seibel A, Neri L, Storti E, Petrovic T, International Liaison Commtee on Lung Ultrasound (ILC-LUS) for International Consensus Conference on Lung Ultrasound (ICC-LUS) (2012) International evidence-based recommendations for point-of-care lung ultrasound. Intensive Care Med 38:577–591
19. Settnes OP, Genner J (1986) Pneumocystis carinii in human lungs at autopsy. Scand J Infect Dis 18:489–496

13

The Assessment of Competency in Thoracic Sonography (ACTS) scale: validation of a tool for point-of-care ultrasound

Scott J. Millington*, Robert T. Arntfield, Robert Jie Guo, Seth Koenig, Pierre Kory, Vicki Noble, Haney Mallemat and Jordan R. Schoenherr

Abstract

Background: The rapid adoption of point-of-care ultrasound (POCUS) has created a need to develop assessment tools to ensure that learners can competently use these technologies. In this study, the authors developed and tested a rating scale to assess the quality of point-of-care thoracic ultrasound studies performed by novices. In Phase 1, the Assessment of Competency in Thoracic Sonography (ACTS) scale was developed based on structured interviews with subject matter experts. The tool was then piloted on a small series of ultrasound studies in Phase 2. In Phase 3 the tool was applied to a sample of 150 POCUS studies performed by ten learners; performance was then assessed by two independent raters.

Results: Evidence for the content validity of the ACTS scale was provided by a consensus exercise wherein experts agreed on the general principles and specific items that make up the scale. The tool demonstrated reasonable inter-rater reliability despite minimal requirements for evaluator training and displayed evidence of good internal structure, with related scale items correlating well with each other. Analysis of the aggregate learning curves suggested a rapid early improvement in learner performance with slower improvement after approximately 25–30 studies.

Conclusions: The ACTS scale provides a straightforward means to assess learner performance. Our results support the conclusion that the tool is an effective means of making valid judgments regarding competency in point-of-care thoracic ultrasound, and that the majority of learner improvement occurs during their first 25–30 practice studies.

Keywords: Point-of-care, Thoracic ultrasound, Assessment tools, Education

Background

The term point-of-care ultrasound (POCUS) refers to a goal-directed ultrasound (US) exam performed directly by the treating physician in order to answer a well-defined question relevant to the immediate care of a patient. In certain clinical circumstances, POCUS has been shown to improve clinical outcomes (as in penetrating thoracic trauma; [1]), to increase patient safety (as with the insertion of central venous catheters; [2]), and to improve diagnostic accuracy over current standards of care (as in the detection of pneumothorax; [3]). A recent international statement written by experts from twelve critical care societies agreed that POCUS should be mandatory in the training of critical care physicians [4]. Despite the increased interest, methods for fostering development of these competencies are highly variable between centers with little agreement on how to train and assess learner proficiency [5].

One method for improving consistency is the development of assessment instruments. The development of an instrument requires that a group of experts come together to formalize their knowledge in a given domain by identifying features that they believe are related to competency. By examining learner performance over a number of training sessions, we can test to see whether experts are correct in their assumptions about the facets

*Correspondence: smillington@toh.ca
Division of Critical Care, University of Ottawa, 501 Smyth Road, Box 207, Ottawa, ON K1H 8L6, Canada

of a competency. Once an assessment instrument has been formalized, it can be used to monitor the development of learner competency and evaluate whether an educational intervention is effective at increasing proficiency. It would also support quality assurance and patient safety initiatives in general by ensuring that scan quality is adequate.

Ultrasound competency and its development

Thoracic ultrasound represents a novel and interesting instrument in the POCUS toolkit [6]. It can, for example, help make the distinction between such clinically similar entities as cardiogenic and non-cardiogenic pulmonary edema [7]. Whereas most other ultrasound subtypes were developed by other specialist groups and later modified for use by acute care physicians, thoracic ultrasound was created and studied primarily by physicians in intensive care units and emergency departments. This fact, coupled with the relatively short history of thoracic ultrasound, means that the modality has been relatively understudied from an educational point of view.

The development of assessment instruments for POCUS has precedents. Using similar methods, we previously developed a scale to assess cardiac POCUS competency [8], demonstrating that cardiac ultrasound competency was associated with two main domains: Image Generation and Image Interpretation. Image Generation reflects a competency involving a learner's knowledge of anatomy in combination with their visuospatial reasoning abilities. In contrast, while Image Interpretation requires that images have been generated successfully, it additionally necessitates clinical knowledge and diagnostic experience. Subsequently, we deployed that same tool to map out the typical cardiac ultrasound learning curves for novices [9]. For these reasons, the adoption of a similar approach in the context of thoracic ultrasound appears principled.

In the present study, we develop a scale capable of rapidly assessing the quality of point-of-care thoracic scans that requires minimal training in its application. As in our previous studies that examined cardiac POCUS we focused on construct validity, defined as the extent to which the feature of a test or scale can adequately measure what it purports to measure [10–13]. We use Messick's [12] validation framework to provide evidence for the ACTS scale's ability to measure the underlying features of POCUS competency. In the context of the present study, we first consider whether experts can reach a consensus on the features of competency in lung ultrasonography and whether multiple independent raters reliably produce similar ratings using the ACTS instrument (content evidence). We then consider how learners' performance for each component of the ACTS scale is related or unrelated to one another (internal structure evidence). For instance, scores obtained from subscales for proximate positions should be strongly related to one another whereas scores obtained from subscales for distal positions should be weakly or unrelated to one another. Finally, as we have developed the ACTS scale to be able to detect changes in competency over the course of training, we should obtain a learning curve that shows evidence of improvements in performance from earlier to later stages of training (response process evidence).

Methods

Phase 1: Developing the ACTS assessment tool

The ACTS scale content was developed in a series of three structured teleconferences with POCUS experts from across North America, most of whom had participated in the development and validation of our previous cardiac tool [8]. These teleconferences identified a comprehensive list of features and dimensions that define lung ultrasound competency (thematic saturation), considered what constitutes both perfect and minimally acceptable performance for thoracic POCUS (standard setting), and identified possible obstacles to implementing the use of lung ultrasound scale.

Following the approach of our previous scale [8], the ACTS tool (Fig. 1) divides assessment into two domains: (1) Image Generation and (2) Image Interpretation (Fig. 2). Image Generation subscale assesses image quality for each of the 8 typical thoracic views on a 6-point scale. Image Interpretation subscale uses a binary pass/fail assessment to decide whether an expert is able to assess each of the 4 common thoracic pathologies (pneumothorax, interstitial syndrome, consolidation, and pleural effusion) based on the images provided.

Additionally, we asked the experts to interpret the images (in absence of any clinical information), providing their opinion on the most likely diagnosis, any secondary diagnoses, and their relative confidence in making these judgments.

Phase 2: Piloting the tool

A pilot ACTS tool was circulated to the same group of six experts and modified based on their feedback. A small series of POCUS studies were then tested by selecting a random sample of ten thoracic exams from the London Health Sciences Center database (London, ON, Canada), removing patient identifiers, and distributing them electronically. Ethics approval was granted by the London Research Ethics Board. After the same ten studies had been scored by each expert, a video conference call was held to review each study in an effort to improve the tool as well as to standardize the criteria used to judge the studies.

Score Sheet

Assessment of Competency in Thoracic Sonography (ACTS) Scale

Date:	Evaluator:
Trainee:	Study #:

Image Generation — Please rate each individual view for image quality based on the following scale:

	Not obtained	Image quality too poor to permit meaningful interpretation		Suboptimal image quality, but basic image interpretation possible		Good image quality, meaningful image interpretation easy	
L1	0	1	2	3	4	5	
L2	0	1	2	3	4	5	
L3	0	1	2	3	4	5	
L4	0	1	2	3	4	5	
R1	0	1	2	3	4	5	
R2	0	1	2	3	4	5	
R3	0	1	2	3	4	5	
R4	0	1	2	3	4	5	/40

Image Interpretation — Based on all the images presented, do you feel able to interpret the following:

	Image quality does not permit meaningful interpretation (right thorax)	Image quality permits meaningful interpretation (right thorax)		Image quality does not permit meaningful interpretation (left thorax)	Image quality permits meaningful interpretation (left thorax)	
Presence or absence of a pneumothorax	0	1		0	1	
Presence or absence of an interstitial syndrome	0	1		0	1	
Presence or absence of a consolidation	0	1		0	1	
Presence or absence of a pleural effusion	0	1		0	1	/8

What would you suspect is the most likely diagnosis?

Primary diagnosis	Normal study		Secondary	Normal study		Confidence Level (50-100 by 10)
(choose one)	Pneumothorax		diagnoses	Pneumothorax		
	Interstitial syndrome		(chose 0-6)	Interstitial syndrome		
	Consolidation			Consolidation		
	Pleural effusion			Pleural effusion		
	Atelectasis			Atelectasis		

Fig. 1 The Assessment of Competency in Thoracic Sonography (ACTS) tool

Phase 3: Tool validation

Thoracic ultrasound studies produced by a group of ten POCUS learners at Western University in London, ON were selected for use in the study. The learners consisted of physician trainees in either emergency medicine or critical care, and were selected based on the criteria of: (1) having had basic training in POCUS, (2) currently participating in the local POCUS training program in London, ON, and (3) having recorded 50 thoracic POCUS studies as part of the local training program. All ultrasound images were stored in the local archiving system (Qpath Software, Telexy Healthcare, Port Coquitlam, BC). A series of representative video clips were extracted by taking the set of available US studies from each learner and sampling their portfolio of thoracic studies at regular intervals. These studies were then anonymized (with both patient and operator information removed), merged into the larger pool of sampled studies from all learners, randomized, and then distributed to the experts for evaluation using the ACTS tool. Each study was evaluated by a pair of experts and all ratings were subsequently pooled for statistical analysis.

Statistical analysis

To investigate the validity of the ACTS scale, we reduced the dataset by obtaining average scores and their standard deviations (Table 1, discussed below). For our analysis of the content of the ACTS Scale, we examined inter-rater reliability between experts when assessing the US studies. High levels of inter-rater reliability would suggest that the ACTS scale is being used in an equivalent manner by raters, and is thus used by multiple raters in a similar manner. Second, we assessed the internal structure of the scale by examining how the eight ACTS scale items were related (Table 2). Our assumption that POCUS competency might be defined by two underlying factors (Image Generation and Image Interpretation) would be supported if ratings of items within a subscale were highly correlated. Finally, learners' POCUS competency should improve over time. If the average learner performance

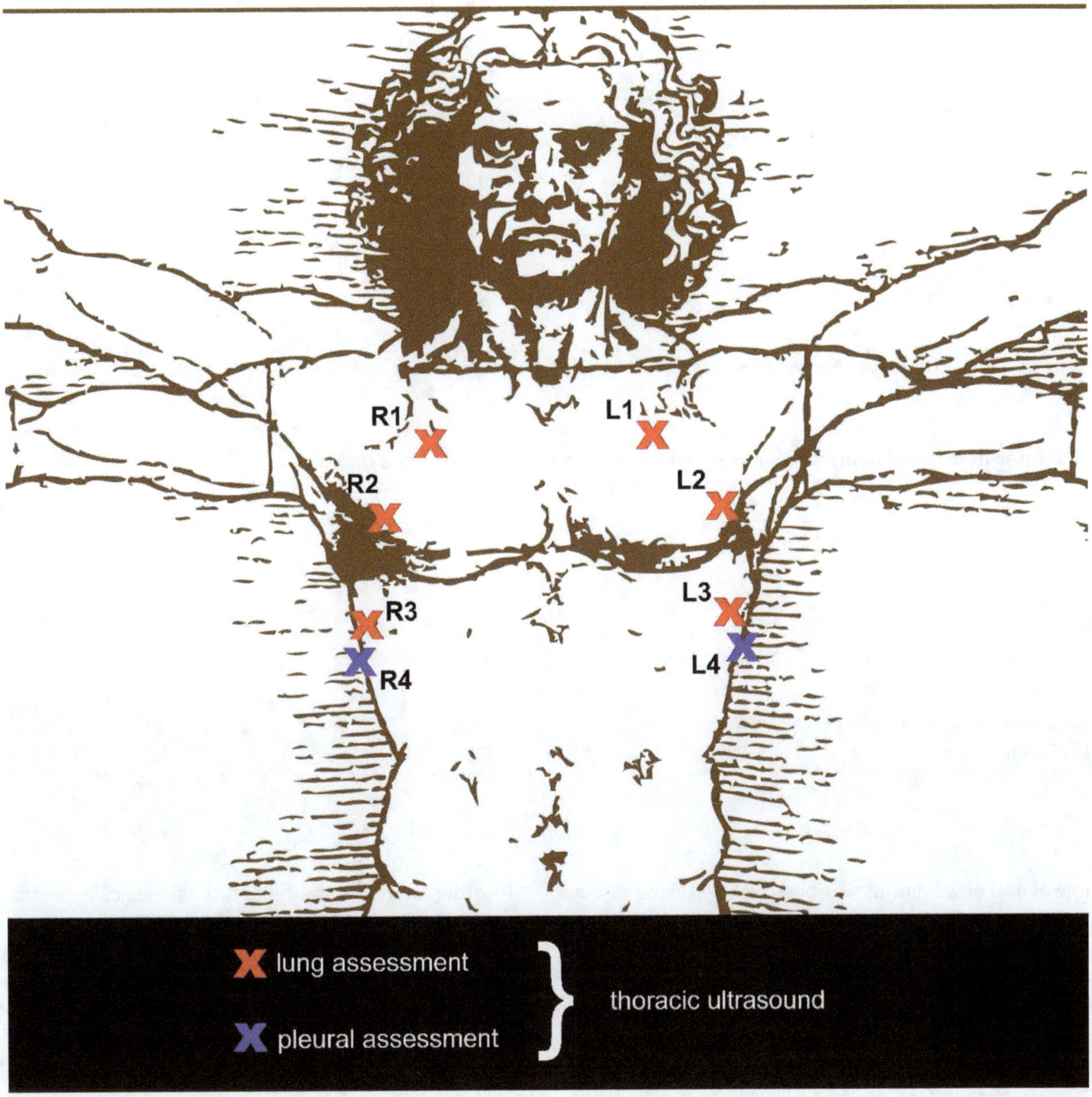

Fig. 2 The eight common view for thoracic ultrasound

increased from earlier to later stages of training, this would provide evidence that the ACTS scale adequately assesses the response process of learners. Taken together, multiple sources of evidence go toward demonstrating the validity of the ACTS Scale.

Results

Content validation and content experts

Evidence for the validity of the content of the ACTS tool was examined in terms of the extent to which experts agreed on the content of the rating scales and the extent to which raters provided comparable ratings on those scales. The structured interviews and subsequent expert discussions revealed that there appeared to be widespread consensus regarding POCUS in general and thoracic POCUS specifically. There was also consensus on Image Generation and Image Interpretation as the two broad determinants of basic thoracic POCUS competency, with the skill set of clinical integration being a necessary but more advanced skill.

Raters and scale reliability

In order to examine the reliability of the ACTS scale, we assessed the extent to which each pair of expert raters produced similar responses (inter-rater reliability). Raters differed for each learner and for each training session. A

Table 1 Descriptive statistics for standardized scores on ACTS subscales for both the right and left analyses

ACTS scale item	Rating (*L*)			Rating (*R*)		
	Mean	Range	SD	Mean	Range	SD
V1	.8173	0–5	.235	.7853	0–5	.278
V2	.7873	0–5	.257	.6673	0–5	.381
V3	.6540	0–5	.320	.6040	0–5	.358
V4	.5993	0–5	.363	.5567	0–5	.387
Pneumothorax	.9500	0–1	.218	.8867	0–1	.318
Interstitial syndrome	.9300	0–1	.256	.8967	0–1	.305
Consolidation	.7067	0–1	.456	.6967	0–1	.460
Pleural effusion	.7367	0–1	.441	.7600	0–1	.428

Ratings are provided in rescaled values (.0–1.0) whereas the range is reported using the range provided on subscale used to assess learners (i.e., 0–5 and 0–1)

Table 2 Inter-item correlations for mean learner RACE ratings collapsed across raters

	1	2	3	4	5	6	7	8
V1_IG	–							
V2_IG	.415**	–						
V3_IG	.181**	.486**	–					
V4_IG	.088	.290**	.639**	–				
Pneumothorax	.487**	.274**	.143*	.042	–			
Interstitial syndrome	.417**	.351**	.322**	.239**	.554**	–		
Consolidation	.183**	.251**	.584**	.559**	.182**	.385**	–	
Pleural effusion	.132*	.190**	.618**	.572**	.157*	.354**	.778**	–

* $p < .05$

** $p < .01$

sample of 150 observations was obtained, by taking fifteen studies from each of the ten learners. These ratings were randomly sampled over the course of the training sessions in order to model an overall learning curve (see below). Given that the Image Generation and Image Interpretation subscales are scored differently (using a 6-point and binary scale, respectively), ratings were rescaled to a range of .0–1.0 in order to compare the two subscales (e.g., items on the Image Interpretation scale that were rated as 0, 1, 2, 3, 4, and 5 would be rescaled to values of .0, .2, .4, .6, .8, and 1.0).

Table 1 presents the basic descriptive statistics for the ACTS subscales, with a few critical results. First, raters used the full scoring range of each of the subscales. Second, comparable values were obtained for both left and right images for the Image Generation subscale items suggesting that learners' performance was nearly equivalent in generating left- and right-sided images. Third, learners received higher ratings for Image Interpretation items for left-side images relative to right-side images, suggesting that right-side images might be more difficult for experts to interpret or for learners to perform.

In order to assess the reliability of the scale, we examine the scores provided by the two raters assigned to each case for each of the learners. The resulting Cronbach's Alpha ($\alpha = .791$) obtained by comparing overall standardized ratings for each learner reflects an acceptable overall level of inter-rater reliability for the ACTS scale as a whole. An assessment of individual subscales revealed that items assessing Image Generation produced a good degree of agreement between raters ($\alpha = .824$) whereas Image Interpretation had an acceptable degree of agreement between raters ($\alpha = .709$).

Internal scale structure

While the previous analysis of correlations between scores from expert raters suggests that the scale was used in a consistent manner across different raters, it leaves unexamined the relationship between the 12 individual scale items (8 Image Generation and 4 Image Interpretation). After average across raters, the mean score for each of the 12 items was included in an inter-item correlation analysis. This analysis was conducted in order to examine whether ACTS items that should logically be related (e.g., imaging Lung View 1 and Lung View 2) will exhibit a stronger correlation than those items that are not as closely related (e.g., imaging Lung View 1 and Lung View 4).

Image Generation subscale items (items 1 through 8) and Image Interpretation subscale items (items 9 through 12) were included together in a correlational analysis. As Table 2 demonstrates, there is evidence that related items tend to strongly and positively correlate with one another. A critical outcome of the ACTS scale is evidenced in the correlations between items in the Image Generation subscale that measured a learner's ability to generate images. Notably, the strength of the correlation decreased as a function of distance from one imaging location to another, as would be expected. We also found that the presence of pleural effusion was correlated with the image quality for viewing positions 3 and 4. As these locations are typical sites where clinicians investigate pleural effusion, it provides additional support for the validity of the ACTS scale.

Learning process and construct validity

To assess whether learners' POCUS competence increased over training, we examined whether there was evidence of change in performance over the course of training. A mean was obtained for each training sessions if available (i.e., the random sampling of learner performance did not always produce ratings for the same sessions for each learner).

First, we examined learning for the overall ACTS score for each ultrasound study collapsing across mean score across subscale components. We selected models into examine whether (1) learning increased systematically over the course of the period of observation (linear function), (2) learning increased rapidly during initial phases of training and stabilized thereafter (power function), and (3) learning proceeded more slowly during initial phases of training, rapidly increased, and then reached a performance asymptote (sigmoid function; where learners improved up to a certain point and then reached a plateau). The three models fit for ACTS scale for overall performance are presented in Fig. 3. While each of the models provided a comparable fit, the power function provided the best fit. This indicates that learners' performance increased rapidly throughout the early stages of in training (roughly sessions 1–25) but that later stages of training (beyond session 35) produced only moderate improvements in performance.

Second, given the observed differences in the Image Generation and Image Interpretation subscales, we analyzed participants learner curves for each of the subcomponents separately (Table 3). For the Image Generation subscale, slightly better fits were obtained for both power and sigmoid functions. Conforming to the results of our previous study examining POCUS competency development [9],

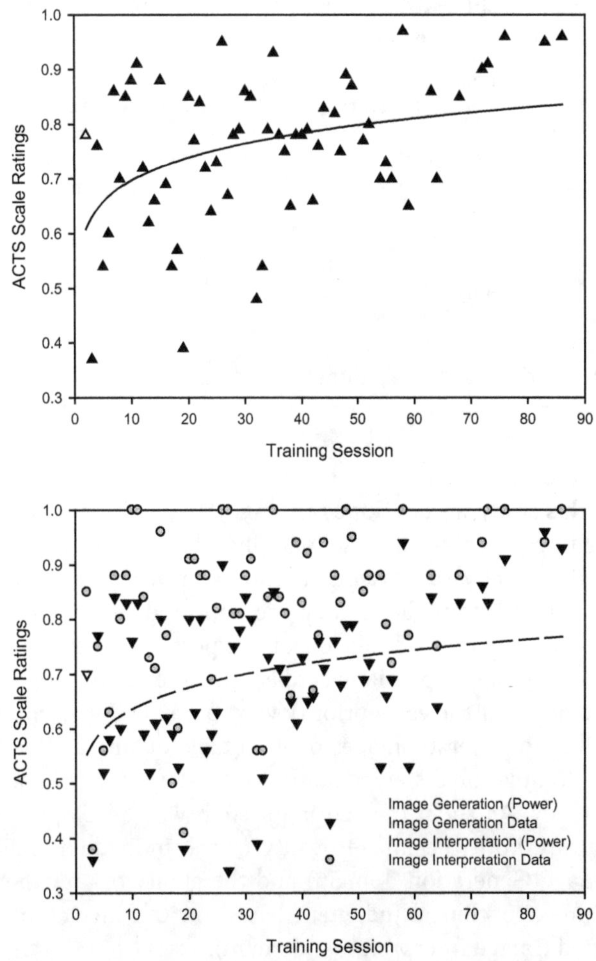

Fig. 3 Learning curves for mean overall performance across ACTS subscales (top) and Image Generation and Image Interpretation subscales (bottom). Best-fit power functions are plotted in each

this might suggest that learners benefit from early training, but after a sufficient number of session their performance no longer improves. Given that the power function provided an equivalent fit to the sigmoid function while using fewer parameters[1], this suggests that the power function reflects a more conservative model of competency development. For the Image Interpretation subscale, the power function also offered the best fit, again suggesting that the abilities that underpin this portion of the scale improve with early training efforts. Thus, given the superior fits of the power functions in the case of both Image Generation and Image Interpretation results, this suggests that the largest effect occurs very early in training (sessions 1–25) and decreases but continued thereafter (beyond session 35). However, additional studies with more learners will need to

[1] The more parameters that are included in a model, the more likely it will fit the data. Models with fewer parameters are therefore preferred on the grounds of parsimony.

Table 3 ***R*-squared measures for curve fits for mean performance for all participants**

	Image Generation score	Image Interpretation score	Overall score
Linear	.1696 (.133)	.1402 (.139)	.1816 (.123)
Power (2)	.2156 (.132)	.2156 (.130)	.1935 (.124)
Sigmoid (4)	.2170 (.131)	.1403 (.142)	.1976 (.124)

Standard error of the estimate is presented in parentheses

be conducted to examine the generalizability of this finding.

Discussion

In this study we developed the ACTS scale, a rapid scoring instrument for lung sonography which can be applied while directly supervising a learner or while reviewing ultrasound scans after they are captured by an image archiving system. Based on our expert interviews, and building on our previous cardiac ultrasound tool [8], we decided that the early priority was to assess the learners' ability to generate images of acceptable quality as this is the foundational step required to develop POCUS competency. As such, the scoring system was developed to capture both the image quality of the individual views (Image Generation domain) and the ability of an expert to make a clinical judgment based on the images provided (Image Interpretation domain).

There are several lines of evidence that provide support for the validity of the ACTS tool, including the high degree of consensus achieved within group of experts assembled. The group of six experts who evaluated the studies received a minimal amount of training, yet still achieved a good level of inter-rater reliability, suggesting that the tool can be used in a wide variety of clinical settings. While individual assessment instruments must be developed based on the demands of the particular clinical environment, ACTS appears to be an effective instrument to monitor the development of competency in lung ultrasonography.

There were strong, positive correlations observed within the measures of the Image Generation domain as well as similar trends within the measures of the Image Interpretation domain. The correlations between items within each of the subscales suggest that these assessment dimensions both make contributions to POCUS competency. Predictably, within the Image Generation subscale, images that were taken closer together (for example View 1 and View 2) were defined by much higher correlations than those images taken further apart (such as View 1 and View 4). This finding also supports the validity of the elements measured by the ACTS tool.

The correlations which were particularly strong can be interpreted clinically in a straightforward manner. For example, the strong correlation seen between the diagnosis of a pneumothorax and the quality of the R1 and L1 images follows from the fact that this condition is usually detected by placing in the ultrasound probe in those positions in typical clinical practice. Similarly, the detection of a pleural effusion correlated well with image quality ratings in the 3rd and 4th positions. Given that these are the typical anatomic locations where clinicians investigate for effusions, it provides further support for ACTS ability to identify lung sonography competency. Moreover, the absence of correlations between certain view positions and the presence of certain pathophysiologies provide additional support. For example, strong correlation between pneumothorax and the 4th scanning position or consolidation and the 1st scanning position would not be expected based on thoracic anatomy, and were not found in our study.

Our curve fitting analysis suggested that learning occurred throughout the course of the training sessions. In comparing three possible models of learning (linear, power, and sigmoid), we observed that a power model provided the best fit for the overall ACTS score as well as the scores for individual subscales. This suggests that learners rapidly acquired lung ultrasonography competencies earlier in training (sessions 1–25) but that competency development leveled off (after approximately session 35). This suggests that while additional training might be beneficial for learners, educators might wish to introduce additional training techniques or change the nature of the feedback provided to learners following 30 practice ultrasound studies. For instance, educators might wish to include simulation that includes diagnostic and treatment elements. Compared to our cardiac assessment tool [8], learners performed better with thoracic ultrasound early in their training. One possible explanation is that the small sample size or the fact that all learners were from a single center yielded an unrepresentative sample. For instance, there might be a self-selection bias wherein learners had better existing visuospatial abilities. Alternatively, previous US experience (cardiac and abdominal ultrasound) might have increased performance in the thoracic POCUS study conducted here. Future studies will need to use more participants and control for individual differences in general and specific clinical experience and knowledge.

Our study has other limitations that should be acknowledged. Given that evidence for validity was obtained in only one context, further work is needed to ensure that the tool is generalizable to other environments. Given that the study was conducted with learners in London, ON, it is entirely possible that the joint influence that educators have on the curriculum and the instrument would make it easier for learners to acquire the specific skills measured by ACTS. The fact that experts were drawn from a number of institutions suggests that this possibility is unlikely, however, it might be the case that the small number of experts (6) lead to a bias sample. As there continues to be disagreement in lung ultrasonography in general [14], this remains a real possibility. Our study assessed only expert ratings and did not incorporate any interpretation data from the learners who generated the actual studies; such a comparison would have been most interesting but was unfortunately unavailable to us. Finally, in our study the binary Image Interpretation subscale performed less well than Image Generation subscale, which was based on a 6-point rating scale. The binary scale was chosen for convenience, but it is certainly possible that lower reliability scores reflect the general disadvantage of checklists relative to general rating scales [15]. An assessment tool based on a rating scale for Image Interpretation as well as Image Generation would might have performed better, albeit at the cost of increased complexity.

Future studies should ideally compare the ACTS scale to other assessment methods such as the Objective Structured Clinical Examination or the Mini Clinical Examination to examine the relationship of our instrument to other instruments (providing evidence for relationship to other variables) as well as the consequences of implementing POCUS assessment on educators and learners (providing evidence of consequences; [12]). A larger study involving multiple centers would also help to allay concerns about generalizability.

Conclusions

Overall, the results of the present study support the use of the ACTS scale to assess learners' competency in point-of-care thoracic ultrasound, and suggests that the majority of learning occurs during the first 25–30 practice studies.

Abbreviations

POCUS: point-of-care ultrasound; ACTS: Assessment of Competency in Thoracic Sonography.

Authors' contributions

SJM: responsible for the design, organization, and primary authorship. JRS: responsible for design and statistical analysis. RTA, PK, VN, SK, and HM: responsible for creation of the scoring tool and study ratings. RJG: responsible for preparation of the scoring tool and the study rating score sheets. All authors read and approved the final manuscript.

Acknowledgements

None.

References

1. Plummer D, Brunette D, Asinger R, Ruiz E (1992) Emergency department echocardiography improves outcome in penetrating cardiac injury. Ann Emerg Med 21(6):709–712
2. McGee DC, Gould MK (2003) Preventing complications of central venous catheterization. N Engl J Med 348:1123–1133
3. Lichtenstein D, Mezière G, Biderman P, Gepner A (1999) The comet-tail artifact: an ultrasound sign ruling out pneumothorax. Intensive Care Med 25(4):383–388
4. Mayo P (2009) American College of Chest Physicians/La Société de Réanimation de Langue Française statement on competence in critical care ultrasonography. Chest 135:1050–1060
5. Quintard H, Philip I, Ichai C (2011) French survey on current use of ultrasound in the critical care unit: ECHOREA. Ann Fr Anesth Reanim 30(11):e69–e73
6. Volpicelli G (2013) Lung sonography. Journal of ultrasound medicine 32:165–171
7. Copetti R, Soldati G, Copetti P (2008) Chest sonography: a useful tool to differentiate acute cardiogenic pulmonary edema from acute respiratory distress syndrome. Cardiovasc Ultrasound 6:16
8. Millington SJ, Arntfield RT, Hewak M, Hamstra SJ, Beaulieu Y, Hibbert B, Koenig S, Kory P, Mayo P, Schoenherr JR (2016) The rapid assessment of competency in echocardiography scale. J Ultrasound Med 35(7):1457–1463
9. Millington SJ, Hewak M, Arntfield RT, Beaulieu Y, Hibbert B, Koenig S, Kory P, Mayo P, Schoenherr JR (2017) Outcomes from extensive training in critical care echocardiography: identifying the optimal number of practice studies required to achieve competency. J Crit Care 40:99–102
10. Cronbach LJ (1975) Beyond the two disciplines of scientific psychology. Am Psychol 30:116–127
11. Kane MT (1992) An argument-based approach to validity. Psychol Bull 112:527–535
12. Messick S (1995) Validation of inferences from persons' responses and performances as scientific inquiry into score meaning. Am Psychol 50:741–749
13. American Educational Research Association (1999) Standards for educational and psychological testing. American Educational Research Association, Washington, DC
14. Volpicelli G et al (2012) International evidence-based recommendations for point-of-care lung ultrasound. Intensive Care Med 38:577–591
15. Regehr G, MacRae H, Reznick R, Szalay D (1998) Comparing the psychometric properties of checklists and global rating scales for assessing performance on an OSCE-format examination. Acad Med 73:993–997

14

The impact of heart, lung and diaphragmatic ultrasound on prediction of failed extubation from mechanical ventilation in critically ill patients: a prospective observational pilot study

Kavi Haji[1,2*], Darsim Haji[3,4], David J. Canty[4,5,6], Alistair G. Royse[7,8], Cameron Green[1] and Colin F. Royse[7,9]

Abstract

Background: Failed extubation from mechanical ventilation in critically ill patients is multifactorial, complex and not well understood. We aimed to identify whether combined transthoracic echocardiography, lung and diaphragmatic ultrasound can predict extubation failure in critically ill patients.

Results: Fifty-three participants who were intubated >48 h and deemed by the treating intensivist ready for extubation underwent a 60-min pre-extubation weaning trial (pressure support $\leq$ 10 cmH_2O and positive end expiratory pressure 5 cmH_2O). Prior to extubation, data collected included ultrasound assessment of left ventricular ejection fraction, left atrial area, early diastolic trans-mitral flow velocity wave (*E*), early diastolic trans-mitral flow velocity wave/late diastolic trans-mitral flow velocity wave (*E/A*), early diastolic trans-mitral flow velocity wave/early diastolic mitral annulus velocity (*E/E′*), interatrial septal motion, lung loss of aeration score and diaphragm movement. At the end of the weaning trial, the rapid shallow breathing index and serum B-type natriuretic peptide concentration were measured. Success and failure of weaning was assessed by defined criteria. Decision to extubate was at the discretion of the treating intensivist. Failure of extubation was defined as re-intubation, non-invasive ventilation or death within 48 h after extubation. Of 53 extubated participants, 11 failed extubation. Failed extubation was associated with diabetes, ischaemic heart disease, higher *E/E′* (OR 1.27, 95% CI 1.05–1.54), left atrial area (OR 1.14, CI 1.02–1.28), fixed rightward curvature of the interatrial septum (OR 12.95, CI 2.73–61.41), and higher loss of aeration score of anterior and lateral regions of the lungs (OR 1.41, CI 1.01–1.82).

Conclusions: Failed extubation in mechanically ventilated patients is more prevalent if markers of left ventricular diastolic dysfunction and loss of lung aeration are present.

Keywords: Weaning, Echocardiography, Ultrasound, Lung, Diaphragm, RSBI

Background

Weaning failure is defined as failing a spontaneous breathing trial or developing a post-extubation respiratory distress that requires re-intubation or non-invasive ventilation within 48 h following extubation [1]. Weaning failure is common and time consuming with approximately 40% of the total ventilation time in "difficult to wean" patients is devoted to weaning [2]. Weaning failure is associated with worse outcome [3], increased risk of myocardial ischaemia [4] and perhaps psychological trauma [5].

Identification of reliable predictors of weaning failure may represent potential avenues of treatment that could

*Correspondence: kevee@bigpond.com
[1] Department of the Intensive Care Unit, Frankton Hospital, PO Box 52, Frankston, VIC 3199, Australia
Full list of author information is available at the end of the article

reduce the incidence of weaning failure and its associated morbidity. Unfortunately, the pathophysiology of weaning failure is complex and is incompletely understood. Known risk factors of weaning failure have considerable crossover, especially those related to the heart, lungs and diaphragm. Weaning is comparable to a cardiac stress exercise where it is likely to increase the heart rate, the pulmonary artery occlusion pressure, which results in myocardial stretch and may increase cardiac output [6]. The myocardial stretch is evidenced by increased release of neurohormone, B-type natriuretic peptide (BNP), which therefore has been suggested as a useful predictor of weaning failure [7]. Known predictors of weaning failure include chronic obstructive airway disease [1], cardiac failure [8–10], lung de-recruitment [11], positive fluid balance [12], pneumonia [12] and diaphragmatic dysfunction [13]. Rapid shallow breathing index (RSBI) is a clinical predictor of failure of weaning from mechanical ventilation and it is widely used in clinical research and in practice [14].

Ultrasound of multiple organ systems is becoming more commonplace in the intensive care unit (ICU) setting. Ultrasound has been used to identify cardiac, respiratory or diaphragmatic risk factors of weaning failure [8, 11, 13]. Further, ultrasound may be helpful in providing a visual assessment of cardiorespiratory state at different phases of weaning [15]. Therefore, a combined structured transthoracic echocardiogram (TTE), lung and diaphragm ultrasound examination added to conventional clinical predictors could be a useful tool to increase the accuracy in predicting weaning outcome and extubation failure. Currently, there are limited data investigating this.

The primary aim of this pilot study was to determine which ultrasound, or clinical and biochemical indicators, were associated with weaning failure. Data from this pilot study will be used to construct future clinical trials.

Methods

Study design and setting

This single-centre, prospective observational pilot study was conducted at a 15-bed, level-III ICU that receives approximately 1500 admissions of medical and surgical presentations per year.

Participants

Recruitment was performed between June 2014 and April 2016, when the primary researcher was available (convenience sampling). Participants aged 18 years or older who were mechanically ventilated for longer than 48 h and considered ready for extubation by the treating intensivist were considered eligible for recruitment. Participants were excluded if they had a diagnosis of brain death, were ventilating through a tracheostomy or if extubation was for palliation. Written informed consent was obtained from the person responsible for decision-making on behalf of the patient.

Summary of study conduct

Participants were considered eligible for inclusion when participants fulfilled the criteria for weaning from mechanical ventilation defined below and authorized by the treating intensivist (Fig. 1). After informed written consent obtained, a 60-min weaning trial was commenced. The primary researcher (KH) performed and documented ultrasound findings of the heart, lungs and diaphragm as defined below, at the beginning of the weaning trial. At the end of the weaning trial, a sample of arterial blood was collected for blood gas analysis and for BNP measurement (The iSTAT Point of Care Analyzer, Abbott Point of Care Inc., Princeton, Ontario, Canada). The primary endpoint of the study was failure of extubation, which was defined as re-intubation or non-invasive ventilation within 48 h after extubation.

Weaning trial

Pressure support is a spontaneous mode of ventilation where the patient breathes spontaneously and the ventilator supports the breathing with a preset pressure value for every breath. Decremented pressure support ventilation is the standard mode of weaning in our unit. Extubation at pressure support up to 10 cmH_2O is an acceptable practice in our unit and a spontaneous breathing trial using T-tube is not mandated for weaning [16–20]. The criteria for eligibility for the weaning trial included resolution or improvement in the disease that led to commencement of mechanical ventilation; FiO_2 $\leq 30\%$; pressure support ≤ 10 cmH_2O; PEEP ≤ 5 cmH_2O; tidal volume ≥ 5 ml/kg; respiratory rate <35 breaths/

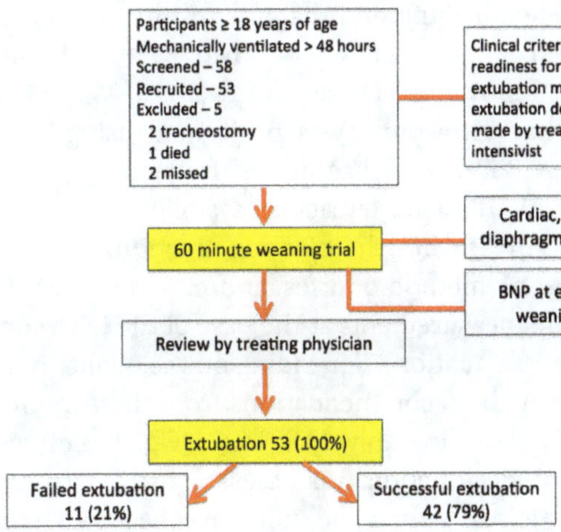

Fig. 1 The participants' flow diagram

min; requirement of low inotropic or vasopressor support; light level of sedation (Richmond Agitation Sedation Score between −2 and +2) [21]; ability to cough; and absence of excessive bronchial secretions. The weaning trial comprised 60 min of pressure support of 0 or ≤ 10 cmH_2O if required, to achieve a respiratory rate < 35 breaths/min and a tidal volume of ≥ 5 ml/kg [16]. Positive end expiratory pressure remained at 5 cmH_2O during the trial.

The weaning trial was considered failed if the following criteria were observed during the trial: excessive diaphoresis, Richmond Agitation and Sedation Score of ≤ −3 or ≥ +3, evidence of increasing respiratory effort (dyspnea, increased accessory muscle activity, thoraco-abdominal paradoxical movement and facial signs of distress), arterial oxygen partial pressure ≤ 60 mmHg or oxygen saturation < 90% on fractional inspired oxygen ≥ 0.4, CO_2 partial arterial pressure > 50 mmHg, or an increase in CO_2 partial arterial pressure by ≥ 8 mmHg, pH < 7.32 or a decrease in pH by ≥ 0.07 pH units, RSBI > 105 breath/min/l, respiratory rate > 35 breaths/min, heart rate > 140 beats/min or increased by ≥ 20%, systolic blood pressure > 180 mmHg or increased by ≥ 20%, systolic blood pressure < 90 mmHg or new cardiac arrhythmias. After the completion of the weaning trial, the treating intensivist reviewed the participant for final assessment before extubation. The treating intensivist was blinded to the ultrasound findings. The decision whether to extubate the participant was determined by the treating intensivist irrespective of the weaning trial outcome. Failed extubation was defined as the requirement for re-intubation, non-invasive ventilatory support or death within 48 h after extubation.

Cardiac ultrasound

Ultrasound was performed by the primary researcher (KH), who held a recognized ultrasound certification and competence in TTE and an appropriate training and experience in lung and diaphragm ultrasound. The ultrasound machine used was a Vivid E9 (GE Healthcare, 9900 Innovation Drive, Wauwatosa, WI 53226, USA). Cardiac ultrasound was performed using sector phased array 3Sc-RS cardiac probe (frequency range of 1.3–4.0 MHz). The left ventricular systolic function was assessed by measuring the ejection fraction, using biplane Simpson's method of discs, and/or acquisition 2-D and M-Mode measurements at the base of the left ventricle (Teichholtz equation), depending on the quality of the images, as per the recommendations from the American Society of Echocardiography (ASE) [22] (Fig. 2). Left ventricular diastolic function was assessed using left atrial area in participants who did not have haemodynamically significant mitral regurgitation or atrial fibrillation (Fig. 2), early diastolic trans-mitral flow velocity wave (*E*), late diastolic trans-mitral flow velocity wave (*A*), early diastolic mitral annulus velocity E' (average septal and lateral E'), *E*/*A*, *E* deceleration time, E/E' (Fig. 3). Additionally, the interatrial septal shape and movement was measured from the parasternal and subcostal short axis, and apical four chamber views, and used as a marker of left atrial filling pressure (Fig. 4) [23–25]. Fixed interatrial septal curvature to the right throughout the cardiac cycle is predictive of a pulmonary artery occlusion pressure > 15 mmHg, while reversal of the septum from right to left during mid-systole (referred to as "mid-systolic reversal") is predictive of a pulmonary artery occlusion pressure of 10–15 mmHg. Marked septal movement and buckling during mid-systole (referred to as "mid-systolic buckling") predicts a pulmonary artery occlusion pressure of < 5 mmHg [24].

Lung and diaphragm ultrasound

Lung and diaphragm ultrasound was performed using the curved array 4C-RS probe (frequency range of 1.8–6.0 MHz).

Lung ultrasound

Lung ultrasound was performed on all participants in a semi-recumbent position at 30°–50° using the six-zone method of each lung as described by Gargani [26] and Volpicelli [27]. The surface anatomy of the lung lobes and lung ultrasound zones are shown in Fig. 5. Each intercostal space was carefully examined by sliding the probe longitudinally over the chest in each region. The exception was the posterior upper zone, where access was limited in mechanically ventilated patients. Moreover, examination of the posterior upper zone was considered to add little information, as the anterior ultrasound examination provided adequate details about the upper lobe of the lung. An aeration score was assigned to each zone based on the presence and degree of aeration loss [11], as shown in Fig. 6. Score 1 represented a normally aerated zone with the absence of/fewer than three B-lines. Score 2 represented moderately aerated zone with three or more discrete B-lines; score 3 represented severe loss of aeration with multiple and fused B-lines; score 4 represented consolidation; score 5 represented consolidation with pleural effusion. Hence, the scoring value of each zone varied from a minimum of one score to a maximum of five scores depending on the degree of the aeration loss. The sum of all zone's score represented the global lung ultrasound score. Bilateral presence of three or more B-lines in two zones or more anteriorly and/or laterally denoted interstitial syndrome suggestive of cardiogenic pulmonary oedema [28], and the score of all zones denoted the overall aeration state.

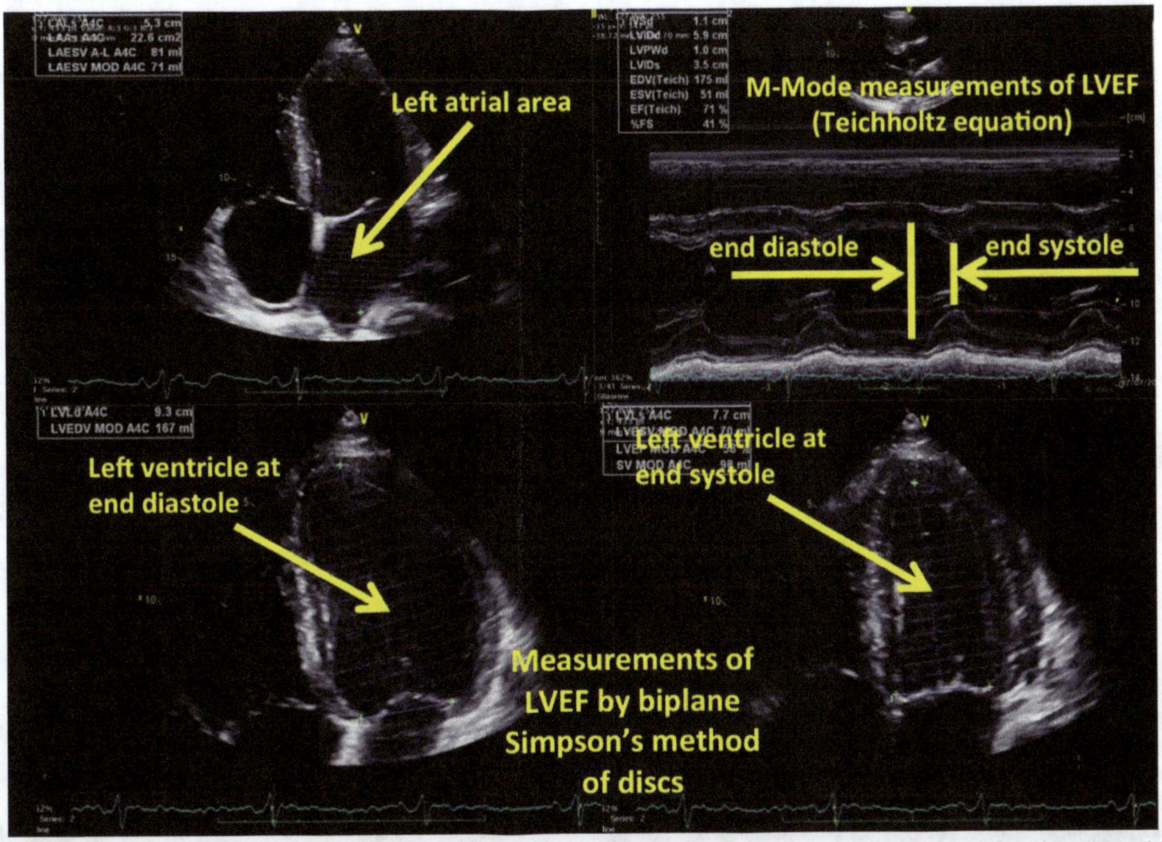

Fig. 2 Echocardiographic assessment of left ventricular systolic function (Simpson's method and Techoltz equation) as defined by Lang et al. [22]

Diaphragmatic ultrasound

The lateral approach was used to image the diaphragm, with the participants in a supine and head-up position at 30°–50° (Fig. 7). The same landmarks and techniques were applied on the right and left hemidiaphragm. The probe was placed laterally and perpendicularly on the lower intercostal spaces of the lateral chest wall between mid- and posterior axillary line [29, 30]. The direction of the ultrasound beam was perpendicular or near perpendicular to the craniocaudal axis during breathing. This provided adequate visualization of the maximum displacement of the diaphragm during breathing. The images of the hemidiaphragm movement were recorded for at least three consecutive respiratory cycles. The range of movement between 2 points (end of inspiration and end of expiration) for all recorded cycles was measured and averaged. The images during forced breaths, sighs and during suctioning were excluded. Diaphragmatic movement of greater than 1 cm represented normal function [31]. Unilateral dysfunction was defined when a unilateral hemidiaphragm movement was less than 1.0 cm; bilateral dysfunction was defined as movement of less than 1.0 cm in both hemidiaphragms.

Reliability of imaging

Reliability of ultrasound measurements of the heart, lungs and diaphragm was assessed by measuring the interobserver variability between two observers with appropriate training and experience in these measurements. Digital images of at least three cardiac cycles and three respiratory cycles for each standard view were assessed off-line using Synapse Cardiovascular software (Fujifilm, Akasaka, Minato, Tokyo, Japan). The mean difference and limits of agreement (±2 SDs of the difference) between the two observers was recorded. We considered the agreement between observers to be acceptable if the limits of agreement were less than 20% of the mean value of the variable being measured for continuous data.

Statistical analysis

Patient characteristics were summarized as n and % for categorical variables and as median and interquartile range for continuous variables. Comparison of quantitative variables was performed using independent samples t test or Mann–Whitney test. Comparison of categorical data was performed using Fisher's exact test. In order to

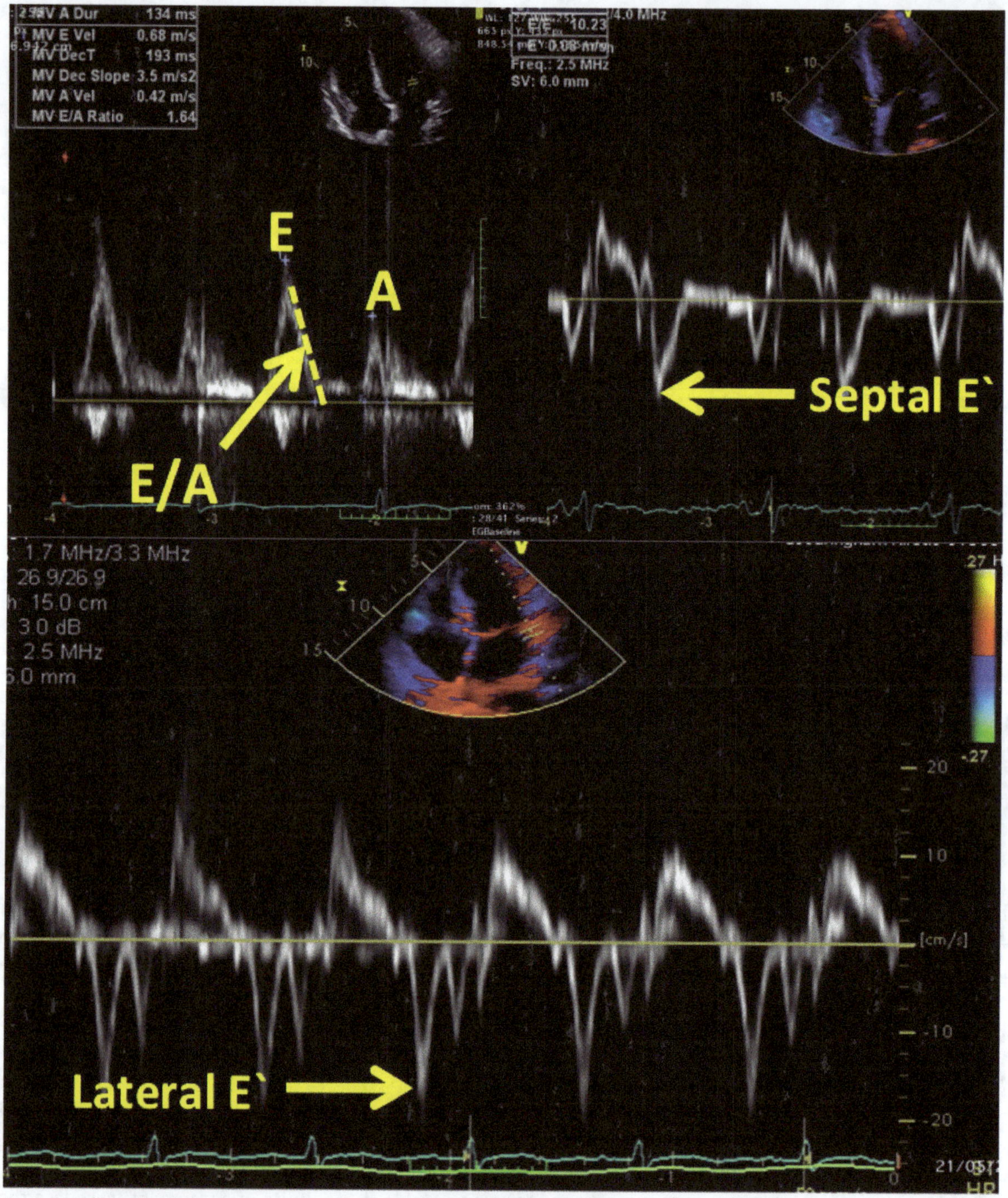

Fig. 3 Examples of Doppler assessments used for assessment of left ventricular diastolic function (trans-mitral inflow and tissue Doppler assessment of the septal and lateral mitral valve annulus). *A*, late diastolic trans-mitral flow velocity wave, *E* early diastolic trans-mitral flow velocity wave, *E′*, early diastolic mitral annulus velocity

determine the key predictors of successful extubation, odds ratio (OR) was obtained for each variable using univariate binary logistic regression. Due to the small sample size and therefore increased risk of Type II error, and also to reduce risk of Type I error due to multiple pairwise comparisons, the p value for significance is defined as $p < 0.01$. As the effect size for the ultrasound endpoints was not known, recruitment was based on a time period not exceeding 2 years, and with a maximum of 80 participants for the pilot study. All analyses were performed in SPSS version 23 (IBM Corp.).

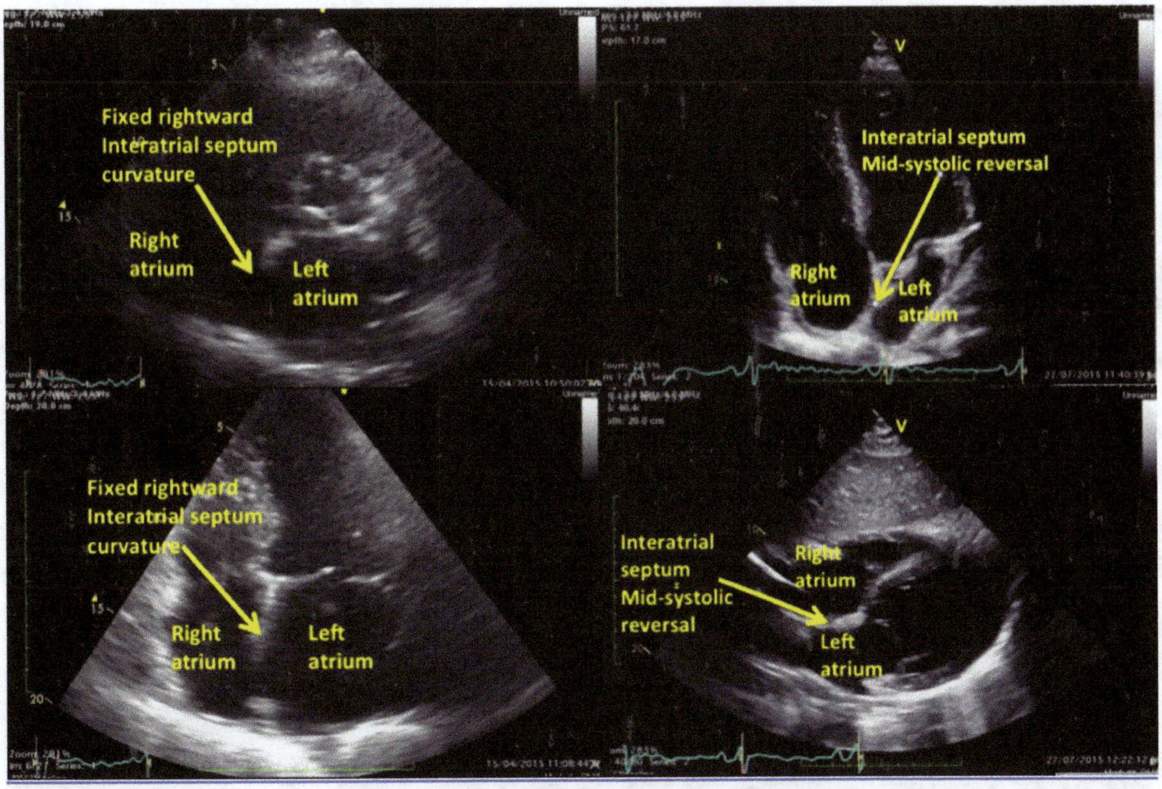

Fig. 4 Interatrial septal movements during the cardiac cycle. Fixed rightward interatrial septum curvature is bowing of the interatrial septal to right throughout the cardiac cycle, and mid-systolic reversal is reversal of the septum from right to left during mid-systole

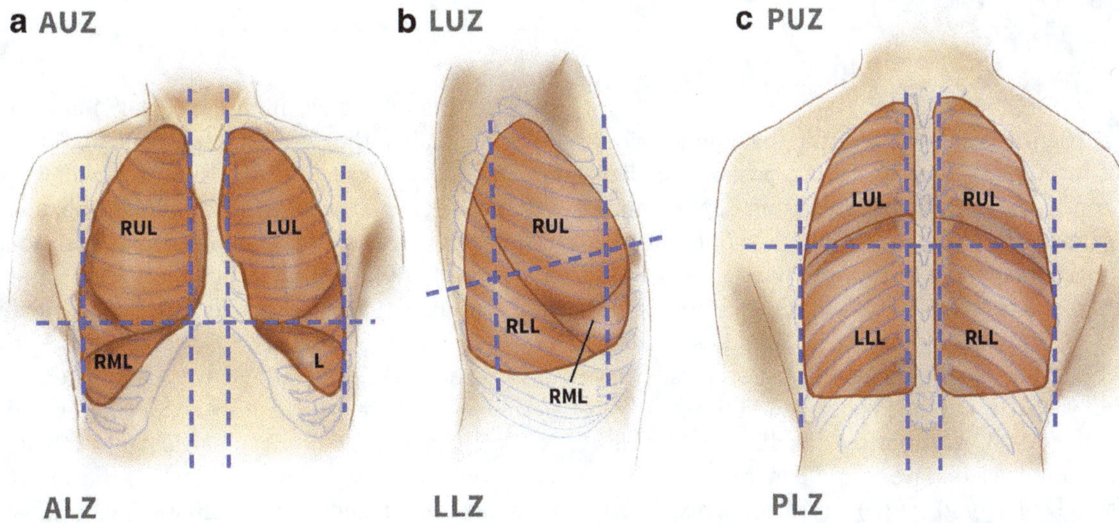

Fig. 5 Surface anatomy of the regions of the lung. Ultrasound surface anatomy: the parasternal, anterior axillary and posterior axillary lines divide the chest wall into anterior, lateral and posterior regions. **a** The anterior region, delineated superiorly by the clavicle, inferiorly by the liver or the spleen, medially by parasternal line and laterally by the anterior axillary line. The anterior region is further divided by an arbitrary line to anterior upper zone and anterior lower zone. **b** The lateral region, delineated superiorly by the axilla, inferiorly by the liver or the spleen, anteriorly by the anterior axillary line and posteriorly by the posterior axillary line. An arbitrary line further divides the lateral region to lateral upper zone and lateral lower zone. **c** The posterior region, delineated by the posterior axillary line laterally and paravertebral line medially. A horizontal arbitrary line at the tip of the scapula further divides the posterior region to upper and lower zone. *ALZ* anterior lower zone, *AUZ* anterior upper zone, *L* lingula, *LLL* left lower lobe, *LLZ* left lower zone, *LUL* left upper lobe, *PLZ* posterior lower zone, *PUZ* posterior upper zone, *RLL* right lower lobe, *RML* right middle lobe, *RUL* right upper lobe

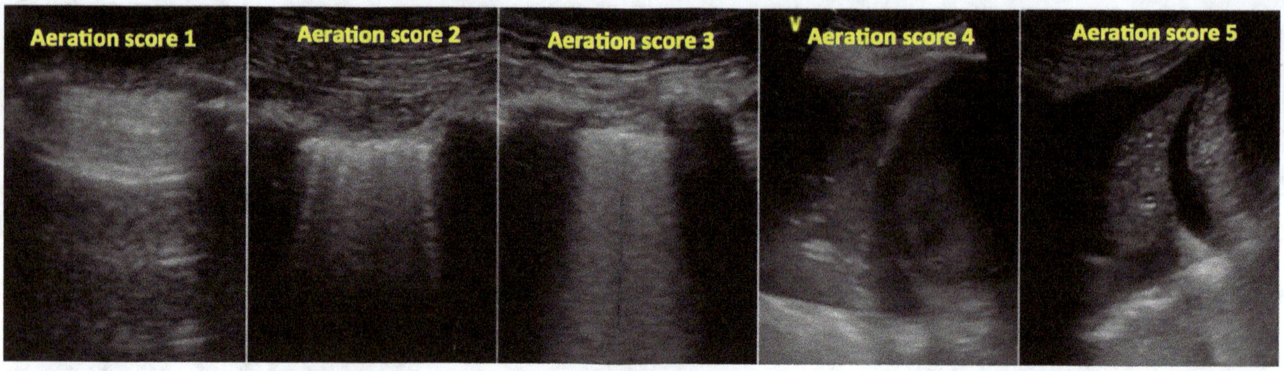

Fig. 6 Lung ultrasound aeration scoring. The pattern and the extent of aeration defect is quantified as follows: A normally aerated or fewer than 3 B-lines scored 1; multiple discrete B-lines scored 2; multiple and fused B-lines scored 3; unaerated consolidated lung scored 4; unaerated consolidation with pleural effusion scored 5. Hence, the maximum score for each half was 5 and the maximum score for the posterior zone was 5

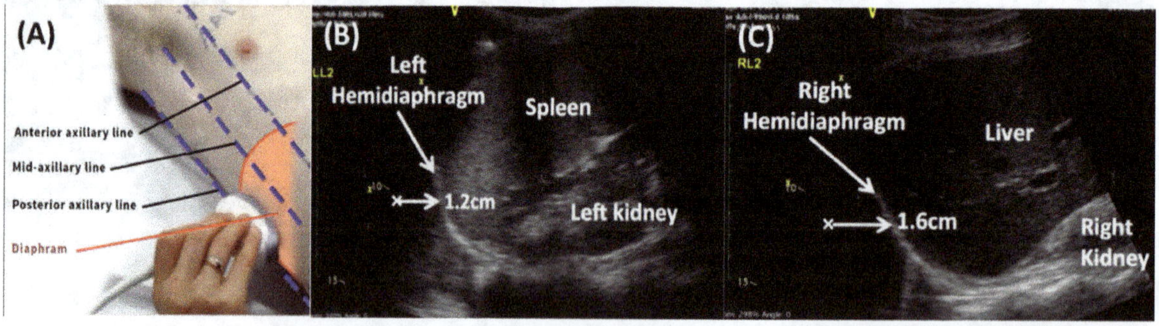

Fig. 7 Ultrasound technique and images of the diaphragm. **A** The location of probe placement on the chest wall for assessment of diaphragm movement. The probe is placed laterally and perpendicularly on the lateral chest wall on the lower intercostal spaces between mid- and posterior axillary line. **B**, **C** The ultrasound images of the left and the right hemidiaphragm and the measurement of the diaphragmatic excursion from end of end inspiration to end expiration

Results

Of the 58 participants screened during the study period, five did not meet inclusion criteria: two participants had a tracheostomy, one participant died from septic shock and two participants were extubated without informing the investigators, and were not recruited. This left 53 participants for data analysis, two-thirds of whom were male. Sepsis (38%) was the most common admission diagnosis. Other diagnoses included post-surgical (gastrointestinal, vascular, musculoskeletal and burns) (15%), drug overdose (13%), gastrointestinal disease (decompensated chronic liver disease, acute pancreatitis, upper gastrointestinal bleeding) (12%), cardiac arrest (8%), neurological disease (status epilepticus, motor neuron disease, encephalitis) (6%) acute cardiogenic pulmonary oedema (4%) and metabolic disorder (hyponatremia and diabetic ketoacidosis) (4%).

All 53 recruited patients followed the weaning trial protocol. All 53 patients received PEEP of 5 cmH_2O. Pressure support received during weaning trial was zero (60%), 5–7 cmH_2O (15%) and 8–10 cmH_2O (25%). Fifty patients passed the weaning trial (94.4%) and three participants failed the weaning trial (5.6%). The treating intensivists, however, decided to extubate all 53 patients. Of the three participants who were extubated despite failing the weaning trial, two participants (systolic blood pressure of 200 mmHg and agitation score of +3) were successfully extubated and one participant (tidal volume 4 ml/kg) failed extubation. Of the 50 participants who passed the weaning trial and were extubated, 40 (80%) participants were successfully extubated. Of the total 53 participants, 11 (20.7%) participants failed extubation over the subsequent 48 h. Two of the 11 (18%) participants that failed extubation were re-intubated and the remaining nine (82%) received non-invasive ventilation. The reasons for failure of extubation as reported by the treating team were pulmonary oedema [7], hospital acquired pneumonia [1], post-operative pain and agitation [1], and deconditioning with insufficient respiratory effort [2].

The participant demographic data are shown in Table 1. Variables that were associated with failed extubation

Table 1 Clinical and biochemical variables of failed and successful extubation groups

	Failed extubation ($n=11$)	Successful extubation ($n=42$)	Unadjusted OR (95% CI)	p value
Characteristics				
Male n (%)	10 (90.9)	24 (57.1)	0.13 (0.01–1.14)	0.06
Age, years median (IQR)	77.0 (65.0–81.0)	63.5 (45.7–73.3.0)	1.05 (0.99–1.11)	0.06
Ideal body weight (kg) median (IQR)	61.0 (54.7–63.9)	62.3 (54.6–66.2)	0.96 (0.87–1.06)	0.44
BMI kg/m^2 median (IQR)	27.0 (23.3–35.1)	27.0 (24.1–31.0)	1.0 (0.9–1.11)	0.95
Ischaemic heart disease n (%)	7 (63.6)	9 (21.4)	6.41 (1.53–26.88)	0.01
Heart failure n (%)	3 (27.3)	5 (11.9)	2.77 (0.54–14.05)	0.21
Diabetes mellitus n (%)	6 (54.5)	9 (21.4)	4.40 (1.08–17.79)	0.03
COPD n (%)	3 (27.3)	6 (14.3)	2.25 (0.46–10.96)	0.31
ICU severity score				
APACHE II median (IQR)	20.0 (17–23)	20.0 (15.0–23.3)	1.06 (0.94–1.20	0.31
APACHE III median (IQR)	82.0 (61.0–97.0)	74.5 (60.5–89.5)	1.02 (0.99–1.04)	0.21
SAPS II median (IQR)	42.0 (33.0–46.0)	46.0 (36.0–57.3)	0.99 (0.94–1.04)	0.72
Weaning trial				
Respiratory rate (breath/min) median (IQR)	24 (18–30)	18 (15–23)	1.14 (1.01–1.27)	0.02
Tidal volume (l) median (IQR)	0.48 (0.39–0.58)	0.51 (0.41–0.75)	0.11 (0.00–5.76)	0.27
Pressure support (cmH$_2$O) median (IQR)	0.0 (0.0–10.0)	0.0 (0.0–7.2)	1.04 (0.89–1.22)	0.58
ICU outcomes				
Extubation failure n (%)				
ICU LOS (day) median (IQR)	10.5 (9.7–17.5)	7.9 (5.5–13.0)	1.14 (0.99–1.25)	0.06
Time from extubation to ICU discharge (days) median (IQR)	4.1 (3.1–7.1)	1.9 (1.0–5.1)	1.13 (0.95–1.34)	0.14
Hospital LOS (day) median (IQR)	19.2 (16.1–33.1)	16.4 (11.2–24.1)	1.00 (0.96–1.04)	0.71
In-hospital mortality n (%)	2 (18.2)	3 (7.1)	0.34 (0.05–2.38)	0.28
Duration of MV (h) median (IQR)	175.0 (99.1–238.5)	130.6 (93.7–180.5)	1.00 (0.99–1.01)	0.11

APACHE acute physiology age and chronic health evaluation, *BMI* body mass index, *BNP* B-type natriuretic peptide, *COAD* chronic obstructive airway disease, *H LOS* hospital length of stay, *ICU LOS* intensive care unit length of stay, *SAPS* simplified acute physiology score, *IQR* interquartile range

included known pre-existing ischemic heart disease (OR 6.41, 95% CI 1.53–26.88, $p=0.01$), pre-existing diabetes mellitus (OR 4.40, 95% CI 1.08–17.79, $p=0.03$), higher respiratory rate (OR 1.14 95% CI 1.01–1.27, $p=0.02$) and RSBI (OR 1.03, 95% CI 1.00–1.06, $p=0.03$). BNP was not associated with success or failure of extubation. There was no group separation for ICU and hospital length of stay. Two participants who failed extubation died and three participants who were successfully extubated died during their hospitalization.

The cardiac, lung and diaphragm ultrasound findings, RSBI and BNP are shown in Table 2. Cardiac ultrasound was un-interpretable in one participant (who was successfully extubated). Failed extubation was associated with echocardiographic markers of left ventricular diastolic dysfunction, including raised left atrial pressure indicated by interatrial septal fixed rightward curvature (OR 12.95, 95% CI 2.73–61.41, $p=0.001$), higher E/E' (OR 1.27, 95% CI 1.05–1.54, $p=0.01$) and larger left atrial area (OR 1.14, 95% CI 1.02–1.28, $p=0.02$).

Higher loss of aeration score of the anterior and the lateral lung regions was associated with failed extubation (OR 1.41, 95% CI 1.01–1.82, $p=0.007$). The magnitude of diaphragmatic movement was not associated with success or failure of extubation.

The interobserver variation showed acceptable agreement. The limits of agreement, using a Bland–Altman approach, were less than 20% of the mean value for all comparisons. There were no critical findings that required immediate disclosure to the treating team for the safety of the participants.

Discussion

Of the clinical and ultrasound indicators in this pilot study, we determined that the most likely parameters which could be useful to help predict failed extubation are those which are related to diastolic dysfunction (left atrial area, E/E', interatrial septal rightward fixed curvature), loss of aeration score of the left and right anterior and lateral regions, and increased RSBI. Interatrial septal fixed curvature and lung ultrasound findings appear promising and may aid in decision-making for extubation, as they are easily and quickly assessed, even in operators with limited echocardiographic experience.

Table 2 Clinical, echocardiographic and respiratory ultrasound variables

Variable	Failed extubation ($n = 11$)	Successful extubation ($n = 42$)	Unadjusted OR (95% CI)	p value
RSBI (breath/min/l) median (IQR)	48.0 (35.1–72.0)	33.5 (25.6–55.4)	1.03 (1.00–1.06)	0.03
BNP (pmole/l) median (IQR)	372 (152–1620)	233 (95–475)	1.0 (0.99–1.00)	0.72
Echocardiographic variables				
LVEF (%) median (IQR)	50 (45–55)	65 (53–65)	0.96 (0.91–1.0)	0.1
E median (IQR)	0.87 (0.68–1.04)	0.83 (0.68–0.99)	5.43 (0.35–85.2)	0.22
E/A median (IQR)	1.20 (0.60–1.64)	1.13 (0.85–1.36)	0.99 (0.38–2.59)	0.99
EDT median (IQR)	175 (125–259)	180 (155–217)	0.99 (0.98–1.01)	0.87
E' median (IQR)	0.07 (0.05–0.11)	0.10 (0.08–0.12)	0.00 (0.00–1.36)	0.052
E/E' median (IQR)	10.9 (8.7–18.0)	7.7 (6.4–10.6)	1.27 (1.05–1.54)	0.01
LAA median (IQR)	25.0 (19.3–32.0)	20.0 (18.0–23.7)	1.14 (1.02–1.28)	0.02
IAS fixed curvature *n* (%)	7 (72.7)	8 (17.1)	12.95 (2.73–61.41)	0.001
Lung ultrasound				
Aeration score of left and right anterior and lateral region (upper and lower zones) median (IQR)	17 (8–20)	11 (8–13)	1.41 (1.01–1.82)	0.007
Aeration score of left and right lungs total median (IQR)	22 (13–28)	18 (13–21)	1.12 (0.99–1.27)	0.06
Diaphragmatic dysfunction *n* (%)				
No diaphragmatic dysfunction	5 (45.5)	24 (57.1)		0.53
Hemidiaphragm dysfunction	4 (36.4)	15 (35.7)	1.28 (0.29–5.53)	0.26
Diaphragm dysfunction	2 (18.2)	3 (7.1)	3.2 (0.41–24.41)	0.49

Normal values of the parameters listed in the table are as follows: RSBI: < 105, BNP < 29 pmol/l, LVEF < 50%, *E* 73 ± 19 cm/s, *A* 69 ± 17 cm/s, *E/A* 1.20 ± 0.20, DT 192 ± 40 ms, E' 12 ± 4 cm/s, E/E' 10 ± 2, hemidiaphragm excursion ≥ 1.0 cm

IAS: interatrial septum; IQR: interquartile range; LAA: left atrial area; LVE/E: left ventricular early diastolic trans-mitral flow velocity; *E* wave: early diastolic mitral annulus velocity E' ratio; LVEF: left ventricular ejection fraction; OR: odds ratio, RSBI: rapid shallow breathing index

However, these results need to be verified in a larger study. The value of combined heart and lung ultrasound is that the physician extends their clinical evaluation to both the cardiac and respiratory systems to identify pathology. In some participants, pathology was confined to either the heart or lungs, and in others, pathology existed in both systems. Further, adding lung findings to heart ultrasound can act as a measure of severity. Systolic or diastolic failure patterns on heart ultrasound, for example, will have a greater severity if there is evidence of interstitial oedema on lung ultrasound, and more so is present in both upper and lower lobes.

Interestingly, participants who were older with diabetes and ischemic heart disease had greater incidence of extubation failure when compared to those who were successful. Such association between weaning failure and diabetes was also reported in a similar study [10]. Although unclear, the association is possibly attributed to left ventricular diastolic failure. This perhaps suggests that older patients, patients with diabetes and or ischaemic heart disease may most benefit from bedside cardiac ultrasound as an adjunct to prediction of their candidacy for ventilatory weaning and endotracheal extubation.

Our study particularly focused on imaging the heart, lung and the diaphragm although only during the weaning trial just before extubation. We believe that ultrasound may provide an opportunity for the intensivist to optimize the patient's cardiac and respiratory function before extubation, and perhaps modify the weaning mechanism, such as transitioning those at risk to non-invasive ventilation before discontinuing the ventilatory support [32, 33].

Our data do not allow us to determine why diastolic dysfunction is associated with weaning failure. However, it is reasonable to assume that patients with raised left atrial pressure may be more likely to develop pulmonary venous congestion as the hemodynamic stress associated with weaning increases. A study by Caille et al. suggested that patients are more likely to fail weaning when their left ventricular ejection fraction is lower than 35% and E/E' is greater than 7.8 [8]. Conversely, Moschietto et al. [10] showed that unlike E/E', ejection fraction had no impact on weaning outcome. Recent published data have demonstrated a positive association between the echocardiographic measurements of diastolic failure, in particular E/E', and weaning failure [8–10, 34]. E/E' is a marker of left atrial pressure, and that of left ventricular diastolic pressure. E/E' correlated well with pulmonary artery occlusion pressure [35, 36]. However, this correlation in the operating room setting was debatable [25].

E/E′ range of cut-off values of 7–14 has been suggested for determining patients at risk of failing weaning from mechanical ventilation [8, 9, 34]. In another study, a higher cut-off value of 14.5 during a spontaneous breathing trial had a sensitivity of 75% and specificity of 95.8% for predicting weaning failure [10].

Fixed rightward curvature of interatrial septum was a prominent finding in the failed extubation group. Assessment of interatrial septal movement is an easy technique to perform to obtain a visual estimation of the left atrial pressure state. Royse et al. [24] found that pulmonary artery occlusion pressure greater than 15 mmHg corresponded to fixed rightward curvature of the interatrial septal movement throughout the cardiac cycle. The findings were supported by an earlier study, where the shape and movement of the interatrial septum were dependent on the gradient between the atria [23]. Interatrial septal movement is easily obtained from a 2-dimensional view of any standard parasternal short axis, apical 4-chamber or subcostal 4-chamber or subcostal short axis.

Left atrial enlargement is an indicator of severity and chronicity of diastolic dysfunction and is associated with increased left atrial pressure [22]. However, left atrial enlargement is non-specific and it is influenced by other factors such as hemodynamically significant mitral valve pathology and atrial fibrillation [37]. There were two participants from the successful group who had atrial flutter during imaging but all participants in the failed group were in sinus rhythm.

Lung ultrasound is a non-invasive and easily performed bedside test. It has clinical and practical advantages over conventional chest radiography [27, 38]. Besides its diagnostic capability, lung ultrasound is useful for monitoring lung aeration during prone positioning [39]. The pattern, location and the extent of loss of aeration on ultrasound identify the pathological process and hence the diagnosis of the respiratory disorder. The loss of aeration scoring method used in this study provides a quantification of the degree of aeration defect, which may be useful in assessing the type, distribution and degree of lung injury. A similar scoring system was used by Soummer et al. [11] for predicting post-extubation distress during a spontaneous breathing trial. Pleural effusion was included in our scoring system, which added to the severity of aeration loss. In this study, an association with worse aeration was found in participants who failed extubation. Moreover, the association was stronger with significantly higher loss of aeration score, when the antero-lateral regions of both lungs were included. This finding may translate to a higher incidence of pulmonary oedema in the failed extubation group, consistent with cardiac failure [26, 28].

Mechanical ventilation may induce diaphragmatic dysfunction from muscle disuse, particularly in prolonged mechanical ventilation [40]. Diaphragmatic disuse leads to protein oxidation via activation of autophagy, lysosome pathway and skeletal muscle proteolysis [41], which subsequently alters the diaphragm contractile property. In a study by Kim et al. [13], the prevalence of diaphragmatic dysfunction was 29% in critically ill patients with no history of neuromuscular or diaphragmatic diseases. In this study, the cut-off diaphragm excursion value for extubation failure was 1.4 cm for the right hemidiaphragm and 1.2 cm for the left hemidiaphragm [13]. Further, patients with diaphragmatic dysfunction had a longer ventilation time, 401 h vs. 90 h in patients with normal diaphragm. In another study, liver and spleen displacement as a surrogate for respiratory sufficiency, in particular diaphragmatic movement, has been shown as predictors for successful extubation when compared to RSBI, spontaneous tidal volume or maximum inspiratory pressure [42]. In contrast to the published evidence about the diaphragmatic role in respiratory weaning outcome, we did not find an association between diaphragm dysfunction and extubation failure. However, due to the small sample size in our study, the role of the diaphragm in weaning needs further exploration.

On current practice, the prediction of successful weaning and readiness for extubation is assessed using clinical and biochemical parameters including the degree of respiratory support, respiratory rate, tidal volume, RSBI and arterial blood gas analysis. RSBI is a surrogate marker of quality of breathing during weaning from mechanical ventilation. It is defined as the ratio between respiratory rate and tidal volume where a value greater than 105 breaths/min/l predicts patients at high risk of failing weaning [14, 43]. However, weaning failure has been associated with RSBI of lower than recommended values [11]. In our study, higher RSBI was weakly associated with failed extubation. BNP is a biochemical marker of cardiac dysfunction. It is a 32-amino acid peptide released into the plasma because of cardiomyocytes overstretch. The role of BNP in weaning from mechanical ventilation is controversial [7, 11, 44]. In our study, there was a weak association with elevated BNP and extubation failure.

This is a pilot study, and therefore it can only be used to identify potentially useful parameters to aid clinical decision-making. The study was based on convenience sampling, which was subject to the availability of the research sonographer. In contrast to some previously published studies, our study protocol did not interfere with the clinician's extubation decision, and all participants proceeded to extubation regardless of weaning trial outcome. In the lung ultrasound, we did not image the postero-superior areas due to difficult windows in supine ventilated patients, and the upper lobe can be visualized from the anterior approach. It is possible, however, that some upper lobe pathology may have been missed. The results of this study can be further tested by a larger prospective study in a high-risk population that perhaps are older with history of diabetes and/or ischemic heart disease and with a clinical diagnosis of cardiac.

Conclusions

Failed extubation in mechanically ventilated patients is more prevalent if markers of left ventricular diastolic dysfunction and loss of lung aeration are present.

Abbreviations

A: late diastolic trans-mitral flow velocity wave; BNP: B-type natriuretic peptide; *E*: early diastolic trans-mitral flow velocity wave; *E/E′*: early diastolic trans-mitral flow velocity wave/early diastolic mitral annulus velocity; ICU: intensive care unit; *E/A*: early diastolic trans-mitral flow velocity wave/late diastolic trans-mitral flow velocity wave; PEEP: positive end expiratory pressure; RSBI: rapid shallow breathing index; TTE: transthoracic echocardiogram.

Authors' contributions

KH designed the study, performed the ultrasound studies, collected and analysed data and wrote the manuscript. CR designed the study, helped in designing, analysing and editing the manuscript. DH interpreted the ultrasound images as the second reviewer and contributed in the final editing. DC, AR and CG contributed in the final editing of the manuscript. All authors read and approved the final manuscript.

Author details

[1] Department of the Intensive Care Unit, Frankton Hospital, PO Box 52, Frankston, VIC 3199, Australia. [2] Faculty of Medicine, Nursing and Health Sciences, Monash University, Melbourne, Australia. [3] Frankston Hospital, Frankston, VIC, Australia. [4] Department of Surgery, University of Melbourne, Melbourne, Australia. [5] Department of Medicine, Health Sciences and Nursing, Monash University, Melbourne, Australia. [6] Royal Melbourne Hospital, Melbourne, Australia. [7] Ultrasound Education Group, Department of Surgery, The University of Melbourne, Melbourne, Australia. [8] Department of Cardiothoracic Surgery, The Royal Melbourne Hospital, Melbourne, Australia. [9] Department of Anaesthesia and Pain Management, The Royal Melbourne Hospital, Melbourne, VIC, Australia.

Acknowledgements

We are grateful for the assistance of many staff at Frankston Hospital who helped in this study. We also thank Sandy Clarke (statistical consulting, The University of Melbourne) who assisted with the statistical analysis.

References

1. Boles JM, Bion J, Connors A, Herridge M, Marsh B, Melot C et al (2007) Weaning from mechanical ventilation. Eur Respir J 29(5):1033–1056. https://doi.org/10.1183/09031936.00010206
2. Esteban A, Ferguson ND, Meade MO, Frutos-Vivar F, Apezteguia C, Brochard L et al (2008) Evolution of mechanical ventilation in response to clinical research. Am J Respir Crit Care Med 177(2):170–177. https://doi.org/10.1164/rccm.200706-893oc
3. Esteban A, Alia I, Tobin MJ, Gil A, Gordo F, Vallverdu I et al (1999) Effect of spontaneous breathing trial duration on outcome of attempts to discontinue mechanical ventilation. Spanish Lung Failure Collaborative Group. Am J Respir Crit Care Med 159(2):512–518. https://doi.org/10.1164/ajrccm.159.2.9803106
4. Hurford WE, Favorito F (1995) Association of myocardial ischemia with failure to wean from mechanical ventilation. Crit Care Med 23(9):1475–1480
5. Jubran A, Lawm G, Duffner LA, Collins EG, Lanuza DM, Hoffman LA et al (2010) Post-traumatic stress disorder after weaning from prolonged mechanical ventilation. Intensive Care Med 36(12):2030–2037. https://doi.org/10.1007/s00134-010-1972-8
6. Lemaire F, Teboul JL, Cinotti L, Giotto G, Abrouk F, Steg G et al (1988) Acute left ventricular dysfunction during unsuccessful weaning from mechanical ventilation. Anesthesiology 69(2):171–179
7. Mekontso-Dessap A, de Prost N, Girou E, Braconnier F, Lemaire F, Brun-Buisson C et al (2006) B-type natriuretic peptide and weaning from mechanical ventilation. Intensive Care Med 32(10):1529–1536. https://doi.org/10.1007/s00134-006-0339-7
8. Caille V, Amiel JB, Charron C, Belliard G, Vieillard-Baron A, Vignon P (2010) Echocardiography: a help in the weaning process. Crit Care 14(3):R120. https://doi.org/10.1186/cc9076
9. Papanikolaou J, Makris D, Saranteas T, Karakitsos D, Zintzaras E, Karabinis A et al (2011) New insights into weaning from mechanical ventilation: left ventricular diastolic dysfunction is a key player. Intensive Care Med. https://doi.org/10.1007/s00134-011-2368-0
10. Moschietto S, Doyen D, Grech L, Dellamonica J, Hyvernat H, Bernardin G (2012) Transthoracic echocardiography with Doppler tissue imaging predicts weaning failure from mechanical ventilation: evolution of the left ventricle relaxation rate during a spontaneous breathing trial is the key factor in weaning outcome. Crit Care 16(3):R81. https://doi.org/10.1186/cc11339
11. Soummer A, Perbet S, Brisson H, Arbelot C, Constantin JM, Lu Q et al (2012) Ultrasound assessment of lung aeration loss during a successful weaning trial predicts postextubation distress*. Crit Care Med 40(7):2064–2072. https://doi.org/10.1097/CCM.0b013e31824e68ae
12. Frutos-Vivar F, Ferguson ND, Esteban A, Epstein SK, Arabi Y, Apezteguia C et al (2006) Risk factors for extubation failure in patients following a successful spontaneous breathing trial. Chest 130(6):1664–1671. https://doi.org/10.1378/chest.130.6.1664
13. Kim WY, Suh HJ, Hong SB, Koh Y, Lim CM (2011) Diaphragm dysfunction assessed by ultrasonography: influence on weaning from mechanical ventilation. Crit Care Med 39(12):2627–2630. https://doi.org/10.1097/CCM.0b013e3182266408
14. Bien Udos S, Souza GF, Campos ES, Farah de Carvalho E, Fernandes MG, Santoro I et al (2015) Maximum inspiratory pressure and rapid shallow breathing index as predictors of successful ventilator weaning. J Phys Ther Sci 27(12):3723–3727. https://doi.org/10.1589/jpts.27.3723
15. Mayo P, Volpicelli G, Lerolle N, Schreiber A, Doelken P, Vieillard-Baron A (2016) Ultrasonography evaluation during the weaning process: the heart, the diaphragm, the pleura and the lung. Intensive Care Med 42(7):1107–1117. https://doi.org/10.1007/s00134-016-4245-3
16. Esteban A, Alia I, Gordo F, Fernandez R, Solsona JF, Vallverdu I et al (1997) Extubation outcome after spontaneous breathing trials with T-tube or pressure support ventilation. The Spanish Lung Failure Collaborative Group. Am J Respir Crit Care Med 156(2 Pt 1):459–465. https://doi.org/10.1164/ajrccm.156.2.9610109
17. Tseng YH, Tseng YC, Hsu HS, Chang SC (2015) Different spontaneous breathing trials in patients with atrial fibrillation. Rev Port Pneumol (2006) 21(5):245–252. https://doi.org/10.1016/j.rppnen.2015.04.007
18. Koksal GM, Sayilgan C, Sen O, Oz H (2004) The effects of different weaning modes on the endocrine stress response. Crit Care 8(1):R31–R34. https://doi.org/10.1186/cc2413
19. Ladeira MT, Vital FM, Andriolo RB, Andriolo BN, Atallah AN, Peccin MS (2014) Pressure support versus T-tube for weaning from mechanical ventilation in adults. Cochrane Database Syst Rev 5:CD006056. https://doi.org/10.1002/14651858.cd006056.pub2
20. Perrigault PF, Pouzeratte YH, Jaber S, Capdevila XJ, Hayot M, Boccara G et al (1999) Changes in occlusion pressure (P01) and breathing pattern during pressure support ventilation. Thorax 54(2):119–123
21. Sessler CN, Gosnell MS, Grap MJ, Brophy GM, O'Neal PV, Keane KA et al (2002) The Richmond Agitation–Sedation Scale: validity and reliability in adult intensive care unit patients. Am J Respir Crit Care Med 166(10):1338–1344. https://doi.org/10.1164/rccm.2107138
22. Lang RM, Badano LP, Mor-Avi V, Afilalo J, Armstrong A, Ernande L et al (2015) Recommendations for cardiac chamber quantification by echocardiography in adults: an update from the American Society of Echocardiography and the European Association of Cardiovascular Imaging. J Am Soc Echocardiogr 28(1):1–39.e14. https://doi.org/10.1016/j.echo.2014
23. Kusumoto FM, Muhiudeen IA, Kuecherer HF, Cahalan MK, Schiller NB (1993) Response of the interatrial septum to transatrial pressure gradients

and its potential for predicting pulmonary capillary wedge pressure: an intraoperative study using transesophageal echocardiography in patients during mechanical ventilation. J Am Coll Cardiol 21(3):721–728
24. Royse CF, Royse AG, Soeding PF, Blake DW (2001) Shape and movement of the interatrial septum predicts change in pulmonary capillary wedge pressure. Ann Thorac Cardiovasc Surg 7(2):79–83
25. Haji DL, Ali MM, Royse A, Canty DJ, Clarke S, Royse CF (2014) Interatrial septum motion but not Doppler assessment predicts elevated pulmonary capillary wedge pressure in patients undergoing cardiac surgery. Anesthesiology 121(4):719–729. https://doi.org/10.1097/aln.0000000000000392
26. Gargani L, Volpicelli G (2014) How I do it: lung ultrasound. Cardiovasc Ultrasound 12:25. https://doi.org/10.1186/1476-7120-12-25
27. Volpicelli G, Elbarbary M, Blaivas M, Lichtenstein DA, Mathis G, Kirkpatrick AW et al (2012) International evidence-based recommendations for point-of-care lung ultrasound. Intensive Care Med 38(4):577–591. https://doi.org/10.1007/s00134-012-2513-4
28. Volpicelli G, Skurzak S, Boero E, Carpinteri G, Tengattini M, Stefanone V et al (2014) Lung ultrasound predicts well extravascular lung water but is of limited usefulness in the prediction of wedge pressure. Anesthesiology 121(2):320–327. https://doi.org/10.1097/aln.0000000000000300
29. Ferrari G, De Filippi G, Elia F, Panero F, Volpicelli G, Apra F (2014) Diaphragm ultrasound as a new index of discontinuation from mechanical ventilation. Crit Ultrasound J 6(1):8. https://doi.org/10.1186/2036-7902-6-8
30. Haji K, Royse A, Tharmaraj D, Haji D, Botha J, Royse C (2015) Diaphragmatic regional displacement assessed by ultrasound and correlated to subphrenic organ movement in the critically ill patients—an observational study. J Crit Care 30(2):439.e7–439.e13. https://doi.org/10.1016/j.jcrc.2014.10.028
31. Boussuges A, Gole Y, Blanc P (2009) Diaphragmatic motion studied by m-mode ultrasonography: methods, reproducibility, and normal values. Chest 135(2):391–400. https://doi.org/10.1378/chest.08-1541
32. Nava S, Hill N (2009) Non-invasive ventilation in acute respiratory failure. Lancet 374(9685):250–259. https://doi.org/10.1016/s0140-6736(09)60496-7
33. Glossop AJ, Shephard N, Bryden DC, Mills GH (2012) Non-invasive ventilation for weaning, avoiding reintubation after extubation and in the postoperative period: a meta-analysis. Br J Anaesth 109(3):305–314. https://doi.org/10.1093/bja/aes270
34. Lamia B, Maizel J, Ochagavia A, Chemla D, Osman D, Richard C et al (2009) Echocardiographic diagnosis of pulmonary artery occlusion pressure elevation during weaning from mechanical ventilation. Crit Care Med 37(5):1696–1701. https://doi.org/10.1097/ccm.0b013e31819f13d0
35. Temporelli PL, Scapellato F, Eleuteri E, Imparato A, Giannuzzi P (2010) Doppler echocardiography in advanced systolic heart failure: a noninvasive alternative to Swan-Ganz catheter. Circ Heart Fail 3(3):387–394. https://doi.org/10.1161/circheartfailure.108.809590
36. Nagueh SF, Middleton KJ, Kopelen HA, Zoghbi WA, Quinones MA (1997) Doppler tissue imaging: a noninvasive technique for evaluation of left ventricular relaxation and estimation of filling pressures. J Am Coll Cardiol 30(6):1527–1533
37. Nagueh SF, Appleton CP, Gillebert TC, Marino PN, Oh JK, Smiseth OA et al (2009) Recommendations for the evaluation of left ventricular diastolic function by echocardiography. Eur J Echocardiogr 10(2):165–193. https://doi.org/10.1093/ejechocard/jep007
38. Lichtenstein D, Goldstein I, Mourgeon E, Cluzel P, Grenier P, Rouby JJ (2004) Comparative diagnostic performances of auscultation, chest radiography, and lung ultrasonography in acute respiratory distress syndrome. Anesthesiology 100(1):9–15
39. Haddam M, Zieleskiewicz L, Perbet S, Baldovini A, Guervilly C, Arbelot C et al (2016) Lung ultrasonography for assessment of oxygenation response to prone position ventilation in ARDS. Intensive Care Med 42(10):1546–1556. https://doi.org/10.1007/s00134-016-4411-7
40. Vassilakopoulos T (2008) Ventilator-induced diaphragm dysfunction: the clinical relevance of animal models. Intensive Care Med 34(1):7–16. https://doi.org/10.1007/s00134-007-0866x
41. Hussain SNA, Mofarrahi M, Sigala I, Kim HC, Vassilakopoulos T, Maltais F et al (2010) Mechanical ventilation-induced diaphragm disuse in humans triggers autophagy. Am J Respir Crit Care Med. 82(11):1377–1386. https://doi.org/10.1164/rccm.201002-0234OC
42. Jiang J, Tsai T, Jerng J, Yu C, Wu H, Yang P (2004) Ultrasonic evaluation of liver/spleen movements and extubation outcome. Chest 126:179–185. https://doi.org/10.1378/chest.126.1.179
43. Tobin MJ, Perez W, Guenther SM, Semmes BJ, Mador MJ, Allen SJ et al (1986) The pattern of breathing during successful and unsuccessful trials of weaning from mechanical ventilation. Am Rev Respir Dis 134(6):1111–1118. https://doi.org/10.1164/arrd.1986.134.6.1111
44. Lara TM, Hajjar LA, de Almeida JP, Fukushima JT, Barbas CS, Rodrigues AR et al (2013) High levels of B-type natriuretic peptide predict weaning failure from mechanical ventilation in adult patients after cardiac surgery. Clinics (Sao Paulo) 68(1):33–38

15

Ultrasound-guided thoracostomy site identification in healthy volunteers

Lindsay A. Taylor*, Michael J. Vitto, Michael Joyce, Jordan Tozer and David P. Evans*

Abstract

Background: Traditional landmark thoracostomy technique has a known complication rate up to 30%. The goal of this study is to determine whether novice providers could more accurately identify the appropriate intercostal site for thoracostomy by ultrasound guidance.

Methods: 33 emergency medicine residents and medical students volunteered to participate in this study during routine thoracostomy tube education. A healthy volunteer was used as the standardized patient for this study. An experienced physician sonographer used ultrasound to locate a site at mid-axillary line between ribs 4 and 5 and marked the site with invisible ink that can only be revealed with a commercially available UV LED light. Participants were asked to identify the thoracostomy site by placing an opaque marker where they would make their incision. The distance from the correct insertion site was measured in rib spaces. The participants were then given a brief hands-on training session using ultrasound to identify the diaphragm and count rib spaces. The participants were then asked to use ultrasound to identify the proper thoracostomy site and mark it with an opaque marker. The distance from the proper insertion site was measured and recorded in rib spaces.

Results: The participants correctly identified the pre-determined intercostal space using palpation 48% (16/33) of the time, versus the ultrasound group who identified the proper intercostal space 91% (30/33) of the time. On average, the traditional technique was placed 0.88 rib spaces away (95 CI 0.43–1.03), while the ultrasound-guided technique was placed 0.09 rib spaces away (95 CI 0.0–0.19) [P = 0.003].

Conclusions: The ability to accurately locate the correct intercostal space for thoracostomy incision was improved under ultrasound guidance. Further studies are warranted to determine if this ultrasound-guided technique will decrease complications with chest tube insertion and improve patient outcomes.

Background

The leading cause of death for individuals in the United States younger than 40 years old is trauma, with approximately 140,000 deaths annually [1]. Of these deaths, thoracic trauma accounts for nearly a quarter of all traumatic deaths [2]. Despite its severity, less than 30% of penetrating chest trauma and 10% of blunt thoracic injuries require thoracostomy [3]. In these patients, thoracostomy tube placement is performed to manage conditions such as pneumothorax, hemothorax, and pleural effusions. The goal of thoracostomy drainage remains unchanged since the time of Hippocrates; however, the procedure itself has changed dramatically since fifth century B.C.E [4]. In 1876, Hewett was the first to use a completely closed intercostal drainage system, [5] but it was not until World War II that tube thoracostomy became common in the treatment of injured patients [6]. From this point, thoracostomy tube placement became a mandatory skill for all providers taking care of trauma patients. Unfortunately, this life-saving procedure has a complication rate up to 30% [7], with complications raging from tube malposition, to bleeding, and organ injury [8–11].

To prevent these risks, training programs design simulations to train their residents on the proper insertion techniques. The classic technique uses landmarks on the body to identify the anatomically correct insertion site to avoid intraperitoneal insertion or lung injury. One study

*Correspondence: Lindsay.Taylor@vcuhealth.org; David.Evans@vcuhealth.org
Virginia Commonwealth University Emergency Medicine, 1250 E Marshall Street, 2nd Floor, Suite 500, P.O. Box 980401, Richmond, VA 23298, USA

evaluated 50 junior physicians' ability to properly identify the chest thoracostomy site using a photograph of a chest wall and showed that only 44% correctly located the 4th–5th intercostal space in the mid-axillary line [12]. Another study had physicians placing a radiopaque marker on a patient's chest wall over the 4th or 5th ICS prior to the patient getting a chest X-ray. This study demonstrated that physicians placed the marker correctly only 36.2% of the time [13]. In both of the aforementioned studies, the most common mistake made by the trainees was placing the marker for thoracostomy insertion too low [12, 13].

In many institutions, thoracic ultrasound is required prior to intervention for suspected pleural fluid, whether simple pleural effusion, hemothorax or other etiology to reduce the risk of iatrogenic complications during pleural interventions [14].

We designed a pilot study to test if ultrasound guidance improved proper thoracostomy site identification over traditional landmark technique in a healthy volunteer.

Methods

Study design

This was a simulation-based study in which observational results were collected during routine thoracostomy tube training of novice providers. The Institutional Review Board approved this study protocol as exempt.

Study population

33 emergency medicine residents volunteered to take part in this study. The participants had varied levels of skill ranging from no experience with thoracostomy placement to senior residents with greater than 10 successful thoracostomy placements. All residents participate in a 16-h ultrasound course at the beginning of their intern (training) year. This course covers echocardiography, thoracic ultrasound, and trauma (eFAST) along with the American College of Emergency Physicians (ACEP) core topics. Following ACEP guidelines, and to ensure the residents are competent in ultrasound, they must perform good-quality scans in several categories upon completion of their training. The categories pertinent to this study include: 25 eFAST, 25 thoracic, and 50 Echocardiograms.

The participants were instructed and evaluated by dedicated clinical ultrasound faculty and received no direct incentive for participating in the study.

Study protocol

A healthy volunteer was used as the standardized patient for this study. The correct thoracostomy site was defined as the mid-axillary line between ribs 4 and 5. The correct site was pre-identified on both sides by two experienced physicians and marked with invisible ink that could only be revealed with a UV LED flashlight.

The study was performed in two stages. The first stage of the study evaluated the participant on the placement of the chest tube using traditional landmarks. After locating the site, the participant was instructed to place a plastic arrow over the chest tube insertion site. The plastic marker was compared to the pre-identified mark using the UV LED light, and if the plastic marker was incorrectly positioned, the difference in ribs spaces was recorded.

The second stage of the study involved a simulation-based approach to teach the participants how to identify the diaphragm as well as identify and count adjacent rib spaces using ultrasound. The participants were given a brief hands-on teaching session using a curvilinear transducer with the indicator pointing cephalad. The transducer was placed at the costophrenic angle on the mid-axillary line as a starting point. Once the diaphragm was identified, the participant was instructed to look for diaphragmatic excursion and track the diaphragm to the near field on the screen where rib shadows would be present (Fig. 1). The ICS adjacent to the first rib cephalad to the diaphragm was designated as ICS zero. Sliding the transducer superiorly 2 additional ribs spaces accurately located the ICS between the 4th and 5th ribs. Once the participant was taught the technique, they were tested. The participant was asked to use the curvilinear transducer to identify the correct ICS and hold the middle of the transducer over the insertion site. The insertion site

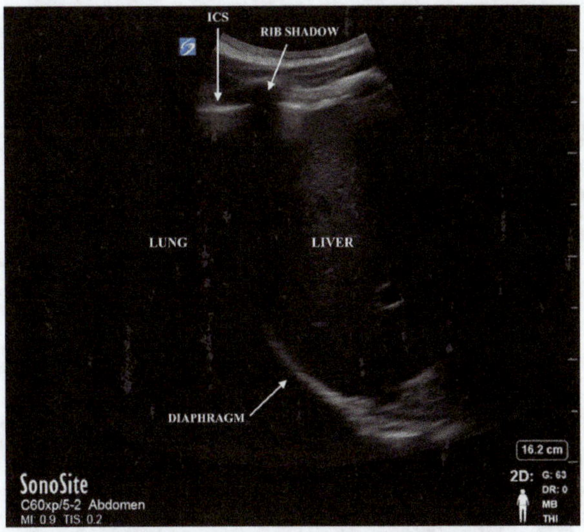

Fig. 1 This is a right upper quadrant ultrasound image at the costophrenic angle demonstrating the starting point of the ultrasound-guided identification of the diaphragm, ribs, and intercostal space

was then compared to the pre-identified site by a UV LED light (Fig. 2).

Equipment

A SonoSite X-Porte ultrasound machine with a curvilinear C60XP 5-2 MHz transducer (SonoSite, Inc, Bothell, WA). TaoTronics 12 UV LED flashlight, model TT-FL001. UV LED flashlight. Reactive invisible ink, nontoxic, fine point pen. Healthy volunteer standardized patient with a BMI of 24.4.

Data collection

The faculty instructors were responsible for recording the data during the study. The number of rib spaces that deviated from the correct ICS was recorded and the data were entered into an Excel spreadsheet (Microsoft Corporation, Redmond, WA). The results were analyzed using a single -ailed student *t* test. After the completion of the study, the participants were asked to fill out a short survey regarding perceived effectiveness of study and its applicability to identify the ideal ICS for thoracostomy placement. The survey choices given to the participant ranged from strongly disagree, disagree, neutral, agree, to strongly agree.

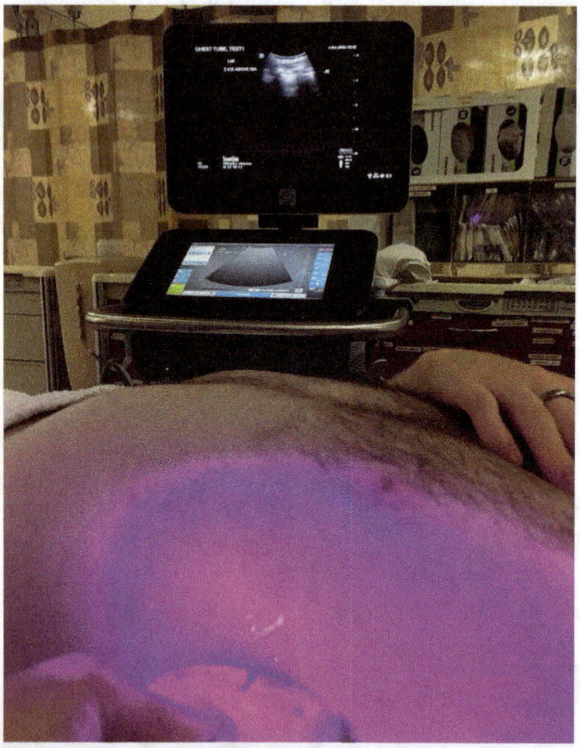

Fig. 2 The curvilinear transducer placement in the correct intercostal space. The LED flashlight has illuminated the landmark (represented by the "X" on the volunteer's skin). On the ultrasound screen in the background, the ICS is demonstrated in the center of the screen between two rib shadows

Results

In the first stage of the study, the landmark-palpated site was accurate at the level of the pre-determined mark 48% (16 of 33) of the time [95 CI 0.43–1.03]. Of these 17 improperly located marks, 12 were 1 ICS off, 3 were 2 ICS off, and 2 were 3 ICS off (Graph 1, Fig. 3). The standard deviation using the traditional technique was 0.88 rib spaces away.

The second stage of the study tested the accuracy of the same 33 participants after a brief hands-on session on identifying the correct ICS under US guidance. The participants correctly identified the pre-determined mark 91% (30 of 33) of the time using ultrasound. Of the 3 improperly located marks, all 3 were 1 ICS off (Graph 1, Fig. 4). The standard deviation using the ultrasound-guided technique was 0.09 rib spaces away (95 CI 0.0–0.19) [$p=0.003$].

Discussion

Chest thoracostomy is a lifesaving procedure in patients with thoracic trauma. Unfortunately, this procedure is not without risks and is associated with significant morbidity and even mortality related to complications of its placement [15–17].

Ultrasonography is a well-established modality with the ability to reduce errors and increase success rate for many emergency medicine procedures [18, 19]. During this study, ultrasound was used to guide placement of the thoracostomy tube and serve as an adjunct to traditional methods in helping to identify the correct ICS, location of the diaphragm and any underlying solid organs.

While other studies challenged learners to place thoracostomy tubes within the "triangle of safety," this study challenged the participants to be more precise and locate the 4th or 5th intercostal space. [12, 20] Of note, the simulated model had normal anatomy with no anatomic variation to the level of his diaphragm; therefore, localizing the precise intercostal space was part of this protocol. This exact methodology may not always apply in real-life situations, as patients may have a variation in the level of the diaphragm secondary to medical conditions such as COPD, phrenic nerve palsy, or increased intraabdominal pressure (e.g., pregnancy or ascites). With this consideration, simply identifying the diaphragm and moving 2–3 intercostal spaces cranially will localize a safe site for tube thoracostomy placement.

Ultrasound showed a significant improvement in the ability to identify the correct thoracostomy site. The traditional landmark technique identified the correct

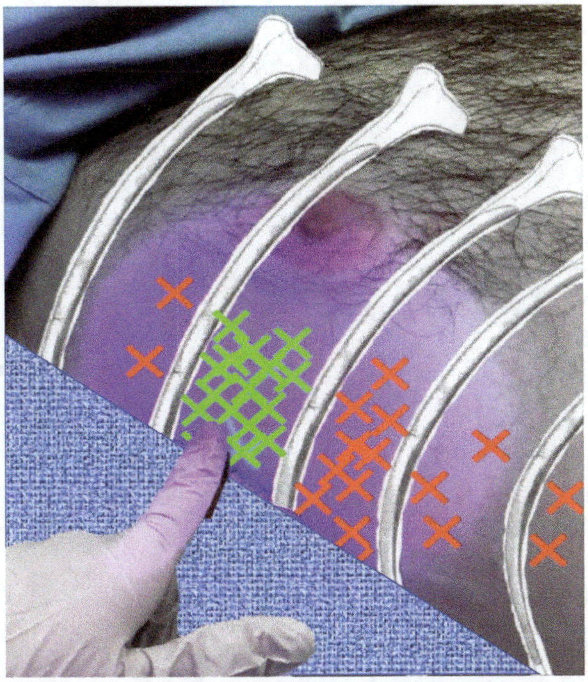

Fig. 3 This is an illustrative representation of the data plotted on the volunteer's chest wall for the landmark-palpated method. The green "X's" represent the correct intercostal space, whereas the red "X's" demonstrate the number of participants who did not place the marker in the correct ICS. The data plotted were illustrated and represented in rib spaces above and below the target

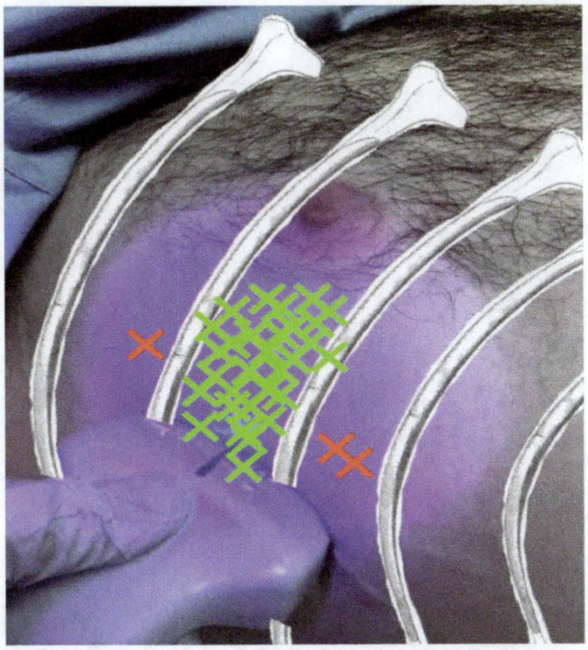

Fig. 4 This is an illustrative representation of the data plotted on the volunteer's chest wall for the ultrasound-guided method. The green "X's" represent the correct intercostal space, whereas the red "X's" demonstrate the number of participants who did not place the transducer in the correct ICS. The data plotted were illustrated and represented in rib spaces above and below the target ICS

thoracostomy site only 48% of the time versus 91% in the ultrasound-guided group.

A post study anonymous survey demonstrated that all participants "agreed" or "strongly agreed" that ultrasound-guided thoracostomy site identification was easy to learn and useful in improving chest thoracostomy site identification. They also "agreed" or "strongly agreed" that they will consider incorporating this adjunct in all patients who require chest thoracostomy, particularly patients with difficult landmarks or a concern for a displaced diaphragm.

For the novice provider, ultrasound can increase the ability to identify the correct intercostal space compared to traditional landmark-guided techniques. Given the expanding use of ultrasound in clinical practice (diagnostic and interventional), this technique may serve as a useful adjunct to the identification of a safe zone for chest thoracostomy. In turn, this interventional ultrasound approach could be added to the ultrasound curricula when teaching critical care ultrasound.

Limitations

This study has several limitations. The simulated nature of the study carried out in a controlled setting is inherently different than the clinical environment in which thoracostomy tubes are placed. Our standardized patient had a normal BMI with palpable landmarks and a normal anatomic location of his diaphragm. It is known that thoracostomy complication rate increases in the obese patient [21]. Despite these limitations, it appears ultrasound could still serve as a useful adjunct to thoracostomy site identification. Another limitation in this study is the lack of subsequent evaluation of the residents to verify if they retained the skills of this educational intervention. Despite the absence of re-evaluation, the residents train at an urban trauma center and perform several eFAST examinations on a clinical shift. This reinforces the skill of identifying the right and left thoracoabdominal interface with each study.

Conclusion

In this pilot study, the ability of novice providers to accurately locate the correct intercostal space for chest tube insertion was improved under ultrasound guidance. The data from this study add to the growing body of evidence that physicians have a high rate of misplaced thoracostomy insertions. This novel technique can greatly improve proper thoracostomy site identification in the clinical setting.

Author contributions

The recognized contribution categories are as follows: 1. Study concept and design, 2. Acquisition of the data, 3. Analysis and interpretation of the data, 4. Drafting of the manuscript, 5. Critical revision of the manuscript for important intellectual content, 6. Statistical expertise, 7. Obtained funding, 8. Administrative, technical, or material support, 9. Study supervision.

Lindsay A. Taylor, MD, RDMS, RDCS 1, 2, 3, 4, 5, 9. Michael J. Vitto, DO, MS, RDMS, RDCS 1, 2, 3, 8, 9. Michael Joyce, MD, RDMS, RDCS 1, 3, 4, 6, 9. Jordan Tozer, MD, RDMS, RDCS 1, 5, 9. David P. Evans, MD, RDMS, RDCS, FACEP 1, 3, 4, 5, 8, 9.

Acknowledgements
Virginia Commonwealth University Emergency Medicine and Emergency Medicine Residency Program.

Meetings Presented: 1. SAEM Mid-Atlantic regional conference March 11th, 2017 Washington, DC, USA. 2. Rao R. Ivatury Trauma Symposium March 29th, 2017, Richmond, VA USA. 3. CORD Academic Assembly April 2017, Ft. Lauderdale, FL USA. 4. SAEM May 17th, 2017 Orlando, FL, USA. This manuscript has not been published anywhere else.

References

1. Meredith JW, Hoth JJ (2007) Thoracic trauma: when and how to intervene. Surg Clin North Am. 87(1):95–118
2. Khandhar SJ, Johnson SB, Calhoon JH (2007) Overview of thoracic trauma in the United States. Thorac Surg Clin. 17(1):1–9
3. American College of Surgeons, Committee on Trauma (2004) Advanced trauma life support course for doctors instructor course manual. American College of Surgeons, Chicago
4. Hippocrates. Writings. In: Hutchins RM, ed. Great books of the western world. Vol. 10. Chicago: Encyclopedia Brittanica; 1952. p. 142
5. Hewett FC (1876) Thoracentesis: the plan of continuous aspiration. Br Med J 1:317
6. Bretts RH, Lees WM (1946) Military thoracic surgery in the forward area. J Thorac Surg 15:44–63
7. Ball CG, Lord J, Laupland KB, Gmora S, Mulloy RH, Ng AK, Schieman C, Kirkpatrick AW (2007) Chest tube complications: How well are we training our residents? Can J Surg 50:6
8. Kesieme EB, Dongo A, Ezemba N, Irekpita E, Jebbin N, Kesieme C (2012) Tube thoracostomy: complications and its management. Pulm Med. 2012:256878
9. Wrightson J, Fysh E, Maskell N, Lee Y (2010) Risk reduction in pleural procedures: sonography simulation and supervision. Curr Opin Pulm Med. 16:340–350
10. Chan L, Reilly KM, Henderson C, Kahn F, Salluzzo RF (1997) Complication rates of tube thoracostomy. Am J Emer Med 15(4):368–370
11. Landay M, Oliver Q, Estrera A, Friese R, Boonswang N, Michael DiMaio J (2006) Lung penetration by thoracostomy tubes. J Thorac Imaging 21(3):197–204
12. Elsayed H, Roberts R, Emadi M, Whittle I, Shackloth M (2010) Chest drain insertion is not a harmless procedure—are we doing it safely? Interact. Cardiovasc Thorac Surg. 11:72
13. Carter Peter, Conroy Sheree, Blakeney Jade, Sood Bimal (2014) Identifying the site for intercostal catheter insertion in the emergency department: is clinical examination reliable? Emerg Med Australas 26(5):450–454
14. Havelock T, Teoh R, Laws D, Gleeson F (2010) Pleural procedures and thoracic ultrasound: British Thoracic Society pleural disease guidelines 2010. Thorax 65(Suppl 2):i61–i76
15. Deneuville M (2002) Morbidity of percutaneous tube thoracostomy in trauma patients. Eur J Cardiothorac Surg 22:673–678
16. McFadden PM, Jones JW (1985) Tube thoracostomy: anatomical considerations, overview of complications, and a proposed technique to avoid complications. Mil Med 150:681–685
17. Shapira OM, Aldea GS, Kupferschmidt J et al (1993) Delayed perforation of the esophagus by a closed thoracostomy tube. Chest 104:1897–1898
18. Hind D, Calvert N, McWilliams R, Davidson A, Paisley S, Beverley C, Thomas S (2003) Ultrasonic locating devices for central venous cannulation: meta-analysis. BMJ 327(7411):361
19. Brass P, Hellmich M, Kolodziej L et al (2015) Ultrasound guidance versus anatomical landmarks for internal jugular vein catheterization. Cochrane Database Syst Rev. 1:011447
20. Griffiths JR (2005) Do junior doctors know where to insert chest drains safely? Postgrad Med J 81(957):456–458
21. Kwiatt M, Tarbox A, Seamon MJ et al (2014) Thoracostomy tubes: a comprehensive review of complications and related topics. Int J Crit Illn Inj Sci 4(2):143–155

16

The implementation of a longitudinal POCUS curriculum for physicians working at rural outpatient clinics in Chiapas, Mexico

Annie Heffernan Rominger[1*], Gerardo Antonio Aguilar Gomez[2] and Patrick Elliott[2]

Abstract

Background: Medical care in resource limited settings is challenging, particularly with limited access to diagnostic and imaging studies. The most portable and cost effective diagnostic imaging in these areas is ultrasound. Ultrasound is a very teachable skill with a short, single intensive training course and hands-on teaching; however, there are limited data on a longitudinal point-of-care ultrasound (POCUS) curriculum in resource limited settings. The goal of this intervention is to develop an effective longitudinal POCUS curriculum for local physicians working in rural clinics in the state of Chiapas, Mexico, and evaluate its effectiveness on patient care.

Methods: This is a 12-month longitudinal ultrasound educational curriculum for local supervising physicians working in rural clinics in Chiapas, Mexico. The 10 clinics are a collaboration of the Mexican government and Compañeros En Salud with limited access to any diagnostic imaging or laboratory studies. The investigators assisted in obtaining four portable ultrasound machines for use in the clinics. Next, they organized four point-of-care ultrasound (POCUS) teaching sessions over a year, each session focusing on several distinct concepts. The sessions included lectures and hands-on teaching with both healthy volunteers and with patients in the various communities. Over the 12 months, the POCUS were logged and the majority of images saved. The logs were analyzed to determine if POCUS affected the medical management of the patients. The primary investigator reviewed 35.2% of the total ultrasounds completed, which was 52.2% of the save images, for quality assurance and feedback.

Results: Over the 12 months, there were 584 ultrasound studies documented. The most common study was a transabdominal obstetric examination (45.5%) followed by abdomen/pelvis (26.6%) and musculoskeletal (5.7%) and skin and soft tissue (5.7%). The use of POCUS changed the patient diagnosis after 194 scans (34%) and changed the clinical management for the patient encounter in 171 (30%) scans. In the 194 scans in which POCUS changed the diagnosis, the clinical management was changed, as a direct result of the scan results, in 152 (78.4%) of those patient encounters.

Conclusion: A longitudinal POCUS educational curriculum is an effective way to equip local physicians in resource limited countries with a tool to improve their clinical management of patients.

Keywords: POCUS education, Global health education, Point-of-care ultrasound (POCUS), Educational curriculum

*Correspondence: anna.rominger@louisville.edu
[1] Department of Pediatrics, Division of Emergency Medicine, University of Louisville, 571 South Floyd Street, Suite 412, Louisville, KY 40202, USA
Full list of author information is available at the end of the article

Background

Medical care in resource-limited settings can present multiple challenges to the timely and accurate clinical diagnoses of patients. Typically, there are limited diagnostic and imaging capabilities available to medical providers. The most accessible diagnostic imaging modalities for primary care and emergency services in underserved areas are radiographs and ultrasounds [1]. If they are not readily available, lengthy transportation for appropriate diagnostic studies can delay treatment and result in increased costs to an already marginalized population [1, 2]. X-ray machines require more space, are more expensive than ultrasound machines, and expose the patients and staff to radiation. Consequently, since 1985, the World Health Organization (WHO) has recommended ultrasound for developing countries because it is portable, inexpensive, non-invasive, safe, and provides immediate information [3, 4].

Becker et al. performed a systematic review of the literature surrounding portable ultrasound use in low and middle income countries. The review included 27 original research articles and 9 case reports, which universally demonstrated effective screening or diagnostic uses of ultrasound for various conditions [5]. Some of these articles included Point-of-Care Ultrasound (POCUS) and others included traditional ultrasound examinations. As a definition, POCUS is performed by the treating physician and is intended to answer a specific question [2]. Diagnoses for which POCUS is suitable should fulfill two criteria: (1) it must be relevant to treatment decision making and (2) it must be easily and accurately recognizable by physicians applying ultrasound without the necessity for extended ultrasound training [6]. Therefore, one key strategy to make a lasting change in resource limited areas is to teach local providers to use POCUS so they can provide a higher level of care to the local people.

Shah et al. conducted an educational intervention in Rwanda to create an effective ultrasound curriculum for the providers at two of the local hospitals [3]. The investigators conducted a 9 week course which included a total of 15 lecture hours and 15–30 scanning hours The clinicians kept logs of their ultrasound studies and indicated that their findings changed the initial patient management in 43% of cases [7]. The most common change in patient management was the decision to perform a surgical procedure following the results of the ultrasound [7]. Overall, the study concluded that ultrasound is a very teachable skill with an intensive training course and hands-on teaching [3].

Another study concluded that ultrasound in low resource settings can provide adequate imaging in screening for placenta previa, fetal malposition, multiple gestations, ectopic pregnancy, obstructed labor, pelvic outlet measurement, and limited fetal anatomy [8]. These are all conditions that would necessitate a cesarean section to protect the life and well-being of both the mother and the neonate. They found that motivated trainees and an intensive and highly abbreviated training course by qualified physicians resulted in the achievement of basic ultrasound skills in much shorter training periods [8]. They also concluded that long-term success of the ultrasound deployment in resource limited areas also requires continuing education [8].

Partners in Health (PIH) is a nonprofit organization that launched Compañeros En Salud (CES) in 2011, which is a group that works with 10 of the rural government clinics in the Sierra Madre region of Chiapas, one of the most marginalized regions of Mexico [9]. Ultrasound is the only imaging modality available to the clinics and the nearest hospital with plain radiography is anywhere from 2 to 6 h away depending on the specific location of the clinic. The local people are very limited financially and traveling many hours away for basic tests or unnecessary referrals can cause a large financial strain on the person and family. Basic POCUS knowledge and skills may greatly aid in the local management of many medical conditions, reduce the number of referrals for imaging, and expedite the care of patients who require transfer for a serious medical or surgical problem.

As described above, short-term ultrasound training programs have proven to deliver adequate knowledge and skills to novices [4]. Most of the previous studies on training programs include a short single and sometimes repeat course taught by an outside group to local providers. Knowledge and skills can deteriorate without continuing education and long term success of an ultrasound program requires it [8]. In addition, a recent article examining POCUS programs in Africa suggests prioritizing longitudinal and sustainable models for training and short courses without ongoing supervision or skill maintenance should be avoided [10]. To the authors' knowledge, there is not an evaluation of the effectiveness of a longitudinal POCUS curriculum in a clinic based resource limited setting. The immediate goal of this program is to develop an effective longitudinal, continuing POCUS curriculum for local CES physicians working in the state of Chiapas, Mexico and determine its effect on patient care in the area.

Methods

This is a longitudinal educational curriculum initiated by the organizers of CES. CES recruits motivated Mexican physicians who are entering a government-required social service year (*pasantes*) to staff each of the 10 rural clinics. The supervisors in the organization are physicians who have completed their social service requirement are responsible for the education of the *pasantes*, administrative responsibilities, arranging transfer of patients, and oversight of the clinics. There are 6–8 supervisors each year and each one oversees 1–3 clinics. The ultrasound curriculum focuses on the supervisors since they are retained in the organization for a longer periods of time, travel between the clinics that they oversee, and are responsible for teaching the *pasantes*.

The instructors for the educational sessions included a Pediatric Emergency Medicine (PEM) physician, an Emergency Medicine (EM) physician, a PEM fellow, and two upper level EM residents from the University of Louisville. An Obstetrician from Harvard University/Brigham and Women's Hospital was the instructor for the session on obstetric ultrasound. Both faculty members from the University of Louisville have extensive bedside ultrasound experience and have taught ultrasound at major national and international conferences.

The course lasted 4 days and it recurred every 3–4 months with different topics at each course. All the material was presented in English because all of the participants were fluent in English. The first 1.5 days were spent in the main offices with lectures (4 h) and hands on training (5 h) on healthy volunteers. The class ratio was 6–10 learners per two instructors. Then, they split up into two groups, each led by one of the ultrasound instructors, and went to the rural community clinics to ultrasound patients with known relevant pathology for the next 2 days (approximately 6–7 h each day). Prior to initiation of the course work, a needs assessment was conducted with the local physicians to determine the most relevant topics and the regional pathologies that are commonly encountered. The curriculum was then adjusted accordingly. All topics were covered over the 12 total months of the curriculum (four sessions). The total lecture time over the four sessions was 16 h and total hands-on time with healthy volunteers was 20 h. In addition, the trainees also received a total of 8 days, 6–7 h per day of hands-on training and bedside POCUS training on patients with known relevant diagnoses over the entire course. This added another 48–56 h of hands-on training to the course. The intent of breaking the course up into multiple sessions was to avoid overwhelming the learners and giving them time to master a couple POCUS topics before moving to the next ones. Multiple trips also allowed the opportunity to review interesting cases, technique, and individual competency from the previous topics. As most supervisors remain in their positions for several years, they re-review the material annually.

The investigators helped CES obtain four refurbished Sonosite nanomaxx ultrasound machines, each with low frequency (phased array) and high frequency (linear) probes. The supervisors were responsible for the ultrasound machines and took turns taking the machines with them to the clinics which they oversaw. Each supervisor had a machine for 2 weeks at a time and brought it to the clinics he or she supervised. While there, they worked with the *pasante* to schedule ultrasounds at the clinic for patients in the community who would benefit from imaging. They could also ultrasound patients if needed as they came into be evaluated. This gave the supervisors the opportunity to show the *pasantes* some concepts and uses of POCUS. Occasionally there would be case when ultrasound was urgently needed in one of the clinics and the supervisors would communicate and coordinate a way to get the machine to that clinic for that specific patient.

The first teaching session was in September 2015 and focused on introduction to ultrasound, care and use of the machine, focused assessment with sonography in trauma (FAST), evaluation of the kidney and bladder, and basic obstetrics. The next session was in February 2016 and it included lung ultrasound, skin and soft tissue, and musculoskeletal. The third session was conducted at the end of April 2016 by an OB/GYN physician and was focused on obstetrics. The fourth session was July 2016 and it reviewed ultrasound basics and then focused on cardiovascular, advanced abdomen, and ocular. The presentations from each session were left with the participants for their reference and review. At the completion of the curriculum, the investigator continued with two trips per year as a review and had 3–4 web based series of cases with images to review and discuss to promote long term competency.

There was an ultrasound log with each machine which documents the type of ultrasound conducted, reason for the study, presumed diagnosis, and if the ultrasound findings confirmed or changed the presumed diagnosis for the patient. The information included the patient's initials, age, gender, and date of study. Lastly, the log contained the initials of the physician performing the ultrasound and site of the study. By providing the type of ultrasounds, it allowed the investigators to track the number of the different studies that were conducted and where more or less time should be spent in the future curriculum. By tracking the number of ultrasounds for each supervisor, the investigators could provide additional resources to those who were not as comfortable using the machines. Every 1–2 months, the supervisors brought the ultrasound logs to the monthly educational conferences where they were compiled from all the clinics, copied, and sent back to the primary investigator for review. The primary investigator transferred the information into a spreadsheet and each study was given a de-identified number and the initials of the person who received the study removed.

De-identified images were loaded onto a Google drive folder for review and feedback. The primary investigator reviewed the images for technique, quality and findings. Feedback was provided at each of the sessions or sooner via email as necessary. The primary investigator was available to review any images urgently if requested for clarification. This educational intervention was reviewed by the University of Louisville Institutional Review Board and deemed to be exempt. In addition, the study was reviewed by CES research committee and received approval to conduct this educational intervention.

Results

It took 6 weeks after the initial session to get the ultrasound logs to all the machines and have consistent recording of the examinations. Therefore, only 10.5 months (December 2015–October 2016) of data were recorded and analyzed. Over the 12 months after the initiation of the curriculum, there were 584 ultrasound studies documented. The most common study was a transabdominal obstetric examination (45.5%) followed by abdomen/pelvis (26.6%), cardiovascular (5.8%), musculoskeletal (5.7%) and skin and soft tissue (5.7%) (Table 1). The number of ultrasounds performed by each supervisor ranged from 27 to 162 (Table 2). There were two supervisors who started their position halfway through the educational curriculum and therefore have less scans.

The use of POCUS changed the diagnosis after 194 scans (34%) and changed the clinical management for the patient encounter in 171 (30%) scans. In the 194 scans in which POCUS changed the diagnosis, the clinical management was changed in 152 (78.4%) of those patient encounters. 113 of the included scans were completed under the direct supervision and feedback of one of the instructors during an educational session, leaving 471 scans completed independently. Of the scans completed without direct supervision, the use of POCUS changed the diagnosis after 33.7% of scans and changed the clinical management for the patient encounter in 30.7% of the scans.

Table 1 The distribution of the types of ultrasound recorded over the study period

Type of ultrasound	Number of ultrasounds (*n*)	Percentage (%)
Obstetric	266	45.5
Abdomen	155	26.6
Cardiac	34	5.8
Breast	34	5.8
Skin and soft tissue	33	5.7
Musculoskeletal	33	5.7
Chest/lungs	17	2.9
Ocular	9	1.5
Thyroid	3	0.5
Total	584	100.0

Table 2 Number of ultrasounds recorded by each supervisor

Physician	Number of ultrasounds (*n*)	Percentage (%)
1	162	27.7
2	109	18.7
3	83	14.2
4	66	11.3
5	58	9.9
6	43	7.4
7	36	6.2
8	27	4.6
Total	584	100.0

Ocular ultrasound changed the diagnosis during the patient encounter most often with 62.5%, followed by skin and soft tissue (45.5%), cardiac (48%), and abdomen/pelvis (43.3%) (Table 3). POCUS changed the clinical management of the patient encounter the most after scans of the thyroid and eyes (both 50%), followed by cardiovascular (43.8%), musculoskeletal (42.4%), abdomen/pelvis (38%), breast (36.4%), and chest/lung (35.3%) (Table 4). The obstetric ultrasounds were the most commonly done and changed the diagnosis in 66 (24.4%) patient encounters and changed the management in 55 (20.2%) patient encounters.

The number of POCUS conducted per month typically spiked after a teaching session with gradual decrease in use over the following months (Fig. 1). Part of the spike was due to the scans completed during the sessions themselves (Fig. 1). The most scans were recorded in September 2016 which is 12 months after the initiation of the educational curriculum and after four educational sessions. In the 5 months after the completion of the educational curriculum, there were 128 scans completed (Fig. 2). There was a drop in scans in February when there was a change in supervisors. It is unclear whether the new supervisors were not logging the ultrasounds, they were not conducting as many ultrasounds, or the data was not entered. Despite this, the group still averaged > 25 scans per month. The most common imaging modalities remained to be obstetrics (56.3%) and abdomen/pelvis (25.1%). It changed diagnosis in 33.6% and changed management in 25.8% of the scans completed over the 5 month period.

Table 3 The frequency for which POCUS changed patient diagnosis in each of the different types of ultrasound examinations

Type of ultrasound	Total studies with data input	Numbers of changed diagnosis	Percent changed diagnosis
Obstetric	262	64	24.4
Abdomen/pelvis	150	65	43.3
Skin and soft tissue	33	15	45.5
Musculoskeletal	33	13	39.4
Breast	33	11	33.3
Cardiovascular	32	15	46.8
Chest/lungs	17	5	29.4
Ocular	8	5	62.5
Thyroid	2	1	50
Missing	15		
Total	584	194	33.2

Table 4 The frequency for which POCUS changed patient clinical management in each of the different types of ultrasound examinations

Type of ultrasound	Total studies with data input	Numbers of changed clinical management	Percentage of changed clinical management
OB	262	53	20.2
Abdomen/pelvis	150	57	38
Skin and soft tissue	33	10	30.3
Musculoskeletal	33	14	42.4
Breast	33	12	36.4
Cardiovascular	32	14	43.8
Chest/lungs	17	6	35.3
Ocular	8	4	50
Thyroid	2	1	50
Missing	14		
Total	584	171	29.2

There were a total of 584 included scans. 113 of the included scans were completed under the direct supervision and feedback of one of the instructors during an educational session, leaving 471 scans completed independently. There were 190 scans which were documented in the ultrasound log but no images were saved for review. Therefore, there were 281 scans that were not obtained under direct supervision of an instructor and had saved images for review. 33% of these scans were randomly selected and reviewed by the primary investigator to confirm the diagnosis and to provide feedback regarding technique. One of the instructors was either present or the primary investigator reviewed the scanned images for 206 of the 394 saved images (52.2%), which is 35.2% of the total 584 scans. There was a disagreement in findings in 4.3% of the images reviewed and none of which affected the clinical management of the patients. There were also 6.5% of scans with inadequate image quality to interpret.

Discussion

The ultrasound use by local physicians following this longitudinal curriculum echoes the conclusions from previous studies that ultrasound is a very teachable and useful skill, particularly in resource limited areas. The previous study by Shah in Rwanda, showed increase ultrasound use 11 weeks after the departure of the ultrasound instructor following the ultrasound course with a high concordance rate of scan interpretation [7]. In US ED residents and faculty, there are improvements of ultrasound knowledge scores 6 months after training suggesting retention of the information [11]. Scores, however, were higher in those who received more hands-on training [11]. The total lecture time in this educational program was similar to previous single, short term educational programs; however, there was almost three times as much hands-on training, which has been shown to result in higher long term skill retention [7, 11]. Similar to the previous findings, the results show that ultrasound use peaks after an educational session; however they decrease to a plateau. After each session's peak, the plateau was higher and higher suggesting more comfort with use following repeated sessions. The highest POCUS use in this study was 12 months after the initial course. Typically, ultrasound use wanes with time but repeated sessions that build on the previous clearly demonstrate an effective strategy for continued POCUS use and clinical application in resource limited settings. In addition, repeated sessions with skill reinforcement and technical review can serve as a revalidation of skills taught in a previous session(s) which is evidenced by a low disagreement rate of scan interpretation [10].

This study demonstrates how training and use of POCUS significantly affects the clinical management and diagnosis of patients in the marginalized region of the Sierra Madre in the state of Chiapas, Mexico. The 584 total scans recorded is a larger sample size than other similar studies since the population was followed for over 12 months. The 34% of patient encounters in which POCUS changed the clinical diagnosis likely prevented delays in care and expedited referral and hospitalization as needed without having to wait for a patient to obtain imaging at another site. In this study, ultrasound changed the management plan in 30% of patients. Although this

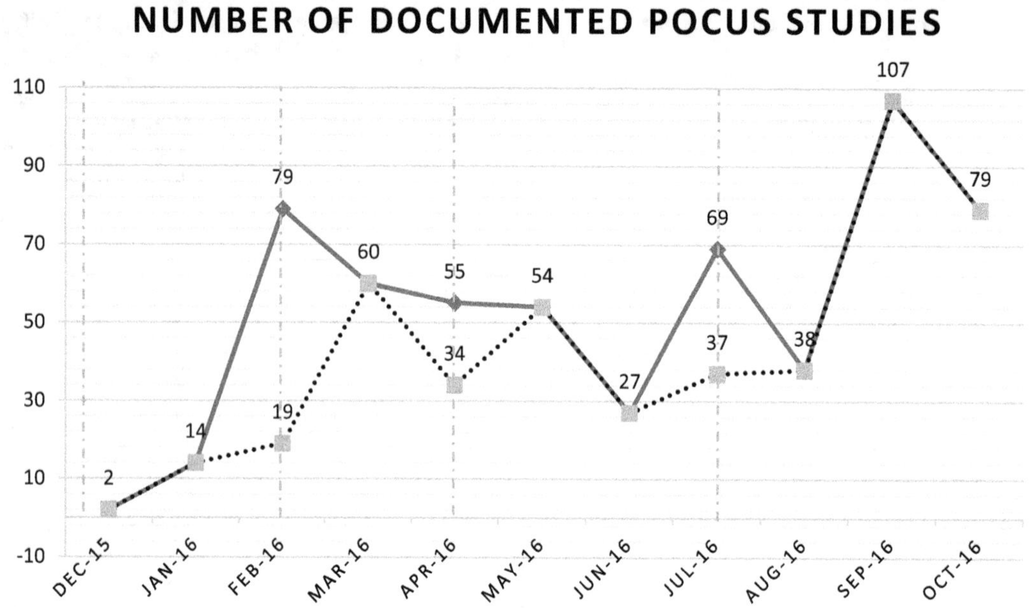

Fig. 1 Linear representation of the total number of documented POCUS studies over the study period. The vertical dashed lines are the dates of the training sessions. The dotted line is the number of unsupervised documented POCUS studies over the study period

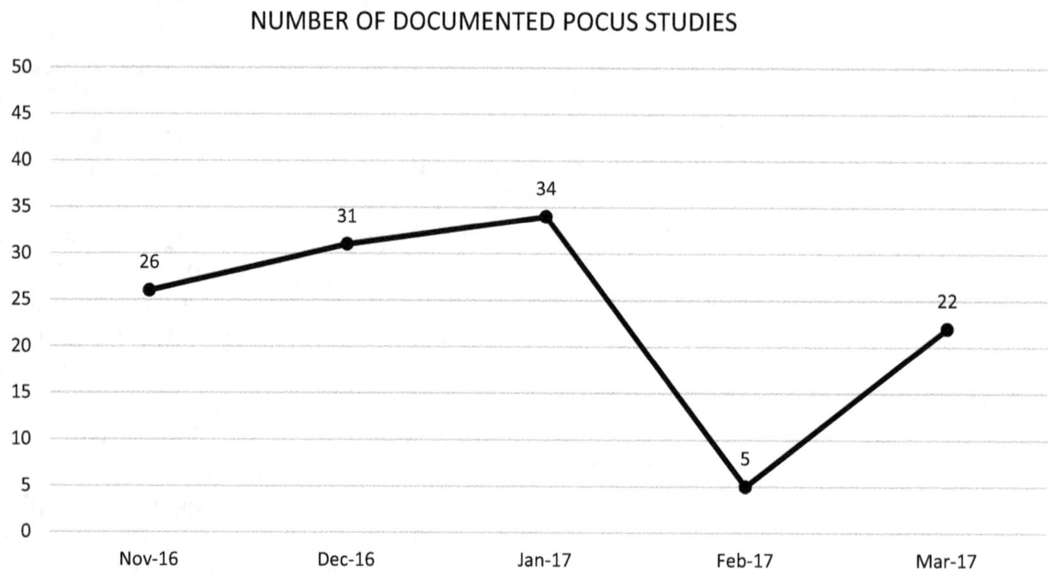

Fig. 2 Linear representation of the total number of documented POCUS studies over the 5 months following the study period

is lower than the findings in Rwanda, which was a hospital based study with higher acuity patients, it shows the significant effect of POCUS in the resource limited primary care clinic based setting. As reported in previous ultrasound studies on inpatients, the remainder of the patients for which POCUS did not change diagnosis or management still benefit from a scan that can confirm a clinical diagnosis and reinforce the current management plan [2].

Similar to previous ultrasound studies in resource limited settings, the most commonly conducted ultrasound was obstetric. The investigators predicted this based on the initial needs assessment so obstetric ultrasound was taught at two educational sessions, including one by an obstetrician. Harris et al. showed that bedside ultrasound in resource limited areas, specifically Nicaragua and Africa is an effective way to identify serious obstetric conditions that can potentially save the life of the woman or the neonate [8]. Over the 12 month study period, some of obstetric POCUS findings that changed the diagnosis include placenta previa, twin pregnancy, molar pregnancy, incomplete spontaneous abortion, subchorionic hemorrhage, abnormal presentation (breech) of the fetus. Although the percent of obstetric scans for which there was change diagnosis is not extremely high, the diagnoses that were detected can be serious and potentially life threatening to the woman or the fetus/neonate in resource limited areas. Maternal and child health is a major health initiative in the developing world and different cultural barriers and traditions present challenges to physicians in these areas [8]. Many women in the region of Chiapas and other resource limited settings have out of hospital deliveries, typically with a traditional birth attendant. By providing the physicians with ultrasounds and appropriate training, they can identify women who are at increased risk of complications and make earlier referral for hospitalized delivery or cesarean section.

Limitations

The major limitation of the analysis of the educational curriculum is an incomplete ultrasound log. The supervisors may not have remembered to record every scan conducted and of those recorded, there were 190 which were not saved. Although this could affect the descriptive data, it would result in the underestimation of the use of ultrasound in the clinics. Since the goal of the curriculum is increase in POCUS use, it does not have an overall impact on the intervention. However, it may have contributed to the primary investigators review of the scans for quality assurance. Another limitation is supervisor turnover during the educational curriculum. There were two supervisors who left for other positions after the first session and two new supervisors were added after the 2nd session. This may have skewed the results since it was not a consistent population of learners throughout the entire curriculum. The two most commonly performed studies were taught during the first session which may have contributed to the large number of these studies and skewed the results.

The investigators did not collect a written or hands-on examination of the course participants to evaluate their improvement in knowledge and skill retention. Although their knowledge would have increased since they reported not having little to no knowledge and experience with ultrasound, having an objective assessment of their knowledge would have been helpful. In addition, a hands-on session would have been helpful to evaluate skill retention. This is another limitation of the evaluation of the educational curriculum. Lastly, although the local physicians were fluent in English, the course was not given in their native language so there may have been comprehension issues that were not apparent during the course.

Conclusion

A longitudinal POCUS educational curriculum is an effective means to teach ultrasound in resource limited settings. It can equip local physicians with a tool to guide their clinical diagnoses and improve their clinical management of patients. In addition, the POCUS program conducted in rural Chiapas, Mexico demonstrates its usefulness in the resource limited outpatient clinic setting.

Abbreviations

POCUS: Point-of-care ultrasound; CES: Compañeros En Salud; PIH: Partners in Health; EM: Emergency Medicine.

Authors' contributions

AR and PE conceived the idea for the longitudinal POCUS curriculum and worked together to design it. PE worked in Mexico to conduct a needs assessment for the design and worked with GA to organize the educational sessions, including scheduling, location, and supplies. AR created and taught the lectures and the hands-on POCUS teaching sessions. PE and GA entered the data from the logs into an electronic format and placed images onto an electronic database. AR reviewed the ultrasound images for concordance and analyzed the data. AR drafted the manuscript and both PE and GA contributed to its revision. AR takes responsibility for the paper as a whole. All authors read and approved the final manuscript.

Author details

[1] Department of Pediatrics, Division of Emergency Medicine, University of Louisville, 571 South Floyd Street, Suite 412, Louisville, KY 40202, USA. [2] Compañeros En Salud, Calle Primera Poniente Sur #25, 30370 Angel Albino Corzo (Jaltenango), Chiapas, Mexico.

Acknowledgements

The authors would like to thank PIH and CES with their support of the ultrasound curriculum. They would also like to thank Sonosite who provided a partial grant for the ultrasound machines through their Soundcaring program.

References

1. Maru DS, Schwarz R, Jason A, Basu S, Sharma A, Moore C (2010) Turning a blind eye: the mobilization of radiology services in resource-poor regions. Glob Health 6:18
2. Stanley A, Wajanga BM, Jaka H et al (2017) The impact of systematic point-of-care ultrasound on management of patients in a resource-limited setting. Am J Trop Med Hyg 96:488–492
3. Shah S, Noble VE, Umulisa I et al (2008) Development of an ultrasound training curriculum in a limited resource international setting: successes and challenges of ultrasound training in rural Rwanda. Int J Emerg Med 1:193–196
4. Via G, Storti E, Spreafico A, Melniker L, Neri L (2012) Point of care ultrasound for sepsis management in resource-limited settings: time for a new paradigm for global health care. Intensive Care Med 38:1405–1407 **(author reply 8-9)**
5. Becker DM, Tafoya CA, Becker SL, Kruger GH, Tafoya MJ, Becker TK (2016) The use of portable ultrasound devices in low- and middle-income countries: a systematic review of the literature. Trop Med Int Health 21:294–311
6. Belard S, Tamarozzi F, Bustinduy AL et al (2016) Point-of-care ultrasound assessment of tropical infectious diseases–a review of applications and perspectives. Am J Trop Med Hyg 94:8–21
7. Shah SP, Epino H, Bukhman G et al (2009) Impact of the introduction of ultrasound services in a limited resource setting: rural Rwanda 2008. BMC Int Health Hum Rights 9:4

8. Harris RD, Marks WM (2009) Compact ultrasound for improving maternal and perinatal care in low-resource settings: review of the potential benefits, implementation challenges, and public health issues. J Ultrasound Med 28:1067–1076
9. Partners in Health. 2013. http://www.pih.org/. Accessed Nov 7 2013
10. Salmon M, Landes M, Hunchak C et al (2017) Getting it right the first time: defining regionally relevant training curricula and provider core competencies for point-of-care ultrasound education on the african continent. Ann Emerg Med 69:218–226
11. Noble VE, Nelson BP, Sutingco AN, Marill KA, Cranmer H (2007) Assessment of knowledge retention and the value of proctored ultrasound exams after the introduction of an emergency ultrasound curriculum. BMC Med Educ 7:40

17

Feasibility study of advanced focused cardiac measurements within the emergency department

Joe Betcher[1*], Al Majkrzak[2], Jim Cranford[3], Ross Kessler[4], Nik Theyyunni[4] and Rob Huang[4]

Abstract

Background: This study aims to compare the increased time needed to perform advanced focused cardiac measurements in the emergency department, including diastolic heart failure evaluation via E/E′, and cardiac output with LVOT/VTI. Patients with pertinent cardiopulmonary symptoms in the emergency department had a focused cardiac ultrasound performed by the emergency department ultrasound team. The ability to obtain basic cardiac windows, evaluate for effusion, systolic ejection fraction, and right-sided heart pressures were recorded. Advanced measurements, along with time to obtain all images and the training level of the provider, were recorded.

Results: Fifty-three patients were enrolled. Basic focused cardiac windows were able to be obtained in 80% of patients. The average 4-window focused cardiac ultrasound took 4 min and 49 s to perform. Diastolic measurements were able to be obtained in 51% of patients, taking an average of 3 min and 17 s. Cardiac output measurements were able to be obtained in 53% of patients, taking an average of 3 min and 8 s.

Conclusion: The ability to obtain these images improved with increasing level of training. Performing both cardiac output and diastolic measurements increased the time with bedside ultrasound by 6 min and 25 s, and were able to be obtained in slightly over half of all ED patients.

Keywords: Ultrasound, Echocardiogram, VTI, Diastolic, Focused cardiac ultrasound, Point of care ultrasound

Background

Focused cardiac ultrasound (FOCUS) has become increasingly utilized by emergency medicine (EM) physicians to evaluate undifferentiated patients within the emergency department (ED). The ability to accurately diagnose patients presenting with acute dyspnea or hypotension has been shown to be aided by use of FOCUS [1–3]. Recent studies have shown that EM physicians are able to interpret complex FOCUS findings with high levels of accuracy [4]. Furthermore, the ability of EM physicians to perform and interpret cardiac findings such as ejection fraction, right heart strain/function, diastolic function, fluid status, valvular dysfunction, and aortic dissection has been studied and proven in the literature [5–12].

Fluid status evaluation is a recommended indication for FOCUS [13]. Although there are multiple methods to evaluate fluid status in the cardiopulmonary patient, including history and physical exam, FOCUS for inferior vena cava measurement, central venous pressure measurement, stroke volume variation, and passive leg raise, there remains no clear foolproof method for this evaluation. Cardiac velocity time integral (VTI) is used to calculate stroke volume in the evaluation of volume responsiveness, and can be measured through basic cardiac windows [14] (Figs. 1, 2). Prior research has shown that EM physicians can perform cardiac VTI measurements accurately [15].

Similarly, the work-up of diastolic heart failure within the ED can be elusive, as the systolic ejection fraction seen on basic windows can appear normal.

*Correspondence: joebetcher@gmail.com
[1] Department of Emergency Medicine, Lake Michigan Emergency Specialists, Mercy Health Muskegon, Muskegon, USA
Full list of author information is available at the end of the article

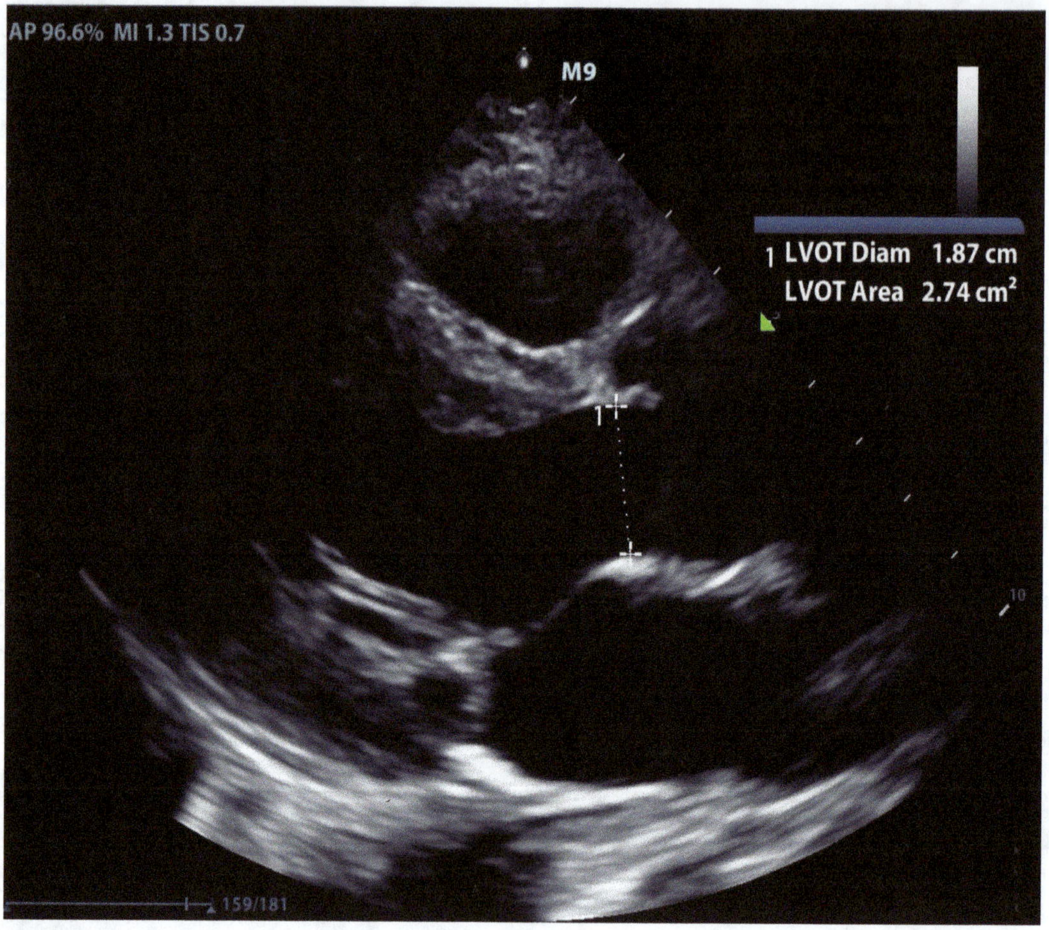

Fig. 1 Measurement of LVOT in PSLV

Approximately 50% of congestive heart failure (CHF) exacerbations are due to diastolic failure, leading to frequent presentations within the ED. EM physicians have also been shown to be able to perform and interpret diastolic CHF measurements with high sensitivity [8] (Figs. 3, 4). Tasked with providing care to many patients simultaneously, FOCUS must be performed efficiently in order to add value in the diagnostic work-up of the patient with cardiopulmonary complaints. Each additional FOCUS measurement adds to the time needed to evaluate each patient. With the recent evidence that EM physicians can perform and interpret complex FOCUS measurements, we sought to prove the feasibility of performing these measurements within the ED. We evaluated both the frequency and speed that physicians at varying skill levels were able to obtain measurements to calculate both VTI and diastolic heart failure. As multiple prior studies have proven that FOCUS impacts decision making, this study only sought to prove feasibility of performance of advanced cardiac measurements, not the impact they have on decision making [16–18].

Methods

This prospective, observational study was conducted in an academic emergency department with a residency training program. The institutional review board approved this study (HUM00113390, 2016). Participation in this study was voluntary and no compensation was offered. Patients were verbally consented prior to inclusion in the study. Patient data were gathered over a 2-month time period. All sonographic images were obtained by Mindray® M9 ultrasound machines (Mindray Ltd., Shenzhen, China) available to the emergency department for regular patient care use. A Mindray phased array (P4-1c) probe was used for obtaining all images.

Patients were selected via a sample of patients who presented to the ED with a chief complaint of chest pain or dyspnea. Patients older than 18 years of age were eligible for the study. When the initial ED provider deemed that FOCUS was necessary in the ED for further aid with narrowing the differential diagnosis, the EM-based ultrasound team was consulted. This team consisted of an ultrasound fellow, along with an EM resident. This team

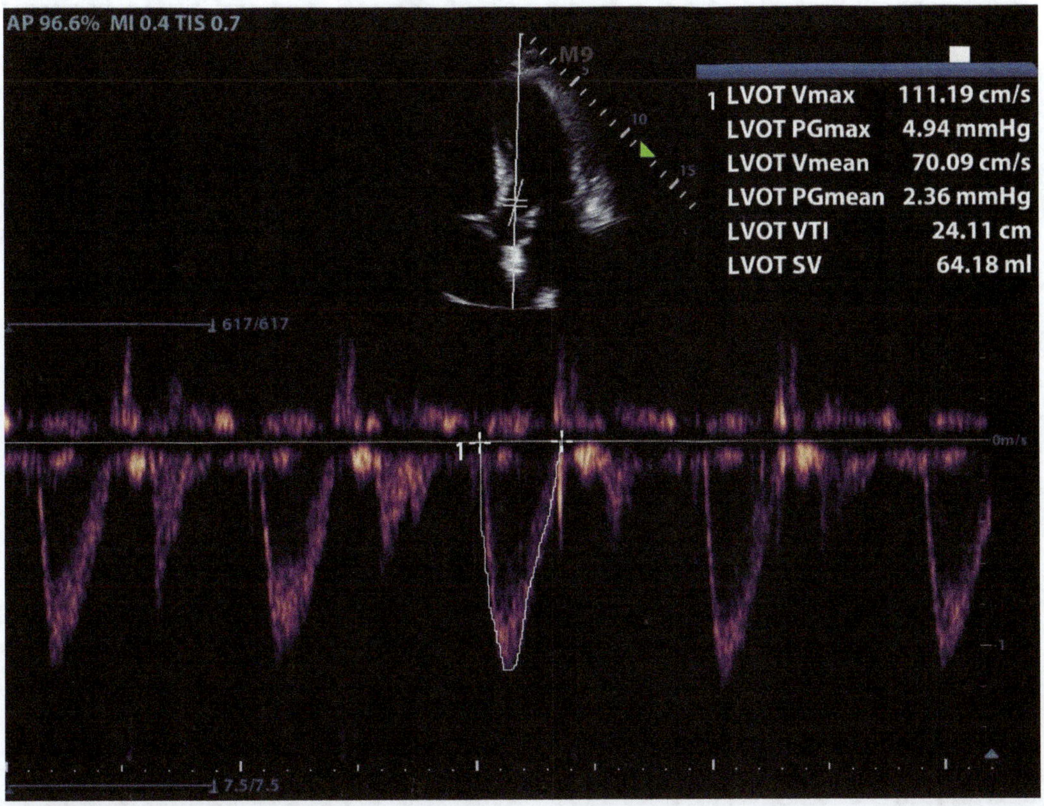

Fig. 2 Measurement of VTI in apical view

was available for 8-h blocks in the ED, from the hours of 12:00 P.M. to 8 P.M., on weekdays. This availability was based on the point of care ultrasound rotation for EM resident education.

Basic demographic information, including the patient's age, weight, and BMI, was gathered. This team then performed FOCUS, and attempted to obtain parasternal long (PSLA), parasternal short (PSSA), apical five-chamber, and subxiphoid views. A gross visual interpretation of the systolic ejection fraction, right ventricular systolic heart strain pertaining to visual interpretation of abnormal ventricular septal movement in the PSSA and apical views, and visual assessment of pericardial effusion was made by the performing resident/fellow. Following this, left ventricular outflow tract (LVOT) diameter in a PSLA, and the VTI in the apical view were obtained, for calculation of stroke volume. Finally, the E and E′ values were obtained in the apical five-chamber view, for measurement of possible diastolic heart failure. The interpretations and measurements were recorded, and reported back to the EM provider. Given that patients were evaluated in real time within the emergency department, while also undergoing further work-up with laboratory studies and other possible imaging studies, only either the resident or fellow performed the ultrasound on the individual patient.

These measurements were chosen as they represent advanced cardiac measurements that require advanced training in FOCUS, yet can potentially aid EM physicians in obtaining complex diagnoses. The time needed to perform LVOT, VTI, E, and E′ was the primary outcome of this study.

Prior to performing the study, residents were given a 20-min didactics on performance of LVOT/VTI and diastolic measurements. They were then allowed to practice on a standardized model prior to performance of any FOCUS on patients with cardiopulmonary complaints. The residents were given hands-on instruction from the fellow on obtaining the advanced cardiac measurements on the standardized model. All residents, varying from Post Graduate Year (PGY) 1–4, had varying amounts of experience with both FOCUS and point of care ultrasound. All residents involved in this study were rotating through a month-long point of care ultrasound rotation as part of their EM residency training. The images and measurements on a patient made by residents were independent from the fellow on the team. Similarly, the ultrasounds performed by the fellows did not have interpretations by the resident.

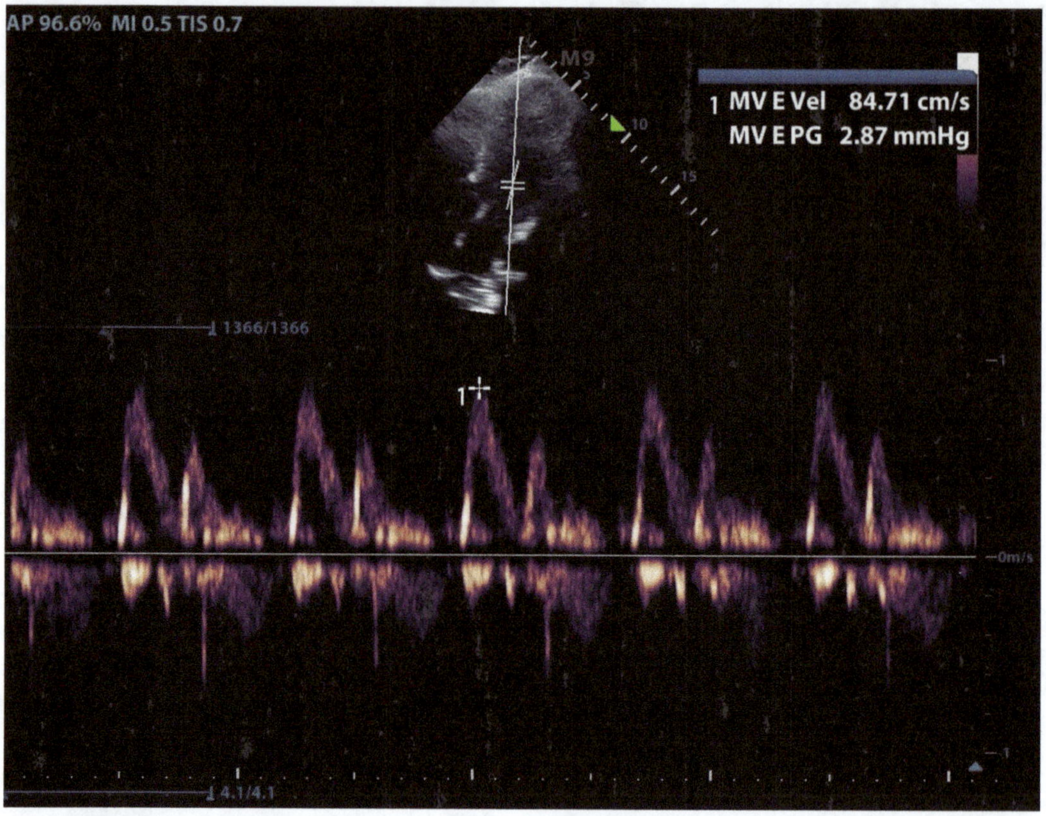

Fig. 3 Measurement of mitral valve E in apical view

The cardiac window images and LVOT/VTI and E/E′ images were then over-read by multiple ultrasound-fellowship trained EM physicians, to determine if images were of suitable quality, as this is the primary outcome of the study. The interpretation and image acquisition had to be complete to be considered adequate. Recorded images were deemed adequate/inadequate based on image gain, depth, appropriate LVOT diameter measurement, appropriate doppler placement for VTI, E, and E′ images, and appropriate doppler waveforms for VTI, E, and E′ images. All criteria for LVOT/VTI/E/E′ needed to be deemed adequate to be considered of appropriate quality. The studies deemed of appropriate quality for use with clinical decision making with regard to LVOT/VTI and E/E′ measurements, by an ultrasound expert were included in the data analysis. These ultrasound-fellowship trained physicians currently practice at the institute performing the study. They did not collect individual data on any patients or assist with any collection of data. The collected data from the residents/fellows was then analyzed by a statistician using a Test of Between-Subjects Effect to evaluate for significance.

Results

A total of 53 patients were enrolled in the study. 19 of these had an ultrasound performed by a junior resident (PGY 1–2), 17 had an ultrasound performed by a senior resident (PGY 3–4), and 17 had an ultrasound performed by an ultrasound fellow. Eight PGY 1–2 residents performed ultrasounds with a mean of 2.4 ultrasounds per resident. Seven PGY 3–4 residents performed ultrasounds with a mean of 2.4 ultrasounds per resident. Two fellows performed ultrasounds with a mean of 8.5 ultrasounds per fellow. The age, weight, and BMI of the patients were similar in characteristics among the 3 provider groups (Table 1).

The level of training was compared with regard to time to obtain 4 windows via a Test of Between-Subjects Effect, and the level of training was found to be statistically significant, $F\,(2,47) = 17.4$, $p < .05$ (Tables 2 and 3).

Following blinded review via emergency medicine ultrasound faculty, junior residents were able to obtain LVOT/VTI/E/E′ measurements in 26% of patients. 79% of the images regarding LVOT/VTI/E/E′ measurements by junior residents were deemed of adequate quality by ultrasound faculty. Junior residents took on average 219 s

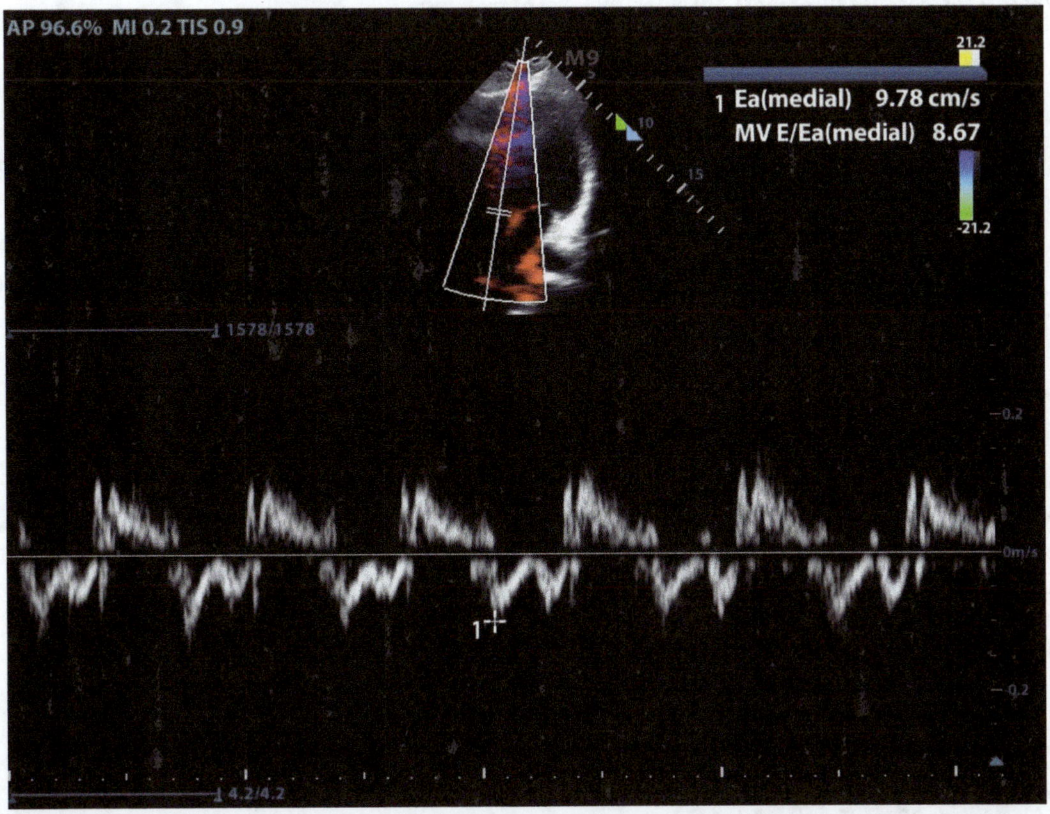

Fig. 4 Measurement of mitral valve E′ in apical view

Table 1 Average patient characteristics

	Age (years)	Weight (kg)	BMI (kg/m²)
Junior resident	55.9	96.5	31.9
Senior resident	59.3	86.0	30.5
Fellow	50.3	84.0	30.1

Table 2 Basic cardiac window obtained by level of training

	% PSLV	% PSSV	% apical	% subxiphoid
Junior resident	68	63	63	79
Senior resident	88	88	88	71
Fellow	88	92	82	82

to perform LVOT/VTI measurements, 249 s to perform E/E′ measurements, and 792 s for the entire FOCUS.

Senior residents were able to obtain LVOT/VTI/E/E′ measurements in 53% of patients. 76% of the images regarding LVOT/VTI/E/E′ measurements by junior residents were deemed of adequate quality by ultrasound faculty. Senior residents took on average 249 s to perform LVOT/VTI measurements, 217 s to perform E/E′ measurements, and 677 s for the entire FOCUS.

Table 3 Time in seconds to obtain cardiac measurements by level of training

	Basic 4 view (s)	LVOT/VTI (s)	E/E′ (s)	Complete echo (s)
Junior resident	400	219	249	792
Senior resident	282	249	217	677
Fellow	193	144	122	446

Fellows were able to obtain LVOT/VTI/E/E′ measurements in 65% of patients. 89% of images regarding LVOT/VTI/E/E′ by fellows were deemed of adequate quality by ultrasound faculty. Fellows took on average 144 s to perform LVOT/VTI measurements, 122 s to perform E/E′ measurements, and 446 s for the entire FOCUS (Table 4).

The level of training was compared with regard to time to obtain LVOT/VTI via a Test of Between-Subjects Effect, and the level of training was found to be statistically significant, $F\ (2,22) = 4.6$, $p < .05$. The level of training was also compared with regard to time to obtain E/E′ via a Test of Between-Subjects Effect, and the level of training was found to be statistically significant, F

Table 4 Advanced cardiac measurements obtained by level of training

	LVOT (%)	VTI (%)	Both LVOT/VTI (%)	E (%)	E′ (%)	Both E/E′ (%)
Junior resident	42	37	37	37	37	37
Senior resident	65	53	53	59	59	59
Fellow	82	65	65	65	65	65

(2,25) = 5.6, $p < .05$. Finally, the level of training was also compared with regard to time to obtain all images and measurements via a Test of Between-Subjects Effect, and the level of training was found to be statistically significant, $F\,(2,23) = 7.6$, $p < .05$.

Discussion

In this study, we evaluated the ability to obtain advanced FOCUS measurements including LVOT/VTI and E′/E′, and the time required to obtain them by an ED physician. The percentage of successful measurements of LVOT/VTI and E/E′ was lower than initially expected. In the previous study by Dinh et al., ED patients that had valvular disease, were unable to lie supine, or were unable to lie in the left lateral decubitus position were excluded, which potentially explains their ability to obtain adequate VTI measurements in 90% of patients [15]. The average patient BMI for all groups in our study was > 30, placing them into the obese category, leading to an increased challenge with obtaining images [19]. Many patients were in respiratory distress, and often on non-invasive or mechanical ventilation. They were frequently unable to assist with any positioning to obtain improved cardiac windows. Performance of the ultrasound was done early in the patient's work-up for the treating ED physician, leaving little time for resuscitation prior to obtaining cardiac windows and measurements. We believe this provides external validity to this study, having patients that were often in critical condition and with an undifferentiated cardiopulmonary diagnosis, which is the rationale for the urgently performed FOCUS within the ED.

To answer the question of 'How fast is fast enough' for obtaining advanced cardiac measurements, this largely depends on the resources available to the EM physician utilizing FOCUS. Acuity level of patients, patients seen per hour, ICU/cardiology consultation availability, and inpatient bed availability are only several of the factors that are taken into account when managing a department and performing a patient's work-up, and subsequently planning for their disposition. Given the widely varying resources within each ED, each provider needs to weigh the pros/cons of performing FOCUS with regard to their efficiency of their work-flow. As the fellows were able to obtain these LVOT/VTI and E/E′ measurements accurately in approximately 2 min in greater than 50% of patients, it is reasonable to perform these when appropriate, based on the provider's resources. While an ultrasound fellow may have more FOCUS experience than most EM physicians, they were still relatively inexperienced in performing these measurements, and we expect that accuracy and time to gather the images would continue to improve, regardless of the provider's prior training. Junior residents were able to obtain the LVOT/VTI and E/E′ measurements in approximately 4 min. In light of diagnostic uncertainty in patients with a complex cardiac history in their ED presentations, these 4 min may be beneficial in starting the correct treatment with regard to their fluid status.

Although frequently discussed in recent Free Open Access Medical Education (FOAM) discussions, these measurements are rarely obtained in the clinical setting within the emergency department [20, 21]. The physicians obtaining these studies were in a teaching setting, and were not responsible for other patient care during the time of FOCUS. Further research is needed to determine if ED physicians are able to perform these measurements while on clinical shifts and responsible for other patient care, and if so, will influence decision making for the critically ill patient.

Our results also indicate a statistically significant increase in success rates with ability to gather adequate measurements as physicians progressed through their training, and also a statistically significant decrease in time to gather those images. While not unexpected that as physicians advance in their training that their skill levels will improve, this helps to demonstrate that ED physicians can improve their ability to perform advanced measurements in FOCUS dramatically with increased training.

Limitations for our project include lack of blinding to the EM physician performing the ultrasound. As our physicians knew they were being evaluated, they may have been more motivated to obtain accurate images. While a previous study by Unluer et al. demonstrated that ED physicians could diagnose diastolic failure with good sensitivity, our study was also largely focused on the time taken to perform these studies, rather than diagnostic accuracy, as our goal was to determine if these measurements are feasible in a busy ED [8]. A more detailed study may track the changes in time needed to perform these by individual physicians as they progress in their skill level with regard to performing advanced cardiac measurements. An additional limitation is with blinded review of the recorded measurements by expert reviewers. Reviewers were asked to approve only images/measurements that were of quality suitable for clinical decision making. This exact level of quality is difficult to quantitate, and will likely vary among expert reviewers.

Conclusion

The scope of FOCUS for EM physicians continues to expand, with patients presenting with increasingly complex cardiopulmonary disease. Their cardiac function and fluid status often remains elusive throughout the beginning of their ED work-up. These advanced cardiac measurements take training to competently perform, and could add additional time to the patient's evaluation with FOCUS, but can be performed in an efficient manner once learned, in the appropriate clinical setting. These measurements performed by ED physicians may become a feasible tool for the critically ill cardiopulmonary patient.

Authors' contributions

JB and RH conceived the study concept. JB and AM recruited participants and obtained ultrasound equipment for the study. JB and AM, coordinated and collected the data, and JC analyzed the data. RK, NT, and RH served as blinded reviewers for the data. JB wrote the first draft. All authors read and approved the final manuscript.

Author details

[1] Department of Emergency Medicine, Lake Michigan Emergency Specialists, Mercy Health Muskegon, Muskegon, USA. [2] Department of Emergency Medicine, Emergency Physicians Medical Group, St. Joseph Mercy Ann Arbor, Ann Arbor, USA. [3] Department of Psychiatry, University of Michigan, Ann Arbor, MI, USA. [4] Department of Emergency Medicine, University of Michigan, Ann Arbor, MI, USA.

References

1. Gallard E, Redonnet JP, Bourcier JE et al (2015) Diagnostic performance of cardiopulmonary ultrasound performed by the emergency physician in the management of acute dyspnea. Am J Emerg Med 33(3):352–358. https://doi.org/10.1016/j.ajem.2014.12.003
2. Mantuani D, Frazee B, Fahimi J, Nagdev A (2016) Point-of-care multi-organ ultrasound improves diagnostic accuracy in adults presenting to the emergency department with acute dyspnea. West J Emerg Med. 17(1):46–53. https://doi.org/10.5811/westjem.2015.11.28525
3. Volpicelli G, Lamorte A, Tullio M et al (2013) Point-of-care multiorgan ultrasonography for the evaluation of undifferentiated hypotension in the emergency department. Intensive Care Med 39(7):1290–1298. https://doi.org/10.1007/s00134-013-2919-7
4. Adhikari S, Fiorello A, Stolz L et al (2014) Ability of emergency physicians with advanced echocardiographic experience at a single center to identify complex echocardiographic abnormalities. Am J Emerg Med 32(4):363–366. https://doi.org/10.1016/j.ajem.2013.12.010
5. Unlüer EE, Karagöz A, Akoğlu H, Bayata S (2014) Visual estimation of bedside echocardiographic ejection fraction by emergency physicians. West J Emerg Med. 15(2):221–226. https://doi.org/10.5811/westjem.2013.9.16185
6. Randazzo MR, Snoey ER, Levitt MA, Binder K (2003) Accuracy of emergency physician assessment of left ventricular ejection fraction and central venous pressure using echocardiography. Acad Emerg Med 10(9):973–977. https://doi.org/10.1197/S1069-6563(03)00317-8
7. Taylor RA, Moore CL (2014) Accuracy of emergency physician-performed limited echocardiography for right ventricular strain. Am J Emerg Med 32(4):371–374. https://doi.org/10.1016/j.ajem.2013.12.043
8. Unluer EE, Bayata S, Postaci N et al (2012) Limited bedside echocardiography by emergency physicians for diagnosis of diastolic heart failure. Emerg Med J. 29:280–283. https://doi.org/10.1136/emj.2011.111229
9. Holst JM, Kilker BA, Wright S, Hoffmann B (2014) Heart failure with preserved ejection fraction. Eur J Emerg Med. 21(6):394–402. https://doi.org/10.1097/MEJ.0000000000000093
10. Fields JM, Lee PA, Jenq KY, Mark DG, Panebianco NL, Dean AJ (2011) The interrater reliability of inferior vena cava ultrasound by bedside clinician sonographers in emergency department patients. Acad Emerg Med 18(1):98–101. https://doi.org/10.1111/j.1553-2712.2010.00952.x
11. Alzahrani H, Woo MY, Johnson C, Pageau P, Millington S, Thiruganasambandamoorthy V (2015) Can severe aortic stenosis be identified by emergency physicians when interpreting a simplified two-view echocardiogram obtained by trained echocardiographers? Crit Ultrasound J. 7(1):5. https://doi.org/10.1186/s13089-015-0022-8
12. Pare JR, Liu R, Moore CL et al (2016) Emergency physician focused cardiac ultrasound improves diagnosis of ascending aortic dissection. Am J Emerg Med 34(3):486–492. https://doi.org/10.1016/j.ajem.2015.12.005
13. Melniker L (2014) International evidence-based recommendations for focused cardiac ultrasound. J Am Soc Echocardiogr. https://doi.org/10.1016/j.echo.2014.05.001
14. Nguyen HB, Losey T, Rasmussen J et al (2006) Interrater reliability of cardiac output measurements by transcutaneous Doppler ultrasound: implications for noninvasive hemodynamic monitoring in the ED. Am J Emerg Med 24(7):828–835. https://doi.org/10.1016/j.ajem.2006.05.012
15. Dinh VA, Ko HS, Rao R et al (2012) Measuring cardiac index with a focused cardiac ultrasound examination in the ED. Am J Emerg Med. https://doi.org/10.1016/j.ajem.2012.03.025
16. Orme RMLE, Oram MP, Mckinstry CE et al (2009) Impact of echocardiography on patient management in the intensive care unit: an audit of district general hospital practice. Br J Anaesth 102(3):340–344. https://doi.org/10.1093/bja/aen378
17. Zieleskiewicz L, Muller L, Lakhal K et al (2015) Point-of-care ultrasound in intensive care units: assessment of 1073 procedures in a multicentric, prospective, observational study. Intensive Care Med 41(9):1638–1647. https://doi.org/10.1007/s00134-015-3952-5
18. Bobbia X, Abou-Badra M, Hansel N et al (2017) Changes in the availability of bedside ultrasound practice in emergency rooms and prehospital settings in France. Anaesth Crit Care Pain Med. https://doi.org/10.1016/j.accpm.2017.06.008
19. Siadecki SD, Frasure SE, Lewiss RE, Saul T (2016) High body mass index is strongly correlated with decreased image quality in focused bedside echocardiography. J Emerg Med 50(2):295–301. https://doi.org/10.1016/j.jemermed.2015.07.023
20. Weingart S (2015) Podcast 162—assessing fluid responsiveness. EMCrit. https://emcrit.org/racc/assessing-fluid-responsiveness/. Accessed 21 Mar 2018
21. Chen C, Swaminathan A (2017) Fluid responsiveness and the six guiding principles of fluid resuscitation. http://rebelem.com/fluid-responsiveness-and-the-six-guiding-principles-of-fluid-resuscitation/. Accessed 22 Mar 2018

18

Feasibility of postural lung recruitment maneuver in children

Cecilia M. Acosta[1], Giovanni Volpicelli[2], Nadia Rudzik[1], Nicolás Venturin[1], Sebastián Gerez[1], Lila Ricci[3], Marcela Natal[3] and Gerardo Tusman[1*]

Abstract

Background: Pulmonary atelectasis in anesthetized children is easily reverted by lung recruitment maneuvers. However, the high airways pressure reached during the maneuver could negatively affect hemodynamics. The aim of this study is to assess the effect and feasibility of a postural lung recruitment maneuver (P-RM); i.e., a new maneuver that opens up the atelectatic lung areas based on changing the child's body position under constant ventilation with moderated driving pressure (12 cmH_2O) and of positive end-expiratory pressure (PEEP, 10 cmH_2O). Forty ASA I–II children, aged 6 months to 7 years, subjected to general anesthesia were studied. Patients were ventilated with volume control mode using standard settings with 5 cmH_2O of PEEP. They were randomized into two groups: (1) control group (C group, $n=20$)—ventilation was turned to pressure control ventilation using a fixed driving pressure of 12 cmH_2O. PEEP was increased from 5 to 10 cmH_2O during 3 min maintaining the supine position. (2) P-RM group ($n=20$)—patients received the same increase in driving pressure and PEEP, but they were placed, respectively, in the left lateral position, in the right lateral position (90 s each), and back again into the supine position after 3 min. Then, ventilation returned to baseline settings in volume control mode. Lung ultrasound-derived aeration score and respiratory compliance were assessed before (T1) and after (T2) 10 cmH_2O of PEEP was applied.

Results: At baseline ventilation (T1), both groups showed similar aeration score (P-RM group 9.9 ± 1.9 vs C group 10.4 ± 1.9; $p=0.463$) and respiratory compliance (P-RM group 15 ± 6 vs C group 14 ± 6 mL/cmH_2O; $p=0.517$). At T2, the aeration score decreased in the P-RM group (1.5 ± 1.6 vs 9.9 ± 2.1; $p<0.001$), but remained without changes in the C group (9.9 ± 2.1; $p=0.221$). Compliance was higher in the P-RM group (18 ± 6 mL/cmH_2O) when compared with the C group (14 ± 5 mL/cmH_2O; $p=0.001$).

Conclusion: Lung aeration and compliance improved only in the group in which a posture change strategy was applied.

Keywords: Atelectasis, Body position, Lung ultrasound, Children, Lung recruitment maneuver

Background

Anesthesia-induced atelectasis is a well-known condition in pediatric patients that is related to perioperative episodes of hypoxemia [1, 2]. The incidence of atelectasis is high and commonly appears in the most dependent lung zones where the trans-pulmonary pressure ($P_L =$ airways pressure − pleural pressure) is the lowest [3, 4]. Mechanical ventilation using standard levels of 5 cmH_2O of positive end-expiratory pressure (PEEP) is generally insufficient to reopen those dependent atelectasis in supine pediatric patients [3, 5]. Contrarily, a brief increase in airways pressures with a lung recruitment maneuver (RM) easily revert atelectasis

*Correspondence: gtusman@hotmail.com
[1] Department of Anesthesiology, Hospital Privado de Comunidad, Córdoba 4545, 7600 Mar del Plata, Buenos Aires, Argentina
Full list of author information is available at the end of the article

because the opening pressure in these dorsal pulmonary areas is overcome [2, 6].

Many studies in healthy and sick children showed that a brief increase in plateau pressure (Pplat) and PEEP during RM is safe [6–8]. However, there are still concerns about the hemodynamic response and the mechanic stress and strain on the lung tissue caused by the maneuver in this population. In order to avoid these concerns, we have described a postural recruitment maneuver (P-RM), i.e., a ventilatory strategy aimed to obtain a lung recruitment effect by changes in body position under constant driving pressure at a moderate level of PEEP [9].

The P-RM is based on the known gravitational effect on P_L. Two principles explain its rationale [9]: one postulates that dorsal atelectasis can be recruited by placing this lung area in the uppermost position, which increases the local P_L. The other principle follows the Laplace's Law, which indicates that, once recruited; a ventral lung area will maintain patency when enough PEEP is applied. Therefore, the proposed P-RM consists to move the patient sequentially in: (1) the left lateral position to recruit atelectasis of the upper right lung; (2) the right lateral position to recruit the left lung atelectasis areas, while keeping open the right lung by applying enough PEEP; and (3) finally back to supine position (Fig. 1). Our preliminary data showed that P-RM using 10 cmH_2O of PEEP and 22 cmH_2O of Pplat was enough to open up atelectasis during anesthesia in children [9].

We hypothesized that the P-RM can re-aerate lung collapse without the need of reaching the high airways pressures obtained in standard RM. The objective of this study was to study the effect and feasibility of P-RM in anesthetized children. Main end-points of the study were lung aeration and respiratory mechanics. The primary outcome was to compare lung aeration assessed by lung ultrasound exams (LUS) between groups. The secondary outcome was to compare respiratory mechanics determined by airways resistance and dynamic respiratory compliance between groups.

Methods

This randomized and controlled trial was performed in the operating theater of a Community Hospital. Ethical approval for this study (IRB #2919/1457/2017) was provided by the Ethical Committee of the Hospital Privado de Comunidad, Mar del Plata, Argentina (ClinicalTrials.gov NCT03141515). Written informed consent was obtained from parents of all subjects participating in the trial. The study started 20 April 2017 and ended 5 January 2018.

Patient's eligibility criteria

We sequentially recruited patients aged 6 months to 5 years undergoing programmed surgeries. Conditions for enrollment were: need for general anesthesia and mechanical ventilator support, American Physical Status Classification (ASA) I–II and baseline pulse oximetry

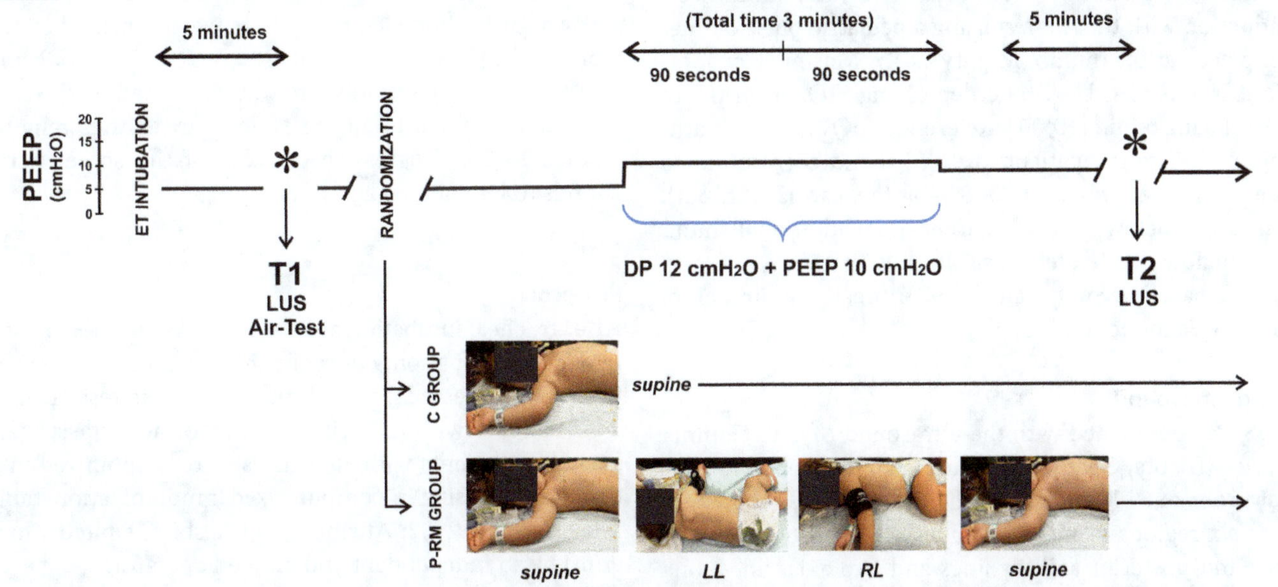

Fig. 1 Diagram of the protocol. Ventilation was switched to pressure control mode using 12 cmH_2O of driving pressure (DP). PEEP was increased from 5 to 10 cmH_2O during 3 min. The control group (C group) remained supine along the protocol while children in the postural recruitment group (P-RM group) were turned to the left lateral position (LL) during 90 s and then to the right lateral (RL) for another 90 s, to finally reach the supine position again. *T1* analysis 5 min after anesthesia induction, *T2* analysis 5 min after treatment, *LUS* lung ultrasound images

saturation (SpO_2) while breathing room air ≥97%. We excluded patients undergoing emergency and thoracic surgeries and patients with pre-existing pulmonary, cardiac or chest wall diseases. After this first selection, we then excluded those patients without LUS evidence of atelectasis after anesthesia induction.

Anesthesia, ventilatory treatment and monitoring

Anesthesia was induced with sevoflurane using a circular system of the GE Aespire workstation (GE Healthcare, Madison, WI, US). Boluses of fentanyl 2 μg kg^{-1} and vecuronium 0.1 mg kg^{-1} were added before tracheal intubation with a cuffed endotracheal tube. Anesthesia was maintained with sevoflurane 0.7 minimum alveolar concentration and remifentanyl 0.3–0.5 μg kg^{-1} min. The lungs were ventilated with a volume control mode using a tidal volume (VT) of 6 mL kg^{-1}, respiratory rate between 20 and 25 bpm, inspiratory-to-expiratory ratio of 1:1.5, 10% of inspiratory pause, PEEP of 5 cmH_2O and a FIO_2 of 0.5.

Standard EKG, non-invasive mean systemic arterial pressure (MAP), capnography, pulse oximetry and respiratory mechanics were monitored with the S5 device (GE Healthcare/Datex-Ohmeda, Helsinki, Finland). Respiratory flow and pressure signals were obtained by a pediatric mainstream gadget placed at the airways opening, from which peak airways pressure (Pip), dynamic respiratory compliance (Cdyn) and respiratory airways resistance (Rrs) were obtained.

Gas exchange evaluated by the Air-test

Arterial oxygenation was evaluated after anesthesia induction with the *Air-test* using a pediatric pulse oximeter placed at the thumb (MightySat Rx, Masimo Corporation, Irvine, CA, USA) and decreasing FIO_2 from 0.5 to 0.21 during 5 min [10, 11]. Reference SpO_2 values breathing air in healthy patients are ≥ 97% and correspond to the anatomical shunt (~ 5–8% of the cardiac output). Any value below 97% is a marker of an additional shunt, presumably due to atelectasis, in those patients who presented baseline SpO_2 values ≥ 97% breathing air before anesthesia induction [12].

Lung ultrasound

LUS was performed with the ultrasound MyLab Gamma device (Esaote, Genova, Italy) using a high-frequency linear probe of 6–12 MHz. Each hemithorax was segmented into six regions using the longitudinal parasternal, anterior and posterior axillary lines and two axial lines, one above the diaphragm and the other 1 cm above the nipples [13]. The ultrasound probe was placed perpendicular to the ribs looking for the standard LUS view, where the pleura and the ventilated lung are visualized between two adjacent ribs (the *bat sign*) [13]. The probe was placed in the oblique position (along the intercostal spaces between ribs) in the areas where the typical atelectatic consolidations were detected. In general, the posterior zones of the lungs are those with the highest incidence of anesthesia-induced atelectasis [3, 4].

A LUS imaging based aeration score was calculated as previously described for children [6]. Briefly, this score is based on four LUS patterns [13–15] investigated in each of the 12 scanned thoracic areas:

1. Normal aeration (*N*): presence of the respiratory movement of the lung image relative to the chest wall (*lung sliding*) and the horizontal artifacts generated by repetition of the linear image of the pleura at regular intervals (*A lines*), with absence of sub-pleural ultrasound parenchymal signs (*B*-lines or consolidations).
2. Moderate loss of lung aeration (*B*1): presence of vertical dynamic lines, originating from the pleural line or from small sub-pleural consolidations, reaching the lowest edge of the screen (*B-lines*).
3. Severe loss of lung aeration (*B*2): multiple coalescent *B*-lines giving the aspect of a "white lung", when the *B*-lines are so intense and numerous to occupy the whole image.
4. Complete loss of aeration (*C*): atelectasis, defined as localized sonographic consolidation, i.e., sub-pleural images with a tissue-like or hypoechoic pattern. Air bronchograms may be observed as bright echogenic branching structures within the consolidated area.

For a given thoracic area, points were allocated to the worst LUS pattern observed: $N=0$, $B1=1$, $B2=2$ and $C=3$. The LUS aeration score was calculated by the sum of points obtained in all the 12 lung areas, thus ranging from 0 to 36. Progressive increase of the score corresponds to loss of lung aeration.

Protocol

After tracheal intubation atelectasis areas were diagnosed by LUS examination, consequences on arterial oxygenation were assessed by performing the Air-test (Fig. 1, T1). Patients without LUS evidence of atelectasis were excluded. Patients with atelectasis were randomized into two groups using a computerized randomization table (StatsDirect v 2.7.2; Altrincham, Cheshire, United Kingdom) by an independent and blinded operator:

- *Control group* (C group, $n=20$). Ventilation was turned to pressure control ventilation using a fixed driving pressure of 12 cmH_2O. PEEP was increased from 5 to 10 cmH_2O along 3 min maintaining the supine position during the whole protocol time.

- *Postural-recruitment maneuver group* (P-RM group, $n=20$). Ventilation was turned to pressure control ventilation using a driving pressure of 12 cmH_2O and PEEP of 10 cmH_2O, but they were immediately and sequentially placed: (1) in the left lateral position (90 s), (2) in the right lateral position (other 90 s), (3) back to the supine position (Fig. 1).

After 3′ maneuver, both groups returned to baseline ventilation adding 8 cmH_2O of PEEP to maintain eventually the recruitment effect. Five minutes later patients were evaluated by LUS at T2 (Fig. 1). The same investigator non-blinded to treatment groups repeated LUS at each step. Respiratory data and hemodynamic parameters were collected at each protocol step.

Statistical analysis

The null hypothesis was that lung aeration score would be similar between groups. Considering a beta-power of 80% and an alpha-error of 5% the statistical power to reject this hypothesis was calculated assuming that atelectasis would be present in 90% of patients in the C group and in only 45% of patients in the RM group [6]. A sample size of 20 patients per group was estimated. Univariate comparisons were performed between and within groups applying the Student's t test. Multiple linear mixed models were adjusted to explain changes in LUS, respiratory and hemodynamic variables related to six predictive factors: age, gender, weight, surgery duration, Air-test and treatment group (fixed effects). The main factor to be analyzed was the proposed treatment.

Data are presented as n (%) for proportions and mean ± SD or median for continuous variables. A p-value < 0.05 was considered statistically significant. All calculations were performed using the R statistical package (R Core Team, 2015, Foundation for Statistical Computing, Vienna, Austria).

Results

Out of the 46 examined patients, six (13%) did not show atelectasis after anesthesia induction and were excluded from the analysis. Forty patients were successfully randomized as observed in the flowchart (Fig. 2).

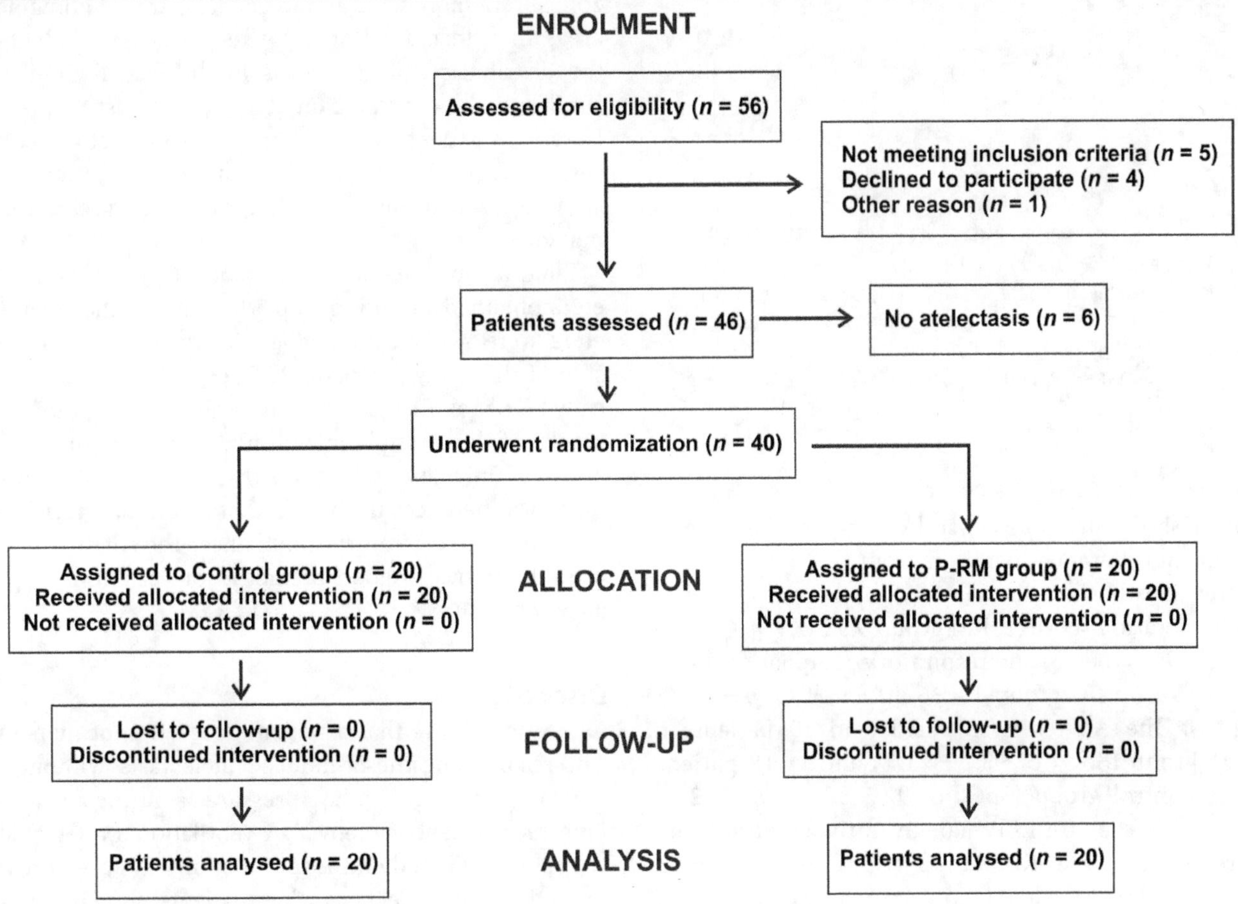

Fig. 2 The CONSORT flow diagram

Table 1 Patient's data

Parameter	C-group, $n = 20$	PR-group, $n = 20$	p value*
Age (months)	38.8 ± 19.1	40.9 ± 16.9	0.708
Male	15 (75)	12 (60)	0.499
Female	5 (25)	8 (40)	
Weight (kg)	15.0 ± 3.9	14.8 ± 3.1	0.891
ASA I	20 (100)	20 (100)	1.00
Duration of anesthesia (min)	59.2 ± 17.9	60.9 ± 18.0	0.767
Type of surgery *n* (%)			
Laparoscopic herniorrhaphy	5 (25)	8 (40)	
Tonsillectomy	7 (35)	8 (40)	
Urological surgery	7 (35)	3 (15)	
Wrist osteosynthesis	0 (0)	1 (5)	
Resection angioma	1 (5)	0 (0)	

* Student's t test

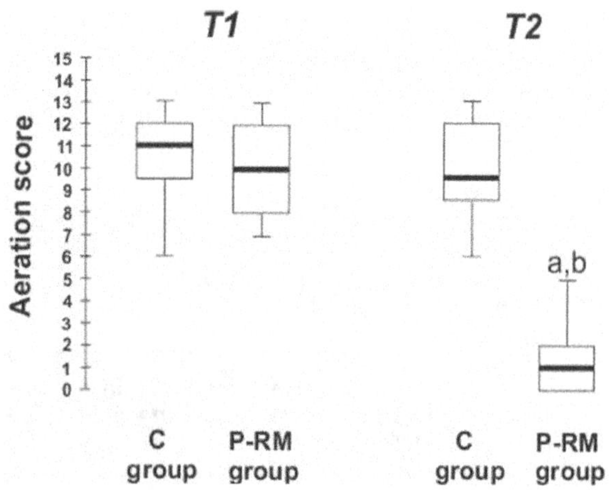

Fig. 3 The aeration score during the study. Box-plot showing the aeration score after anesthesia induction (T1) and after 3 min of 10 cmH_2O of PEEP in the control (C group) and postural recruitment maneuver (P-RM group) groups. Inter-group comparison, Student's *t* test: **a** C group vs P-RM group at T2, $p < 0.0001$. **b** P-RM group T1 vs T2, $p < 0.0001$

Table 1 shows patient's general characteristics without significant differences between groups.

After anesthesia induction (T1), both groups showed similar aeration score (P-RM group 9.9 ± 1.9 vs C group 10.4 ± 1.9; $p = 0.463$) and respiratory compliance (P-RM group 15 ± 6 vs C group 14 ± 6 mL/cmH_2O; $p = 0.517$) (Fig. 3). The Air-test was positive in 19 patients of P-RM group (SpO_2 of 93.7 ± 2.0%) and in 18 patients of the control group (SpO_2 of 92.5 ± 2.3%; $p = 0.248$). At T2 after the 10-PEEP maneuver, the aeration score decreased in the P-RM group (1.5 ± 1.6 vs 9.9 ± 2.1; $p < 0.001$), but remained without changes in the C group (9.9 ± 2.1; $p = 0.221$). Compliance was higher in the P-RM group (18 ± 6 mL/cmH_2O) compared with the C group (14 ± 5 mL/cmH_2O; $p = 0.001$—Table 2).

Figure 4 shows LUS images of one representative patient per group during the protocol. The distribution of LUS-diagnosed atelectasis is shown in Fig. 5. All patients in the C group presented atelectasis in dependent pulmonary zones at T1 and T2. These lung atelectatic zones were more common in caudal, para-diaphragmatic areas than in cranial areas. After anesthesia induction, the distribution of atelectasis in the P-RM group was similar to the control group. However, most of the atelectasis in patients of P-RM group resolved at the end of surgery (Fig. 5). Only four patients of this latter group showed residual atelectasis after the postural recruitment maneuver.

Table 2 shows hemodynamics and respiratory parameters obtained in both groups. In general, those parameters were statistically similar between groups at each step of the study protocol. $PETCO_2$ values were statistically higher at T1 than at T2 in both studied groups. The results of the multiple mixed models are summarized in Table 3. The main finding was that the P-RM caused significant differences in the score of aeration, arterial oxygenation and respiratory compliance. The Air-test, on the other hand, was a good predictor for variations in peak airway pressure.

Discussion

Our study shows that a postural recruitment maneuver can resolve anesthesia-induced atelectasis without the need to reach high airways pressure as during a standard lung recruitment maneuver. A ventilation strategy using the same PEEP and end-inspiratory airways pressure had null effects on atelectasis when patients remained in the supine position. These findings confirm our previous data

Table 2 Hemodynamics and respiratory variables

Parameter	C group			P-RM group			*p* value-between groups at T2
	T1	*p* value Intra-group	T2	T1	*p* value Intra-group	T2	
Heart rate (bpm)	102 ± 15	0.033	99 ± 14	95 ± 14	0.928	97 ± 14	0.678
MAP (mmHg)	58 ± 7	0.338	58 ± 6	58 ± 6	0.763	59 ± 6	0.597
SpO_2 (%)	98.5 ± 0.8	0.500	98.4 ± 1.1	98.8 ± 0.7	0.996	99.3 ± 0.5	0.002
$PETCO_2$ (mmHg)	45 ± 3	0.006	42 ± 4	47 ± 4	< 0.0001	39 ± 3	0.005
Pip (cmH_2O)	15 ± 2	0.002	17 ± 1	14 ± 2	0.003	16 ± 2	0.855
PEEP (cmH_2O)	5	–	8	5	–	8	–
Cdyn (cmH_2O)	14 ± 6	0.579	14 ± 5	15 ± 6	0.001	18 ± 6	0.0002
Rrs (cmH_2O/L^{-1})	33 ± 8	0.941	36 ± 11	33 ± 10	0.833	35 ± 12	0.839

T1 after anesthesia induction, *T2* after 10 cmH_2O of PEEP in the control group (C group) and in the postural recruitment maneuver group (P-RM group), *MAP* mean arterial blood pressure, *SpO_2* pulse oximetry hemoglobin saturation, *$PETCO_2$* end-tidal partial pressure of carbon dioxide, *Pip* peak inspiratory pressure, *PEEP* positive end-expiratory pressure, *Cdyn* dynamic respiratory compliance, *Rrs* respiratory airways resistance. Intra-group comparison at T1 = all *p* ns

on the postural recruitment effect [9] and reinforce the feasibility and reproducibility of the P-RM in ventilated pediatric patients with healthy lungs in the clinical field.

Four patients in the P-RM group presented residual atelectasis in the left lower para-diaphragmatic areas (Fig. 5). Previous data showed the high incidence of atelectasis in anesthetized children in this specific lung zone, which could be caused by the pressure that the weight of the heart exerts over the left inferior lobe [4]. Thus, the end-inspiratory airways pressure used during the P-RM and/or the level of PEEP applied after the P-RM were not enough to overcome the alveolar opening and closing pressure, respectively [6]. We hypothesize these patients might need application of higher end-inspiratory airways pressure/PEEP or/and a longer time ventilating in the right lateral posture, to fully resolve this residual lung collapse.

The clinical implication of our results is the chance to treat lung collapse without the need for inducing prolonged high airways pressure. Moderate level of PEEP together with slight increment in end-inspiratory airways pressure for only 3 min was enough to reach complete lung aeration in almost all our patients. The postural change was easy to perform in children. P-RM should be applied when atelectasis appears after anesthesia induction and to resolve any residual atelectasis at the end of surgery. Other potential clinical advantages of P-RM could be the theoretically minor hemodynamics repercussion and less stress on the lung tissue when compared with standard RM performed at higher airways pressure.

Normalizing lung aeration in the perioperative period could be important for patient's care because: (1) shunt induced by atelectasis is related to hypoxemia, whose incidence in children is high during the perioperative period [1, 16]. (2) Atelectasis constitutes, by definition, a common postoperative pulmonary complication that potentially induces other more severe complications like pneumonia and ventilator-induced lung injury [17–19]. Therefore, resolving atelectasis seems to be a reasonable therapeutic goal in the perioperative period.

Potential mechanisms explaining the postural recruitment effect

Gravity creates a vertical gradient of P_L that decreases in the dependent lung areas [20]. Anesthesia-induced atelectasis are mainly caused by a compressive mechanism, where P_L in the dependent parts of the lungs is low and not enough to offset the compressive forces of thoracic and abdominal content densities, including the weight of the lungs themselves. This vertical gradient of P_L (P_L in the superior areas minus P_L in the bases divided by lung's height) changes with body mass and posture. Agostoni and D'angelo showed that this gradient ranged from 0.24 cmH_2O/cm of height in rams to > 0.8 cmH_2O/cm in rats, which demonstrates that the smaller is the animal the higher is the vertical P_L gradient [21]. According to this body mass effect demonstrated in animals, it is calculated that adults (similar to mean weight of rams = 75 kg) may potentially have a P_L gradient close to 0.2 cmH_2O/cm. Children of different sizes would have a gradient between 0.4 cmH_2O/cm (similar to weight of small dogs = 15 kg) to 0.6 cmH_2O/cm (similar to weight of larger dogs = 30 kg) [21]. The same authors showed in rabbits that the P_L gradient increased when body position was changed from supine (0.55 cmH_2O/cm) to the lateral position (0.73 cmH_2O/cm) [22]. These experimental data demonstrate that the lateral position causes higher P_L in the most ventral lung areas than what could be obtained in the same areas in the supine position, mainly because

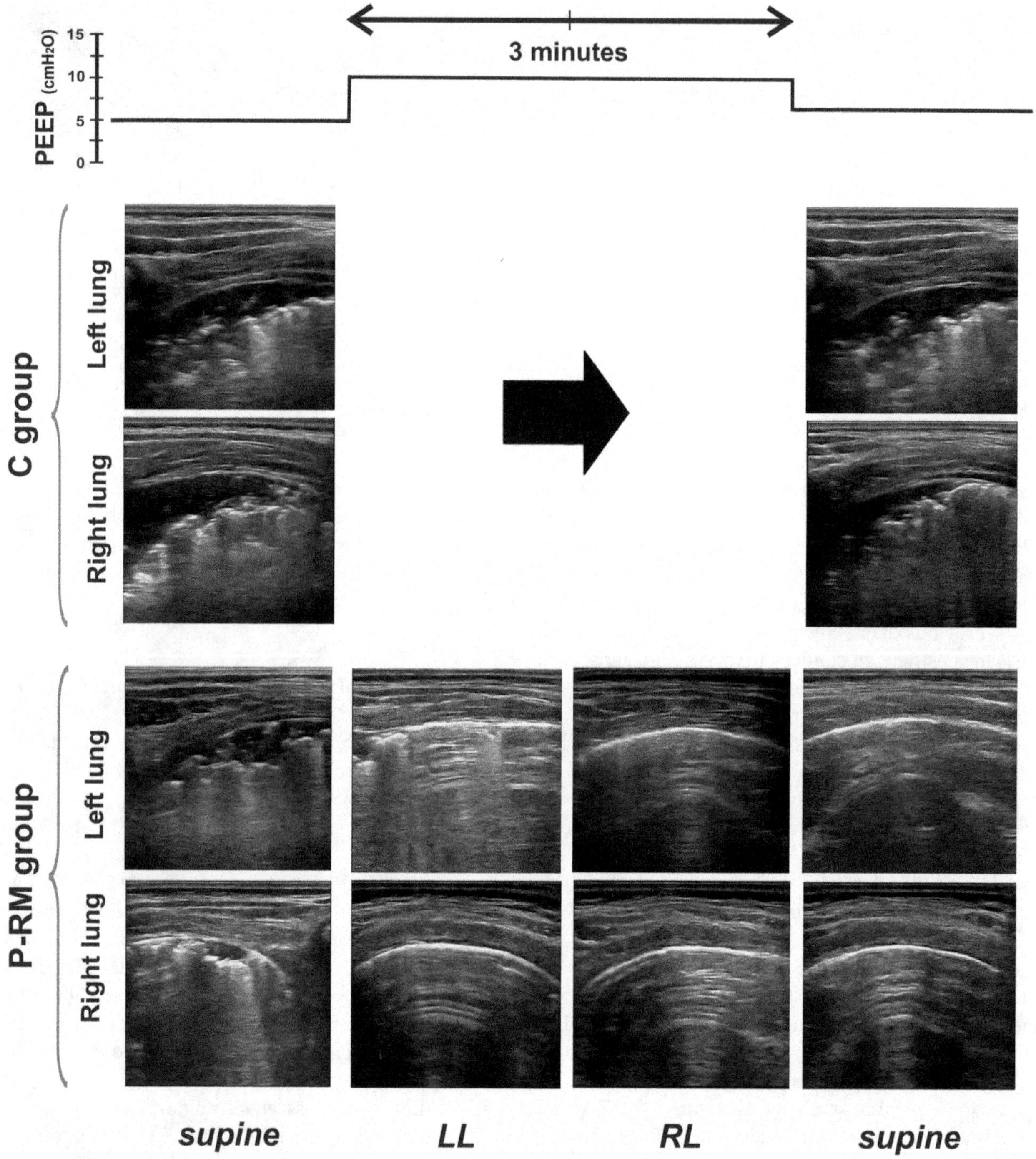

Fig. 4 Example of the protocol in one representative patient per group. LUS images were assessed in the posterior areas in supine (dorsal lung) and in the uppermost areas in the lateral positions (ventral lung). *C group* control patients, *P-RM* postural recruitment patients, *LL* left lateral, *RL* right lateral position. Note typical atelectasis with air bronchograms before the 10-PEEP maneuver in both groups and how only the P-RM resolved it

the thoracic right-to-left distance is longer than the anterior–posterior [9].

The change in body positions during positive pressure mechanical ventilation have been extensively used in pediatric patients with different results [23–26]. The physiological and clinical effects of body positioning on lung function depend on the distribution of perfusion and ventilation. The distribution of ventilation is highly variable in spontaneous breathing children at different positional changes [27]. Conversely, in mechanically ventilated children in lateral position, the distribution of ventilation was more homogeneous between lungs

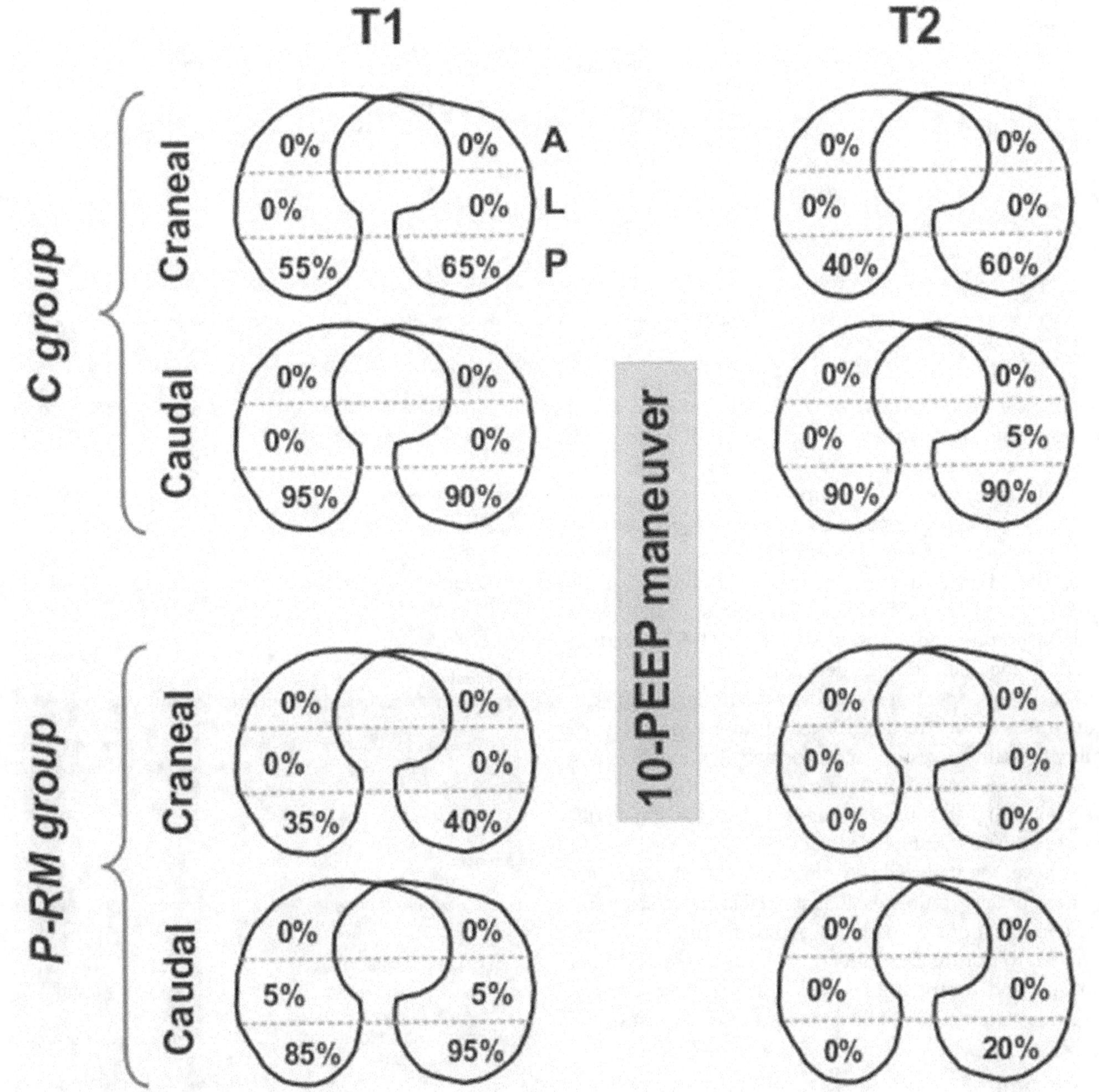

Fig. 5 Distribution of atelectasis between groups along the study. *C group* control patients, *P-RM* postural recruitment patients, *A* anterior, *L* lateral, *P* posterior lung zones assessed by lung ultrasound. Cranial = axial cut representing the superior thoracic area above a horizontal line crossing the nipples. Caudal = axial cut representing the inferior thoracic area below a horizontal line crossing the nipples. % = the percent of all patients per group that presented atelectasis in a particular lung zone

when using PEEP [28]. PEEP improved the ventilation in nondependent lung and increased both, functional residual capacity and PaO_2. Thus, the lateral position can explain the recruitment effect using normal range of end-inspiratory airways pressure. P_L becomes larger in the nondependent lung areas due to gravity while PEEP distributes ventilation to the superior lung areas. Then, once recruited, these areas remain "open" with 10 cmH_2O of PEEP, according to the Laplace's law, and these nondependent areas become "dependent" during the change in the opposite lateral decubitus.

Limitations

The P-RM was tested in preliminary patients using different durations and levels of PEEP and end-inspiratory airways pressure. The present study was not designed to

Table 3 Multiple mixed models

Response	Predictive factors				
	Treatment	Age/weight	Gender	Surgery time	Air-test
Score of aeration	< 0.0001	0.477	0.316	0.286	0.264
Heart rate (bpm)	0.298	0.005	0.882	0.441	0.102
MAP (mmHg)	0.940	0.316	0.966	0.241	0.180
SpO_2 (%)	< 0.0001	0.879	0.013	0.104	0.601
$PETCO_2$ (mmHg)	0.407	0.748	0.643	0.794	0.360
Cdyn (mL/cmH_2O)	0.064	0.104	0.791	0.797	0.428
Pip (cmH_2O)	0.584	0.454	0.565	0.524	< 0.0001

MAP mean arterial blood pressure, *SpO_2* pulse oximetry hemoglobin saturation, *$PETCO_2$* end-tidal partial pressure of carbon dioxide, *Cdyn* dynamic respiratory compliance, *Pip* peak inspiratory pressure

analyze the best combination between time and target pressures, but it was ideated just as a proof of concept. In fact, four patients in the P-RM group present some residual atelectasis despite improvement of lung aeration (Fig. 5). The lung opening and closing pressures vary among patients, which means that the P-RM (as well as standard RM) should be personalized to avoid unrealistic and potential harmful higher airways pressure [29]. Next studies should be done to optimize the P-RM settings and its individualization guided by LUS.

LUS is an operator-dependent technique that can induce bias in our results. To avoid inter-observer variability the same investigator performed all scans. Besides, LUS assessment using linear probe of 6–12 MHz in children gives high-resolution images that can diagnose different patterns with high accuracy [13].

We have not analyzed the effect of P-RM after surgery or the repercussion of residual atelectasis in post-operative complications or patient's outcome. This study was designed to test the feasibility of the postural recruitment concept, and future studies with specific protocols and large populations should be done for these purposes.

Conclusions

Atelectasis commonly observed in healthy pediatric anesthetized patients is better resolved by a P-RM than by an isolated increase in PEEP. In our study, an increase in PEEP at constant driving pressure maintained for a short time was enough to open up the lungs and keep them open only when combined with sequential changes in body posture. This study confirms the feasibility and efficacy of a P-RM in children with anesthesia-induced atelectasis.

Abbreviations

ASA: American Physical Status Classification; Cdyn: Dynamic respiratory compliance; LUS: Lung ultrasound; MAP: Mean arterial blood pressure; PEEP: Positive end-expiratory pressure; $PETCO_2$: End-tidal partial pressure of carbon dioxide; Pip: Peak inspiratory pressure; P_L: Trans-pulmonary pressure; Pplat: Plateau pressure; P-RM: Postural lung recruitment maneuver; RM: Lung recruitment maneuver; Rrs: Respiratory airways resistance; SpO_2: Pulse oximetry hemoglobin saturation; VT: Tidal volume.

Acknowledgements

Not applicable.

Authors' contributions

Conception and design: CMA, GV and GT. Collection of data: CMA, NR, NV, SG and GT. Statistical analysis: LR and MN. Drafting: CMA, GV and GT. All authors read and approved the final manuscript.

Author details

[1] Department of Anesthesiology, Hospital Privado de Comunidad, Córdoba 4545, 7600 Mar del Plata, Buenos Aires, Argentina. [2] Department of Emergency Medicine, San Luigi Gonzaga University Hospital, Orbassano, Torino, Italy. [3] Department of Mathematics, Facultad de Ciencias Exactas, Universidad Nacional de Mar del Plata, Mar del Plata, Argentina.

References

1. de Graaff JC, Bijker JB, Kappen TH et al (2013) Incidence of intraoperative hypoxemia in children in relation to age. Anesth Analg 117:169–175
2. Habre W, Disma N, Virag K et al (2017) Incidence of severe critical events in paediatric anaesthesia (APRICOT): a prospective multicentre observational study in 261 hospitals in Europe. Lancet Respir Med 5:412–425
3. Damgaard-Pedersen K, Qvist T (1980) Pediatric pulmonary CT-scanning. Anaesthesia-induced changes. Pediatr Radiol 9:145–148
4. Tusman G, Bohm SH, Tempra A et al (2003) Effects of recruitment maneuver on atelectasis in anesthetized children. Anesthesiology 98:14–22
5. Serafini G, Cornara G, Cavalloro F et al (1999) Pulmonary atelectasis during paediatric anaesthesia: CT scan evaluation and effect of positive end expiratory pressure (PEEP). Pediatr Anesth 9:225–228
6. Acosta CM, Sara T, Carpinella M et al (2018) Lung recruitment maneouvre reverts lung collapse induced by capnoperitoneum and anesthesia in children: A randomized, controlled study. Eur J Anesthesiol 35:573–580
7. Duff JP, Rosychuk RJ, Joffe AR (2007) The safety and efficacy of sustained inflations as a lung recruitment maneuver in pediatric intensive care unit patients. Intensive Care Med 33:1778–1786
8. Cruces P, Donoso A, Valenzuela J et al (2013) Respiratory and hemodynamic effects of a stepwise lung recruitment maneuver in pediatric ARDS: a feasibility study. Pediatr Pulmonol 48:1135–1143
9. Tusman G, Acosta CM, Böhm SH et al (2017) Postural lung recruitment assessed by lung ultrasound in mechanically ventilated children. Crit Ultrasound J 9:22
10. Sapsford DJ, Jones JG (1995) The PIO2 vs SpO2 diagram: a non-invasive measurement of pulmonary oxygen exchange. Eur J Anaesth 12:375–386
11. Rowe L, Jones JG, Quine D et al (2010) A simplified method for deriving shunt and reduced V_A/Q in infants. Arch Dis Child Fetal Neonatal Ed 95:F47–F52

12. Ferrando C, Romero C, Tusman G et al (2017) The accuracy of postoperative, non-invasive Air-Test to diagnose atelectasis in healthy patients after surgery: a prospective, diagnostic pilot study. BMJ Open 7:e015560
13. Acosta CM, Maidana GA, Jacovitti D et al (2014) Accuracy of transthoracic lung ultrasound for diagnosing anesthesia-induced atelectasis in children. Anesthesiology 120:1370–1379
14. Volpicelli G, Elbarbary M, Blaivas M (2012) Conference reports and expert panel: international evidence-based recommendations for point-of-care lung ultrasound. Intensive Care Med 38:577–591
15. Soummer A, Perbet S, Brisson H et al (2012) Ultrasound assessment of lung aeration loss during a successful weaning trial predicts postextubation distress. Crit Care Med 40:2064–2072
16. Xue FS, Huang YG, Tong SY et al (1996) A comparative study of early postoperative hypoxemia in infants, children and adults undergoing elective plastic surgery. Anesth Analg 83:709–715
17. Mamie C, Habre W, Delhumeau C et al (2004) Incidence and risk factors of perioperative respiratory adverse events in children undergoing elective surgery. Pediatr Anesth 14:218–224
18. Roeleveld PP, Guijt D, Kuijper EJ et al (2011) Ventilator-induced pneumonia in children after cardiac surgery in The Netherlands. Intensive Care Med 37:1656–1663
19. Tusman G, Bohm SH, Warner DO et al (2012) Atelectasis and perioperative pulmonary complications in high-risk patients. Curr Opin Anaesthesiol 25:1–10
20. D'angelo E, Bonanni MV, Michelini S et al (1970) Topography of the pleural Surface pressure in rabbits and dogs. Respir Physiol 8:204–209
21. Agostoni E, D'angelo E (1970) Comparative features of the transpulmonary pressure. Respir Physiol 11:76–83
22. Agostoni E, D'angelo E, Bonanni MV (1970) The effect of the abdomen on the vertical gradient of pleural pressure. Respir Physiol 8:332–346
23. Heaf DP, Helms P, Gordon I et al (1983) Postural effects on gas exchange in infants. N Engl J Med 308:1505–1508
24. Schlessel JS, Rappa HA, Lesser M et al (1993) Pulmonary mechanics and gas exchange: effect of lateral positioning during recovery from respiratory distress syndrome. Pediatr Pulmonol 15:36–40
25. Brunherotti MAA, Martinez EZ, Martinez FE (2014) Effect of body position on preterm newborns receiving continuous positive airways pressure. Acta Paediatr 103:e101–e105
26. Balaguer A, Roqué M (2007) Infant position in neonates receiving mechanical ventilation. Cochare Library. https://doi.org/10.1002/14651858.CD003668.pub.2
27. Luton-Smith AR, Argent AC, Rimensberger PC et al (2014) Challenging a paradigm: positional changes in ventilation distribution are highly variable in healthy infants and children. Pediatr Pulmonol 49:764–771
28. Schibler A, Henning R (2002) Positive end-expiratory pressure and ventilation inhomogeneity in mechanically ventilated children. Pediatr Crit Care Med 3:124–128
29. Tusman G, Acosta CM, Costantini M (2016) Ultrasonography for the assessment of lung recruitment maneuvers. Crit Ultrasound J 8:8

19

Strain analysis for the identification of hypertensive cardiac end-organ damage in the emergency department

Pavitra Kotini-Shah[1*], Susana Cuadros[2], Felix Huang[1] and Joseph S. Colla[1]

Abstract

Hypertensive emergency is a life-threatening state. End-organ damage affecting the heart accounts for up to 52% of hypertensive emergencies commonly encountered in the emergency department. Recent evidence indicates that strain echocardiography with computerized speckle-tracking is more sensitive at identifying hypertension induced changes in the left ventricle (LV) mechanical function than traditional 2-D echocardiography. We present a case demonstrating the use of emergency physician performed point-of-care strain echocardiography to identify and quantify LV mechanical dysfunction during a hypertensive crisis and to monitor improvement over 6 h.

Background

An estimated 26% of ED patients will have an elevated BP with half of these patients having a BP > 160/100 [1, 2]. Distinguishing hypertensive urgency and emergency is challenging as both conditions involve marked elevation of blood pressure (BP, i.e., systolic BP ≥ 180 and/or diastolic BP ≥ 120). Hypertensive emergency is a life-threatening state with evidence of end-organ damage, as opposed to hypertensive urgency, and requires rapid reduction in BP [3, 4]. The heart is the most common organ affected, accounting for 52% of hypertensive emergencies [3]. Strain echocardiography is a relatively new way to measure left ventricular (LV) mechanical function. Unlike conventional 2D echocardiography which relies on visual estimation to assess cardiac contractility, strain echocardiography utilizes computerized speckle-tracking to measure actual tissue deformation of the myocardium. Strain can be measured in the longitudinal, radial and circumferential planes of the left ventricle (LV). Peak longitudinal strain (PLS) is a measurement of the overall longitudinal deformation of the left ventricle from diastole to systole. PLS can be measured from clips captured from standard apical views of the heart [5]. Longitudinal strain has been shown to be more sensitive at identifying hypertensive changes in LV mechanical function than ejection fraction (EF), fractional shortening, mitral E/A ratio, and tissue Doppler mitral annular velocity [5, 6]. Normal strain measurements range from − 15 to − 22% [7]. We present a case where emergency physician (EP) performed point-of-care PLS analysis is used to monitor improvement in LV mechanical function over time for a patient with hypertensive cardiac emergency.

*Correspondence: pkotini@uic.edu; pkotini@gmail.com
[1] Department of Emergency Medicine, University of Illinois at Chicago, 808 S. Wood Street (MC 724), Chicago, IL 60612, USA
Full list of author information is available at the end of the article

Case report

A 41-year-old woman with past medical history of peripartum cardiomyopathy, mitral regurgitation, and hypertension was referred to the emergency department (ED) due to severely elevated blood pressure. Patient reports a one week history of dyspnea, mild chest pressure with exertion, and stated that she had similar symptoms before with her pulmonary embolism more than 10 years ago. Three days prior to the onset of her symptoms, the patient had stopped taking her prescribed hydrochlorothiazide (HCTZ) due to increased urinary frequency, but maintained compliance with losartan. Vital signs at presentation were temperature 37.2 °C, BP 218/150, heart rate 121, respiratory rate 16, and pulse oximetry 100% on room air. On exam, the patient was well-appearing and in no apparent distress. The patient's lungs were clear to auscultation and she had no S3, jugular vein distention, or lower extremity edema. The remainder of the physical exam was unremarkable. Further testing included labs, an electrocardiogram (EKG), a chest radiograph, and bedside echocardiogram (BSE) performed by ultrasound trained EPs. An apical four-chamber was obtained to calculate peak longitudinal strain (PLS) using only this view. Two initial troponin levels were mildly elevated at 0.08 μg/L, but down-trended thereafter to 0.05 μg/L. There was mild cardiomegaly and increased pulmonary vasculature on chest x-ray, and a new left bundle branch block (LBBB) on EKG. At the time of the initial BSE, BP was 252/163 [mean arterial pressure (MAP) = 170)] and PLS was − 3.5% (Fig. 1). The EF was not calculated, but estimated to be mildly reduced. Six hours later, the BP was 171/94 (MAP = 123) and a repeat BSE was performed and PLS was recalculated. Between the first and second BSE, the patient had received a total of 60 mg IV labetalol, 25 mg PO HCTZ, 40 mg IV furosemide, and was on a nitroglycerine drip at 40 mcg/min. The MAP had been reduced by 27% and the PLS improved to − 14% (Fig. 2). Repeat EKG after the IV medications continued to show a persistent LBBB. The patient was admitted to the cardiac intensive care unit for hypertensive emergency and acute coronary syndrome rule-out. Follow-up outpatient notes indicate that the patient was discharged home the following day and did not get readmitted to the hospital within 30 days.

Figure 1 reflects the patient before hypertension treatment and Fig. 2 reflects the patient after treatment. Both Figs. 1 and 2 are quad displays of an apical 4-chamber image demonstrating peak longitudinal strain (PLS) of the left ventricle (white arrow). In each figure, top left image (A) is a 2D depiction showing the color coding for each left ventricle (LV) segment and the PLS in the 4-chamber view; bottom left image (B) displays the peak systolic strain for each of the six LV segments in the 4-chamber view; top right image (C) displays strain (*y*-axis) plotted over time (*x*-axis) for each of the six color-coded LV segments in a linear graphical display. The white dotted line shows the average of the six strain curves; bottom right image (D) shows the anatomical M-mode display depicting instantaneous strain for the 4-chamber plane with each LV segment color-coded on

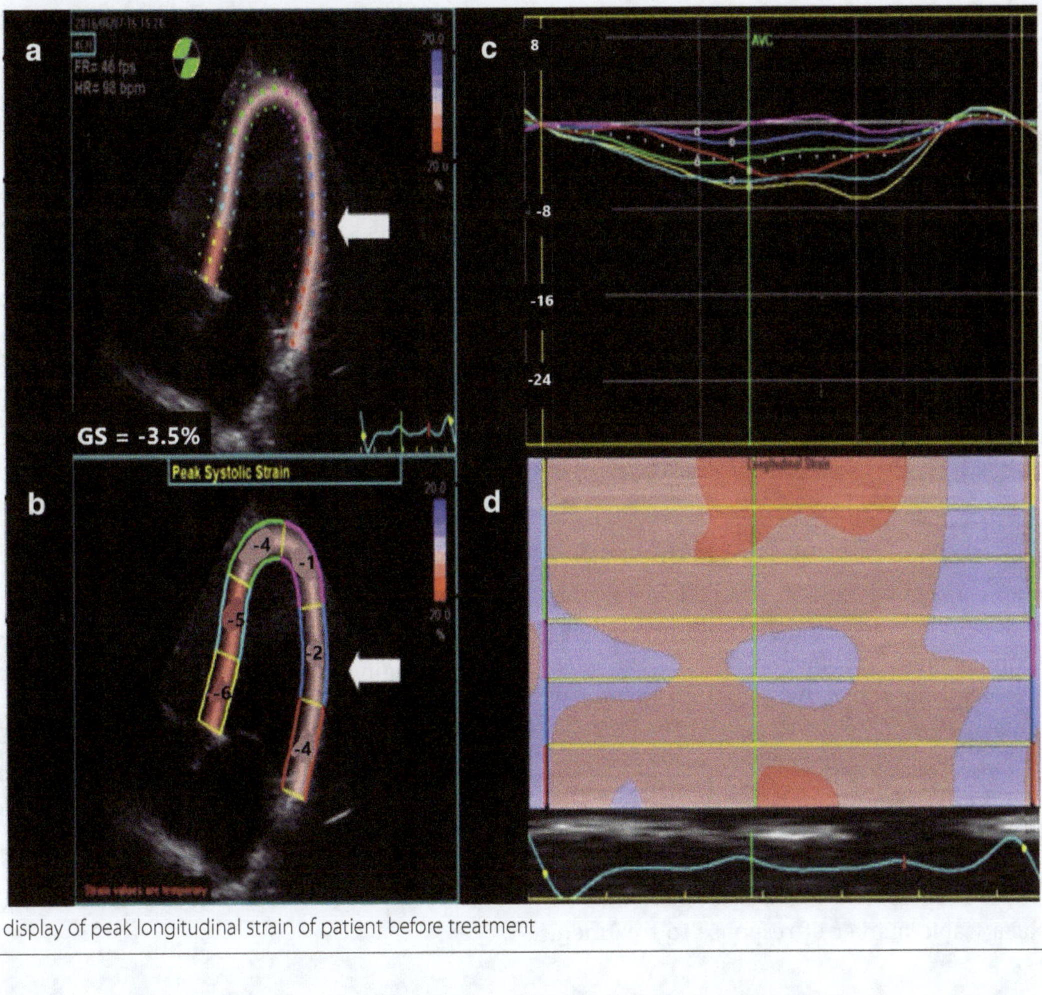

Fig. 1 Quad display of peak longitudinal strain of patient before treatment

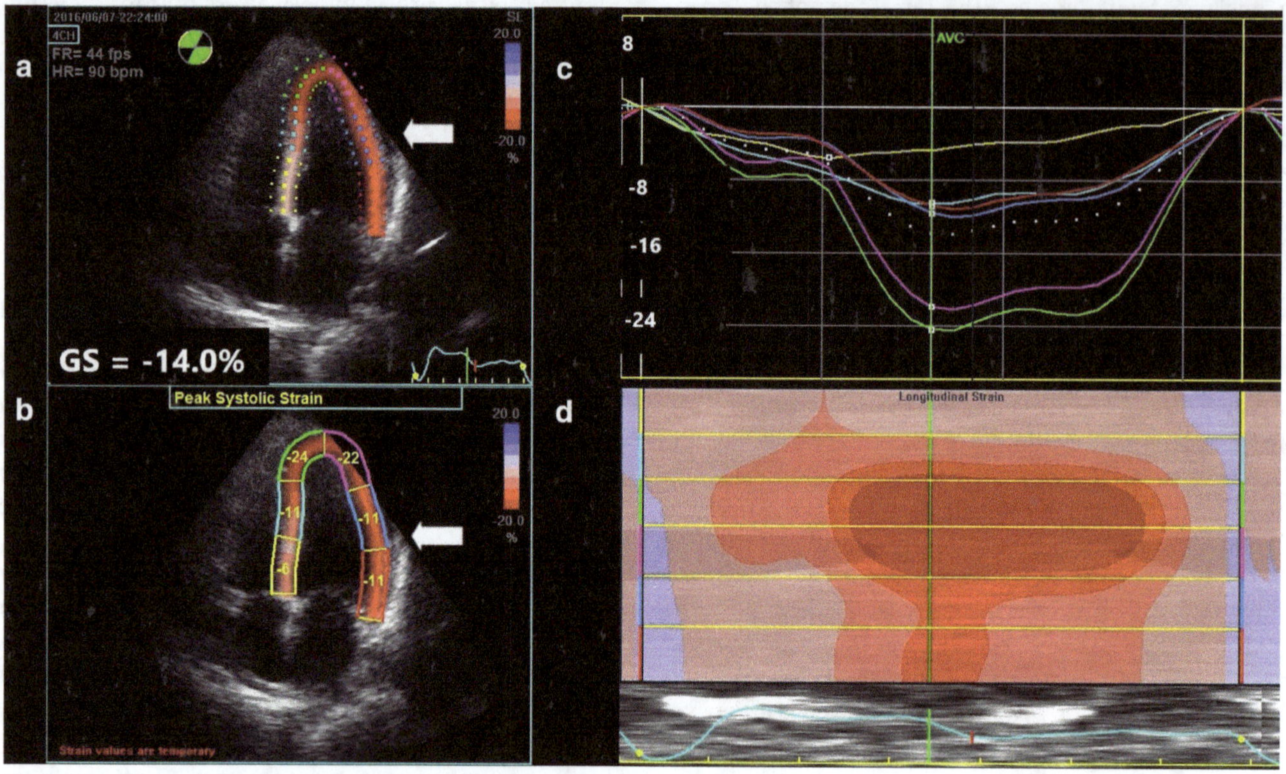

Fig. 2 Quad display of peak longitudinal strain of patient after treatment

the *y*-axis, where the red color represents more negative strain.

Discussion

Hypertensive emergency is a life-threatening disease with visits more than doubling from 2006 to 2013 [8]. Identification of cardiac end-organ damage requires high clinical suspicion and correlation with abnormalities in either EKG, cardiac markers or chest X-ray [9]. Two-dimensional transthoracic echocardiography is helpful, but requires more time to complete, and is not available to emergency departments at all hours. In addition, the delay from image acquisition by a technologist and image interpretation by a cardiologist limits its usefulness for monitoring cardiac function in the ED [10]. Once a good sonographic apical window is obtained at the bedside, an objective computer-generated strain percentage can be acquired by using speckle tracking software, eliminating the need for subjective visual estimation of EF. This advantage of strain analysis will likely decrease rates of LV EF misinterpretation. Furthermore, longitudinal strain provides information about both diastolic and systolic function and does not require complex Doppler measurements to estimate diastolic dysfunction [6, 11].

In the ED, it has been demonstrated that strain imaging can be used as a viable marker of response to treatment of acute heart failure, using ED re-admissions as a marker of adverse outcome [10, 12]. Strain analysis is also a viable method to monitor improvement of LV mechanical function after treatment of systemic hypertension [6, 11, 13, 14]. This case report supports recent papers suggesting potential role for strain analysis in evaluating heart disease in the ED setting.

Our patient demonstrated a three-fold improvement in LV strain, approaching a normal LV strain value, after antihypertensive and pre-load reducing treatment were given. Despite the improvement in PLS value observed within 6 h, the LBBB on EKG did not improve until the next morning. This suggests that the improvement in the electrical conductivity of the heart lagged behind the improvement of the mechanical deformation of the myocardium in this patient. Prior studies have suggested that strain imaging can detect alterations in the LV mechanics at the earliest phase of hypertensive disease even in asymptomatic patients [13]. However, this case is the first to document that subtle adaptive changes of the myocardium may precede changes depicted by conventional screening modalities such as EKG.

Conclusion

Peak longitudinal strain analysis shows promise as an objective parameter for emergency physicians to monitor improvement of LV function during treatment for hypertensive cardiac emergency. This case report is the first to demonstrate a novel clinical application of this echocardiographic tool in the ED. Further study and documentation of PLS along the spectrum of hypertension is needed to better understand the myocardial dynamics at the patient's bedside.

Abbreviations

BP: blood pressure; BSE: bedside echocardiogram; EP: emergency physician; ED: emergency department; EF: ejection fraction; EKG: electrocardiogram; PLS: peak longitudinal strain; HCTZ: hydrochlorothiazide; LBBB: left bundle branch block; LV: left ventricle; MAP: mean arterial pressure.

Authors' contributions

PKS obtained the follow-up sonographic images, performed the PLS analysis, created the figures, performed chart review on the patient, drafted the initial outline of the manuscript, and contributed significantly to manuscript revisions. JSC conceived the study, obtained the initial sonographic images, verified the PLS analysis, and contributed substantially to the editing and revision of the manuscript. SC created the initial draft and performed the literature review. FH contributed significantly to the drafting and editing of the manuscript. All authors contributed equally to the conceptualization of the manuscript. All authors read and approved the final manuscript.

Author details

[1] Department of Emergency Medicine, University of Illinois at Chicago, 808 S. Wood Street (MC 724), Chicago, IL 60612, USA. [2] University of Illinois at Chicago, College of Medicine, Chicago, USA.

Acknowledgements

None.

References

1. Svenson JE, Repplinger M (2008) Hypertension in the ED: still an unrecognized problem. Am J Emerg Med 26:913–917
2. Karras DJ, Ufberg JW, Heilpern KL et al (2005) Elevated blood pressure in urban emergency department patients. Acad Emerg Med 12:835–843
3. Grech AK (2015) Hypertensive crisis-the acute take. BJMP 8:a823
4. Zampaglione B, Pascale C, Marchisio M et al (1996) Hypertensive urgencies and emergencies: prevalence and clinical presentation. Hypertension 27:144–147
5. Gorcsan J III, Tanaka H (2011) Echocardiographic assessment of myocardial strain. J Am Coll Cardiol 58:1401–1413
6. Alam M, Zhang L, Stampehl M et al (2013) Usefulness of speckle tracking echocardiography in hypertensive crisis and the effect of medical treatment. Am J Cardiol 12:260–265
7. Yingchoncharoen T, Agarwal S, Popovic Z et al (2013) Normal ranges of left ventricular strain: a meta-analysis. J Am Soc Echocardiogr 26:185–191
8. Janke AT, McNaughton CD, Brody AM et al (2016) Trends in the incidence of hypertensive emergencies in US emergency departments from 2006 to 2013. J Am Heart Assoc 5:e004511
9. Martindale JL, Wakai A, Collins SP et al (2016) Diagnosing acute heart failure in the emergency department: a systematic review and meta-analysis. Acad Emerg Med 23:1553–2712
10. Favot M, Courage C, Ehrman R et al (2016) Strain echocardiography in acute cardiovascular diseases. West J Emerg Med 17:54–60
11. Imbalzano E, Zito C, Carerj S et al (2011) Left ventricular function in hypertension: new insight by speckle tracking echocardiography. Echocardiography 28:649–657
12. Favot M, Gowland L, Ehrman R et al (2016) Point-of-care strain echocardiography in acute heart failure. Am J Emerg Med 34:2222–2249
13. Cheng S, Shah AM, Albisu JP et al (2014) Reversibility of left ventricular mechanical dysfunction in patients with hypertensive heart disease. J Hypertens 32:2479–2487
14. Celic V, Tadic M, Suzic-Lazic J et al (2014) Two- and three-dimensional speckle tracking analysis of the relation between myocardial deformation and functional capacity in patients with systemic hypertension. Am J Cardiol 113:832–839

20

A randomised crossover study to compare the cross-sectional and longitudinal approaches to ultrasound-guided peripheral venepuncture in a model

James Griffiths[1], Amadeus Carnegie[1,3*], Richard Kendall[2] and Rajeev Madan[2]

Abstract

Background: Ultrasound-guided peripheral intravenous access may present an alternative to central or intraosseous access in patients with difficult peripheral veins. Using venepuncture of a phantom model as a proxy, we investigated whether novice ultrasound users should adopt a cross-sectional or longitudinal approach when learning to access peripheral veins under ultrasound guidance. This result would inform the development of a structured training method for this procedure.

Methods: We conducted a randomised controlled trial of 30 medical students. Subjects received 35 min of training, then attempted to aspirate 1 ml of synthetic blood from a deep vein in a training model under ultrasound guidance. Subjects attempted both the cross-sectional and longitudinal approaches. Group 1 used cross-sectional first, followed by longitudinal. Group 2 used longitudinal first, then cross-sectional. We measured the time from first puncture of the model's skin to aspiration of fluid, and the number of attempts required. Subjects also reported difficulty ratings for each approach. Paired sample *t*-tests were used for statistical analysis.

Results: The mean number of attempts was 1.13 using the cross-sectional approach, compared with 1.30 using the longitudinal approach ($p = 0.17$). Mean time to aspiration of fluid was 45.1 s using the cross-sectional approach and 52.8 s using the longitudinal approach ($p = 0.43$). The mean difficulty score out of 10 was 3.97 for the cross-sectional approach and 3.93 for the longitudinal approach ($p = 0.95$).

Conclusions: We found no significant difference in effectiveness between the cross-sectional and longitudinal approaches to ultrasound-guided venepuncture when performed on a model. We believe that both approaches should be included when teaching ultrasound-guided peripheral vascular access. To confirm which approach would be best in clinical practice, we advocate future testing of both approaches on patients.

Keywords: Ultrasound, Ultrasound education, Venepuncture, Emergency medicine, Emergency ultrasound, Ultrasound guided

Background

Achieving intravenous (IV) access is one of the most common, and most important, clinical skills used in hospital medicine. In the majority of patients, such vascular access is provided by a peripheral intravenous (PIV) cannula. Traditionally, PIV access is achieved by a landmark-and-palpation approach; however, locating a suitable vein by this method is not always straightforward.

Finding and accessing a peripheral vessel in patients with a history of IV drug abuse, severe obesity or chronic medical problems can be impossible using the landmark-and-palpation approach alone. Failure rates for this skill range from 9 to 56% [1]. The alternative in such cases is commonly a central line insertion.

*Correspondence: caa47@cam.ac.uk
[3] Robinson College, Grange Road, Cambridge CB3 9AN, UK
Full list of author information is available at the end of the article

While effective, central venous access is not without risks and is often inappropriate for patients requiring only a short duration of IV treatment. Catheter-related sepsis, arterial puncture, pneumothorax and arrhythmias are all recognised complications of central venous access, and can cause significant morbidity and mortality for these patients [2].

The increasing portability of ultrasound machines has led to a surge in the availability of point-of-care ultrasound (PoCUS) in the hospital environment. Ultrasound-guided central venous access is now considered the standard of care, improving both success rates and reducing complications such as arterial puncture [3]. It has been suggested that the use of ultrasound to guide the cannulation of the deep brachial or basilic veins in patients with difficult peripheral access may improve success rates and, ultimately, patient outcomes [4, 5].

Ultrasound-guided peripheral vascular access is a safe alternative to central line placement and could be used instead in up to 85% of patients classified as having difficult IV access [6]. Training students and staff to locate and access deep peripheral veins under ultrasound guidance may therefore lead to fewer central line placements and, consequently, a reduced incidence of central line-related complications.

There are two commonly used approaches for ultrasound-guided PIV access: the cross-sectional approach (short-axis or out-of-plane approach) and the longitudinal approach (long-axis or in-plane approach). Previous studies have shown that it is possible to teach this skill to novice ultrasound users effectively, using a single 30-min didactic training session [7, 8]. It is unclear as to whether novices find it easier to learn and effectively perform the cross-sectional approach or the longitudinal approach, and there is no consensus which approach should be taught. We devised this trial to identify which approach (or approaches) ought to be taught to novices and to help inform the development of a structured learning package.

We chose to conduct a prospective randomised controlled trial using medical students in order to answer this question. It has been demonstrated that previously ultrasound-naïve medical students are able to use ultrasound to guide peripheral vascular access on real patients after a single training session [9]. It has also been demonstrated that simulation-based training using a dedicated ultrasound phantom can lead to improved levels of skill when applied to real clinical practice [10]. However, we appreciate that we did not follow up phantom training with testing on patients. As such, we advocate testing with patients in future.

As we were testing the efficacy of novices, we used phantom models to simulate patients. Due to the construction of these phantom models, cannula lines tended to kink when inserted; thus, failure reflected the model limitations rather than the skill of the novice. To overcome this, we instead aimed for venepuncture, with the students required to aspirate 1 ml of fluid. This gave the benefit of requiring the students to correctly identify, locate and puncture the vein, while removing any failure bias due to the firm material of the model. We feel that as the main purpose of ultrasound guidance is to aid in locating and puncturing the vein, venepuncture acted as an adequate proxy for peripheral venous access.

Methods

Study design

We conducted a prospective randomised controlled trial to compare the effectiveness of the cross-sectional and longitudinal approaches to ultrasound-guided peripheral venepuncture when employed by novice ultrasound users. The study was reviewed and approved by the Cambridge Psychology Research Ethics Committee. All subjects gave written, informed consent before taking part in the study.

Study setting and population

We recruited a convenience sample of 30 senior medical students at Cambridge University. Six sessions were held over the course of 2 weeks. There were five places available per session, and students were free to choose which session they attended. None of the students had used ultrasound to guide vascular access or venepuncture prior to this study. Nine of the 30 students reported having previously handled an ultrasound machine. All 30 of the students reported having at least some ultrasound teaching in the past.

Study protocol

Each subject was randomly assigned to either the 'cross-sectional first' group ($n = 14$) or the 'longitudinal first' group ($n = 16$) prior to attending a session. This randomisation was performed according to the table generated by 'Research Randomizer', an online random assignment programme [11].

At each session, the group of five students was given a 30-min structured didactic teaching session in the form of an oral presentation. All teaching sessions were delivered by the same individual and covered:

- The value of ultrasound guidance in patients with difficult peripheral access;
- The basic physics behind ultrasound;
- Operation of the portable ultrasound machine;
- Interpretation of the image;
- A tutorial on how to use ultrasound to guide peripheral venepuncture.

Both the cross-sectional and longitudinal approaches were covered during this teaching session, and each approach was given equal coverage. A video walkthrough at the end of the presentation covered both approaches to the technique.

After the teaching presentation, all subjects were given an opportunity to practise using a Toshiba Viamo portable ultrasound machine to scan the blood vessels in the upper limbs of a human model. Subjects were taught how to operate the machine, and how to discriminate arteries from veins. Each subject was allowed 5 min practice with the machine and was asked to practise visualising vessels in both cross-sectional and longitudinal planes. Subjects were allowed to observe one another during this practice opportunity.

Subjects then underwent the study alone with the study coordinator. They were asked to use a 21-gauge needle and syringe to aspirate 1 ml of synthetic blood from a Blue Phantom (Kirkland, WA, USA) ultrasound training model under ultrasound guidance (Additional file 1). Subjects randomised to the 'cross-sectional first' group were required to use only the cross-sectional approach at this stage (Additional file 2). Likewise, the subjects randomised to the 'longitudinal first' group were required to use only the longitudinal approach for this task (Additional file 3). After succeeding, each subject was given a new needle and required to aspirate another 1 ml of synthetic blood from the model, this time using the approach that they had not tried previously. This crossover study design was employed to control for the effect of practice on performance.

Measures

The time that elapsed from first puncture of the model's skin to successful aspiration of 1 ml of synthetic blood into the syringe was measured. Also recorded was the number of attempts required successful aspiration i.e. the total number of times the needle passed through the model's skin before aspiration of fluid. After attempting both approaches, subjects were asked to rate the difficulty of each approach using a pair of 11-point visual analogue scales (Figs. 1 and 2).

Data analysis

Paired sample *t*-tests with 95% confidence intervals (95% CI) were used for the statistical analysis. Data were analysed using IBM SPSS Statistics 21 (IBM Corp., Armonk, NY, USA) [12]. Three separate paired sample *t*-tests were used to compare the cross-sectional and longitudinal approaches in terms of

a. Mean time required;
b. Mean number of attempts required;
c. Mean difficulty rating.

Students were said to have 'failed' if more than three minutes had elapsed between first pass of the needle and aspiration of the fluid, or if three or more attempts were required. Students exceeding three needle passes were assigned the maximum value of three attempts, and students exceeding 3 min were assigned the maximum value of 180 s. This was decided on in advance, and was done for the purpose of statistical analysis in order to prevent excessive skewing of results by outliers.

Results

The data for all 30 subjects were analysed. No student was excluded from the data analysis.

The mean time from first puncture of the model's skin to successful aspiration using the cross-sectional approach was 45.1 s (95% CI 29.4 to 0.9 s). The mean time required using the longitudinal approach was 52.8 s (95% CI 36.7 to 69.0). Performing a paired samples t test, we found that the difference of 7.7 s (95% CI −12.1 to 27.4) was not statistically significant ($p = 0.43$).

The mean number of skin punctures required using the cross-sectional approach was 1.13 (95% CI 0.94 to 1.32).

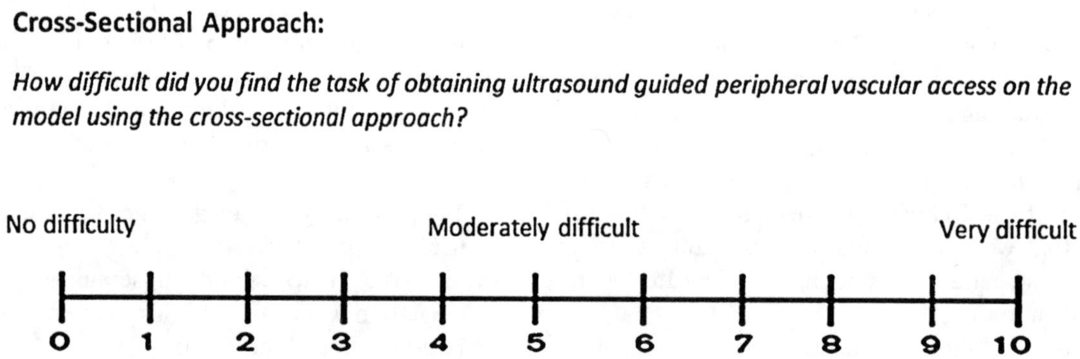

Fig. 1 11-point visual analogue scale to assess and quantify how difficult subjects found the task of aspirating 1 ml of synthetic blood using the cross-sectional approach

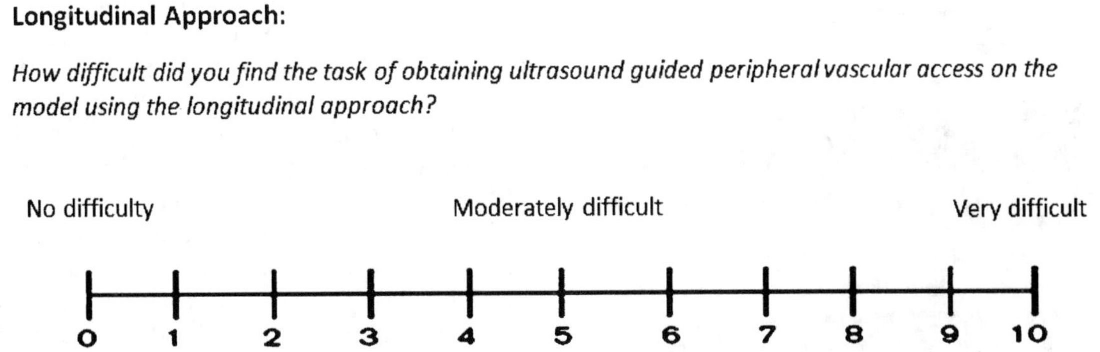

Fig. 2 11-point visual analogue scale to assess and quantify how difficult subjects found the task of aspirating 1 ml of synthetic blood using the longitudinal approach

The mean number of skin punctures required with the longitudinal approach was 1.30 (95% CI 1.08 to 1.52). Paired sample t-tests demonstrated that this difference of 0.17 skin punctures (95% CI −0.08 to 0.41) was not statistically significant ($p = 0.17$).

The mean perceived difficulty score reported for the cross-sectional approach was 3.97 out of 10 (95% CI 3.10 to 4.83). The mean perceived difficulty for the longitudinal approach was 3.93 out of 10 (95% CI 3.21 to 4.65). The difference in mean perceived difficulty of 0.04 out of 10 (95% CI −0.95 to 1.01) was not statistically significant ($p = 0.95$).

All the results are summarised in Table 1.

For graphical representations of the results, see Figs. 3, 4 and 5.

Discussion

Since the first emergency department observational study of the use of ultrasound to establish peripheral vascular access in 1999, [5] the availability of both ultrasound equipment and the ultrasound expertise of emergency physicians has expanded considerably. In many emergency departments, ultrasound is being increasingly utilised to obtain PIV access in patients where attempts using the traditional landmark-and-palpation technique have failed [2].

Table 1 Table to show the mean scores and 95% confidence limits for each of the three variables we measured, sorted by approach

	Cross-sectional	Longitudinal
Mean no. of skin punctures	1.13 ± 0.19	1.30 ± 0.22
Mean time (seconds)	45.1 ± 15.8	52.8 ± 16.2
Mean difficulty (out of 10)	3.97 ± 0.87	3.93 ± 0.72

The mean score recorded in each box was generated from the 30 individual scores collected for that condition, as each subject attempted each condition once (i.e. $n = 30$ for each box)

Ultrasound-guided PIV cannulation is also being utilised in other settings such as intensive care units [13]. Use of ultrasound provides a very real alternative to more invasive approaches such as central venous access, [6, 13] external jugular vein, [14] venous cutdown or intraosseous access. In addition, ultrasound-guided PIV cannulation has been shown not to pose a significant infection risk [15].

With regard to the efficacy of ultrasound-guided PIV cannulation over a traditional landmark-and-palpation

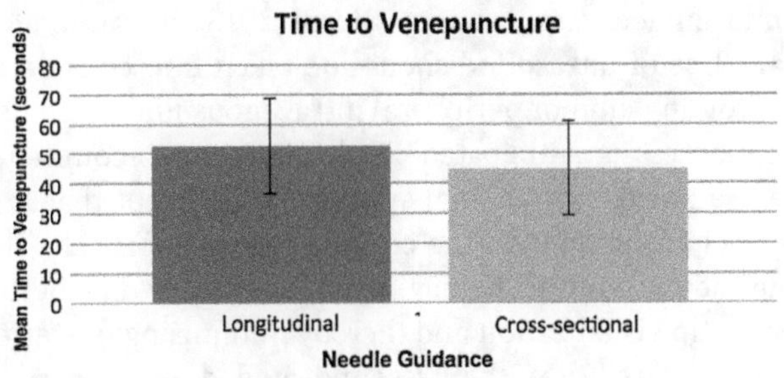

Fig. 3 Graph showing the mean time required to achieve successful venepuncture for each of the two approaches. *Error bars* represent the 95% confidence limits of the means

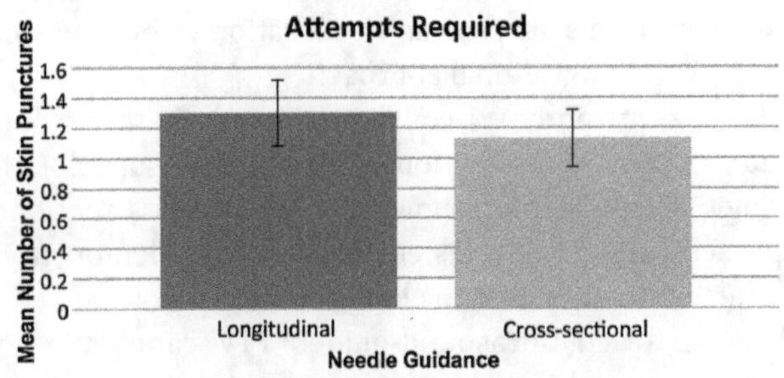

Fig. 4 Graph showing the mean number of skin punctures required to achieve successful venepuncture for each of the two approaches. *Error bars* represent the 95% confidence limits of the means

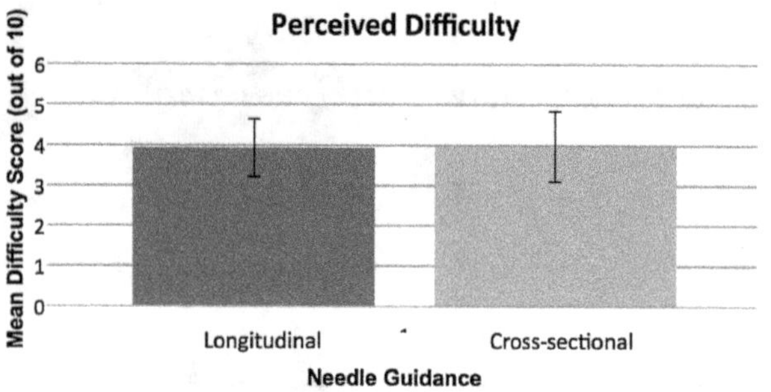

Fig. 5 Graph showing the mean perceived difficulty rating for each of the two approaches. *Error bars* represent the 95% confidence limits of the means

technique, the literature is conflicting. Whist Constantino found that ultrasound was more successful than traditional techniques [16], not all the literature is positive. Several studies have failed to show any advantage of ultrasound-guided peripheral vascular access over a traditional technique [17, 18]. A study in children under 10 years also failed to show any statistical advantage of ultrasound over a traditional approach [19].

Although ultrasound-guided PIV cannulation has not been shown to be better than traditional techniques in all patients, there is evidence to support its use in difficult patients or where traditional techniques have failed. The international evidence-based recommendations on ultrasound-guided vascular access from 2013 recommended that, "Use of ultrasound should be taken into consideration for any kind of peripheral intravenous line when difficult access is anticipated" [20]. They also recommend the use of the longitudinal approach but accept that it is more challenging than the cross-sectional approach. The longitudinal approach may be safer by allowing better needle tip visualization and thereby minimising posterior wall puncture [8]. With ultrasound-guided central venous access, it can be difficult to distinguish between the vein and the artery in longitudinal view, with a greater risk of arterial puncture with the longitudinal approach. The cross-sectional approach allows identification of not just the vessel to be punctured (the vein) but also the vessel to be avoided (the artery). This visualisation of both vessels is lost with a longitudinal approach.

There is currently no consensus as to whether a longitudinal or a cross-sectional approach is superior. In a single study Mahler showed that the cross-sectional approach was slightly faster, but failed to demonstrate any further benefit over the longitudinal approach [21].

How to teach ultrasound-guided PIV cannulation is less well covered in the literature. After a short training package, perceived difficulty of obtaining peripheral vascular access was reduced in a cohort of emergency nurses [4]. A study involving utilisation of ultrasound to aid PIV access learning by medical students using just the short-axis approach showed no difference in terms of obtaining PIV access, but the ultrasound group did perceive the experience as easier and felt they had gained more knowledge of the mechanics of placing an IV cannula [9].

There has been some focus on how best to teach this skill and also which approach is best (cross-sectional versus longitudinal). Blaivas et al. [7] found a clear superiority of the cross-sectional approach over the longitudinal approach in terms of time taken from placing the ultrasound probe and needle to successful vascular access. Interestingly, our study generated some quite different results, and failed to show a difference despite our sample size being almost twice that used by Blaivas and colleagues. (30 subjects, compared to 17 subjects).

Our study has a number of limitations that should be acknowledged. Firstly, our subjects were required to access simulated vessels in an ultrasound phantom, as opposed to the real vessels in a living human patient. The task of aspirating fluid from a model under ultrasound guidance is undoubtedly easier than taking real blood from a patient, as our subjects did not have to attend to the model's concerns or discomfort during the procedure. Additionally, the deep peripheral veins in real patients are unlikely to be as straight as the vessels in our inanimate phantom. Acquiring and maintaining an adequate longitudinal view of a tortuous vein in a real patient is likely to be considerably more difficult than obtaining a good longitudinal view in our model. As such it is difficult to extrapolate our findings to clinical practice, and this study does not provide evidence of benefit of one approach over the other in clinical practice. The findings are limited to the training of novices using a phantom model.

It should also be noted that our study measured only whether our subjects could achieve venepuncture, while in reality the insertion of a PIV cannula requires an additional step in which the catheter is inserted into the vessel following venepuncture. We appreciate that venepuncture does not include all the difficulties of cannulation, for example, confirmation of patency and the increased risk of puncturing of the posterior wall. However, as the purpose of ultrasound is to guide the user in locating the vessel rather than the technique of cannulation, we considered it an adequate proxy.

This study has demonstrated that, in novice ultrasound users, neither the longitudinal nor transverse approach showed a clear superiority when ultrasound-guided venepuncture was attempted in a model. More research is needed to definitively answer the question of whether the cross-sectional or longitudinal approach is more effective when teaching this skill to novice ultrasound users.

Future researchers may wish to have subjects attempt the technique on human subjects to produce results that translate clearly to real clinical practice. However, considering the clear benefits of peripheral venous access (as demonstrated in other studies), the most pertinent point may be to increase teaching of ultrasound-guided peripheral venous access in general, regardless of approach [2, 3]. Until such times as this question is resolved, we believe that both the longitudinal and cross-sectional approaches have value, and that both techniques should be included when developing a training programme to teach this useful clinical skill.

Additional files

Additional file 1. Blue Phantom ultrasound model.

Additional file 2. Cross-sectional ultrasound image of needle in phantom.

Additional file 3. Longitudinal ultrasound image of needle in phantom.

Abbreviations

PIV: peripheral intravenous; IV: intravenous.

Authors' contributions

JG and RK conceived and designed the study. JG had primary responsibility for the planning and data analysis of the study and drafted the original manuscript. All authors contributed in editing the manuscript. All authors read and approved the final manuscript.

Author details

[1] School of Clinical Medicine, University of Cambridge, Cambridge, UK. [2] Emergency Department, Cambridge University Hospitals NHS Foundation Trust, Cambridge, UK. [3] Robinson College, Grange Road, Cambridge CB3 9AN, UK.

Acknowledgements

The authors thank the medical students of the University of Cambridge who took part in the study. We also thank the University of Cambridge Clinical School for the use of its facilities.

References

1. Jacobson AF, Winslow EH (2005) Variables influencing intravenous catheter insertion difficulty and failure: an analysis of 339 intravenous catheter insertions. Heart Lung J Acute Crit Care. 34(5):345–359
2. Shokoohi H, Boniface K, McCarthy M et al (2013) Ultrasound-guided peripheral intravenous access program is associated with a marked reduction in central venous catheter use in non-critically ill emergency department patients. Ann Emerg Med 61(2):198–203
3. Atkinson P, Boyle A, Robinson S, Campbell-Hewson G (2005) Should ultrasound guidance be used for central venous catheterisation in the emergency department? Emerg Med J 22:158–164
4. Blaivas M, Lyon M (2006) The effect of ultrasound guidance on the perceived difficulty of emergency nurse-obtained peripheral IV access. J Emerg Med 31(4):407–410
5. Keyes LE, Frazee BW, Snoey ER et al (1999) Ultrasound-guided brachial and basilic vein cannulation in emergency department patients with difficult intravenous access. Ann Emerg Med 34(6):711–714
6. Au AK, Rotte MJ, Grzybowski RJ et al (2012) Decrease in central venous catheter placement due to use of ultrasound guidance for peripheral intravenous catheters. Am J Emerg Med 30(9):1950–1954
7. Blaivas M, Brannam L, Fernandez E (2003) Short-axis versus long-axis approaches for teaching ultrasound-guided vascular access on a new inanimate model. Acad Emerg Med 10(12):1307–1311
8. Stone MB, Moon C, Sutijono D et al (2010) Needle tip visualization during ultrasound-guided vascular access: short-axis vs long-axis approach. Am J Emerg Med 28(3):343–347
9. Osborn SR, Borhart J, Antonis MS (2012) Medical students benefit from the use of ultrasound when learning peripheral IV techniques. Crit Ultrasound J 4:2
10. Andreatta P, Chen Y, Marsh M et al (2011) Simulation-based training improves applied clinical placement of ultrasound-guided PICCs. Support Care Cancer 19(4):539–543
11. Urbaniak GC, Plous S (2013). Research randomizer (Version 4.0) [Computer software]. http://www.randomizer.org/. Accessed 29 Apr 2014
12. IBM Corp (2012) IBM SPSS Statistics for Windows, Version 21.0. Armonk, IBM Corp
13. Gregg SC, Murthi SB, Sisley AC et al (2010) Ultrasound-guided peripheral intravenous access in the intensive care unit. J Crit Care 25(3):514–519
14. Constantino TG, Kirtz JF, Satz WA (2010) Ultrasound-guided peripheral venous access vs. the external jugular vein as the initial approach to the patient with difficult vascular access. J Emerg Med 39(4):462–467
15. Adhikari S, Blaivas M, Morrison D et al (2010) Comparison of infection rates among ultrasound-guided versus traditionally placed peripheral intravenous lines. J Ultrasound Med 29(5):741–747
16. Constantio TG, Parikh AK, Satz WA et al (2004) Ultrasonography-guided peripheral intravenous access versus traditional approaches in patients with difficult intravenous access. Ann Emerg Med 46(5):456–461
17. Bauman M, Braude D, Crandall C (2009) Ultrasound-guidance vs. standard technique in difficult vascular access patients by ED technicians. Am J Emerg Med 27(2):135–140
18. Stein J, George B, River G et al (2009) Ultrasonographically guided peripheral intravenous cannulation in emergency department patients with difficult intravenous access: a randomized trial. Ann Emerg Med 54(1):33–40
19. Doniger SJ, Ishimine P, Fox JC et al (2009) Randomized controlled trial of ultrasound-guided peripheral intravenous catheter placement versus traditional techniques in difficult access pediatric patients. Pediatr Emerg Care 25(3):154–159
20. Lamperti M, Bodenham AR, Pittiruti M et al (2012) International evidence-based recommendations on ultrasound-guided vascular access. Intensive Care Med 38:1105–1117
21. Mahler SA, Wang H, Lester C et al (2011) Short- vs long-axis approach to ultrasound-guided peripheral intravenous access: a prospective randomized study. Am J Emerg Med 29:1194–1197

21

Doppler images of intra-pulmonary shunt within atelectasis in anesthetized children

Cecilia M. Acosta[1*], Gerardo Tusman[1], Mauro Costantini[1], Camila Echevarría[2], Sergio Pollioto[3], Diego Abrego[3], Fernando Suarez-Sipmann[4,5] and Stephan H. Böhm[6]

Abstract

Background: Doppler images of pulmonary vessels in pulmonary diseases associated with subpleural consolidations have been described. Color Doppler easily identifies such vessels within consolidations while spectral Doppler analysis allows the differentiation between pulmonary and bronchial arteries. Thus, Doppler helps in diagnosing the nature of consolidations. To our knowledge, Doppler analysis of pulmonary vessels within anesthesia-induced atelectasis has never been described before. The aim of this case series is to demonstrate the ability of lung ultrasound to detect the shunting of blood within atelectatic lung areas in anesthetized children.

Findings: Three anesthetized and mechanically ventilated children were scanned in the supine position using a high-resolution linear probe of 6–12 MHz. Once subpleural consolidations were detected in the most dependent posterior lung regions, the probe was rotated such that its long axis followed the intercostal space. In this oblique position, color Doppler mapping was performed to detect blood flow within the consolidation. Thereafter, pulsed waved spectral Doppler was applied in the previously identified vessels during a short expiratory pause, which prevented interferences from respiratory motion. Different flow patterns were identified which corresponded to both, pulmonary and bronchial vessels. Finally, a lung recruitment maneuver was performed which leads to the complete resolution of the aforementioned consolidation thereby confirming the pathophysiological entity of anesthesia-induced atelectasis.

Conclusions: Lung ultrasound is a non-invasive imaging tool that not only enables the diagnosis of anesthesia-induced atelectasis in pediatric patients but also analysis of shunting blood within this consolidation.

Keywords: Atelectasis, Intra-pulmonary shunt, Children, Lung ultrasound, Recruitment maneuvers

Background

Anesthesia-induced atelectasis is a well-known entity observed in approximately 68–100% of pediatric patients undergoing general anesthesia [1–4]. The collapse of dependent lung zones starts with anesthesia induction but can persist for hours after surgery. Anesthesia-related atelectasis have a number of negative clinical consequences such as the impairment of arterial blood oxygenation and lung mechanics [5–7] as well as the predisposition for ventilator-associated lung injury caused by tidal recruitment (i.e., the repetitive opening and closing of unstable lung units during mechanical ventilation) and tidal overdistension of the non-atelectatic regions [8–10].

Lung ultrasound (LUS) has demonstrated its high sensitivity and specificity for diagnosing the entity of anesthesia-induced atelectasis in mechanically ventilated patients [11, 12]. LUS can also reveal tidal recruitment occurring mainly at the boundary of atelectatic lung tissue and its complete resolution after an appropriate lung recruitment maneuver [13].

The use of Doppler for the study of pulmonary vessels within consolidated lung areas has already been reported by several authors [14–16]. Yuan et al. [15] described the role of Doppler in many pulmonary diseases such as infarction, pneumonia, pulmonary sequestration,

*Correspondence: ceacosta77@icloud.com
[1] Department of Anesthesia, Hospital Privado de Comunidad, Córdoba 4545, 7600 Mar Del Plata, Buenos Aires, Argentina
Full list of author information is available at the end of the article

abscesses and tumors. The same authors described different flow patterns in pulmonary vessels and proposed that such patterns may be helpful in differentiating malignant tumors from benign consolidations such as pneumonias, abscesses or obstructive atelectasis [14]. Using Doppler, Görg et al. [16] described the dual arterial supply within different kinds of consolidations. They discriminated pulmonary from bronchial vessels by the pattern of the spectral flow signal.

Even though it has been known that intra-pulmonary shunting is the main reason for the deterioration of gas exchange in anesthesia-induced atelectasis, the visualization of shunting blood usually requires technologies such as PET, SPECT or arteriography. As opposed to these complex diagnostic tools, the examination of pulmonary vessels within consolidated lung areas by Doppler is simple, non-invasive, non-ionizing and perfectly suitable to assess shunt at the bedside [14, 15]. Furthermore, Doppler is capable of differentiating pulmonary from bronchial vessels within a lung consolidation [16]. However, to our knowledge, Doppler has never before been used to visualize the intra-pulmonary shunting of blood within anesthesia-induced atelectasis. Therefore, the aim of this case series is to provide the first evidence of shunt in anesthetized mechanically ventilated children, in whom high-resolution images of atelectasis can easily be obtained using a linear high-frequency probe.

Sonographic diagnosis of anesthesia-induced atelectasis in the operating room and evidence of intra-pulmonary shunt

Three pediatric patients aged two months, one year and four years of age undergoing general anesthesia for abdominal laparoscopic surgery were analyzed. A protective ventilation strategy was applied using volume-controlled ventilation with a tidal volume of 6 ml/kg ideal body weight, a positive end-expiratory pressure (PEEP) of 5 cmH_2O, an inspiration/expiration (I:E) ratio of 1:1 and FIO_2 of 0.5. Respiratory rate was adjusted to keep end-tidal CO_2 between 35 and 40 mm Hg.

LUS assessment was performed with the portable echograph MicroMaxx (Sonosite, Bothell, WA, USA) using a linear probe of 6–12 MHz. Patients were examined in the supine position placing the probe longitudinally as recommended by expert consensus [17]. Given the small size of the chest of neonates or infants, LUS examination of each hemithorax was performed in three regions—anterior, lateral and posterior [18] (Fig. 1).

Subpleural consolidations were identified as atelectasis when they were associated with the following signs [11]: absence of lung sliding and A-lines, presence of multiple spaced B-lines or coalescent B-lines born in subpleural consolidation, static air bronchograms and the presence of a pulse sign. The finding of tidal recruitment within the consolidation reinforced the diagnosis of atelectasis. Finally, the reversal of the consolidation by the recruitment maneuver confirmed the entity of anesthesia-induced atelectasis [13].

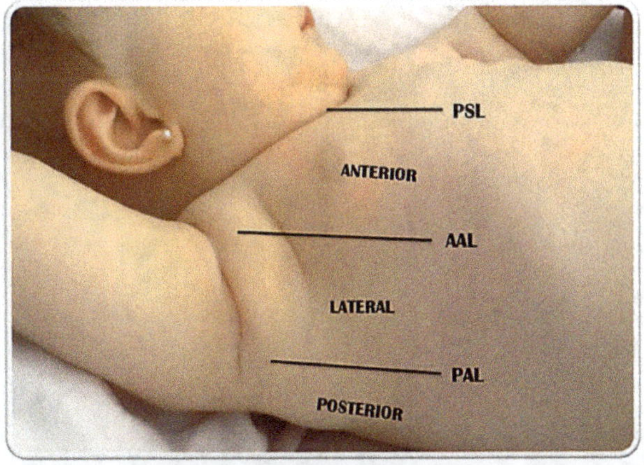

Fig. 1 Each hemithorax was divided into three regions: anterior, lateral, and posterior regions corresponding to the anatomical landmarks of the *parasternal line*, *anterior* and *posterior axillary lines*. *AAL* anterior axillary line; *PAL* posterior axillary line and *PSL* parasternal line

Atelectasis should be distinguished from other types of consolidation like pneumonia and pulmonary embolism. Pneumonia appears as a consolidation with irregular and somewhat blurred margins, commonly associated with dynamic tree-shaped air bronchograms and pleural effusion. The sonographic signs of pulmonary embolism consist of generally two or more small pleural based, hypoechoic consolidations with sharp margins and without central vascularization. Importantly, these two kinds of consolidations cannot be reverted by a lung recruitment maneuver.

Once subpleural consolidations were detected in the most dependent lung areas, the probe was rotated to overcome the acoustic shadows of the ribs and an oblique intercostal view was used for further analysis (Fig. 2a, b).

Color Doppler ultrasound detected pulmonary vessels within consolidated lung areas [14–16]. Most vessels showed a radial anatomical configuration (Fig. 2; Additional file 1: Video 1). Later on, pulsed wave spectral Doppler analysis was performed by positioning the sample volume into the center of the lumen of the detected vessel and by placing the ultrasound beam as parallel to the axial flow ($\leq 60°$) as possible [14]. To avoid interferences from mechanical ventilation, spectral Doppler analysis was done during an expiratory hold and spectral waveforms of similar shape were sampled from at least five consecutive cardiac cycles.

We observed two different arterial flow patterns within atelectatic areas (Fig. 3):

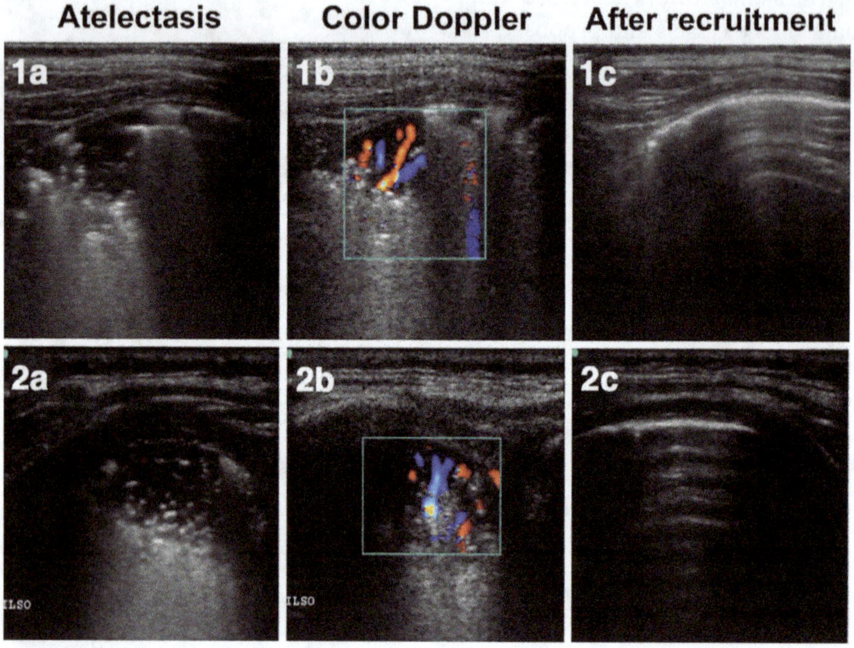

Fig. 2 Color Doppler images of intra-pulmonary shunt. The images belong to two mechanically ventilated anesthetized children: (1) 1 year old and (2) 2 months old. **a** Atelectasis is observed as subpleural consolidations with air bronchograms and coalescent B-lines. **b** Color Doppler revealed lung vessels within the atelectasis showing a radial distribution to the lung periphery. **c** Normal lung tissue after successful treatment of the atelectasis by a recruitment maneuver, the normal aeration prevents the pulmonary vessels from being seen by lung sonography. These images correspond to the Additional file 1: Video 1

- A high-impedance flow signal. This flow pattern originates from a pulmonary artery because as activation of the local hypoxic pulmonary vasoconstriction reflex results in high impedance [19].
- A low-impedance monophasic flow signal that corresponded to bronchial arteries [19].

Finally, we performed a lung recruitment maneuver as previously described [13, 20]. The maneuver consisted of a brief and controlled step-wise increase in airway pressure aiming at re-expanding the atelectasis. The maneuver started from 5 cmH_2O of PEEP that was then increased in 5 cmH_2O steps until airway opening pressure of 30 cmH_20 was reached. At this point, LUS images confirmed the resolution of atelectasis, with the subsequent improvement in lung aeration. Thereafter, a step-wise decrease in PEEP allowed the detection of the minimum level that prevented the reappearance of atelectasis seen in the LUS images. The complete resolution of dependent lung atelectasis by the recruitment maneuver was confirmed 5 min after this maneuver by longitudinal and oblique LUS examination in three regions in each hemithorax, anterior, lateral y posterior; leading to the diagnosis of anesthesia-induced atelectasis [4] (Fig. 2; Additional file 1: Video 1). The normally aerated lung tissue now reflected the ultrasound beam such that intrapulmonary vessels were no longer detectable.

Commentary

In this case series, we are presenting Doppler images of blood shunting within anesthesia-induced atelectasis in mechanically ventilated children. Doppler analysis of these lung vessels was similar to the one already described for different types of lung consolidations.

This finding has two important implications: (1) *academic/educational*, since we are not aware of any previous study that presented Doppler images of shunt within consolidated lungs of anesthetized children; (2) *clinical*, which is related to the potential analysis of blood flow in vessels within lung consolidations. Thus, color and spectral Doppler confirm the existence of shunt while the Doppler flow pattern could provide a general idea about the vascular origin of those vessels (arterial vs. venous–bronchial vs. pulmonary). The spectral Doppler analysis of pulmonary vessels could be useful to assess the impact of hypoxic pulmonary vasoconstriction on arterial oxygenation or right ventricular afterload. The role of Doppler analysis of pulmonary and bronchial flow within atelectasis should be evaluated in new protocols.

Therefore, many questions arise: are these regional changes in vascular flow representative of the blood flow pattern within the main pulmonary arteries? Do atelectasis have negative effects on right heart function? Can blood flow throughout the shunt pathways be manipulated by vasoactive drugs? Surely, future studies should

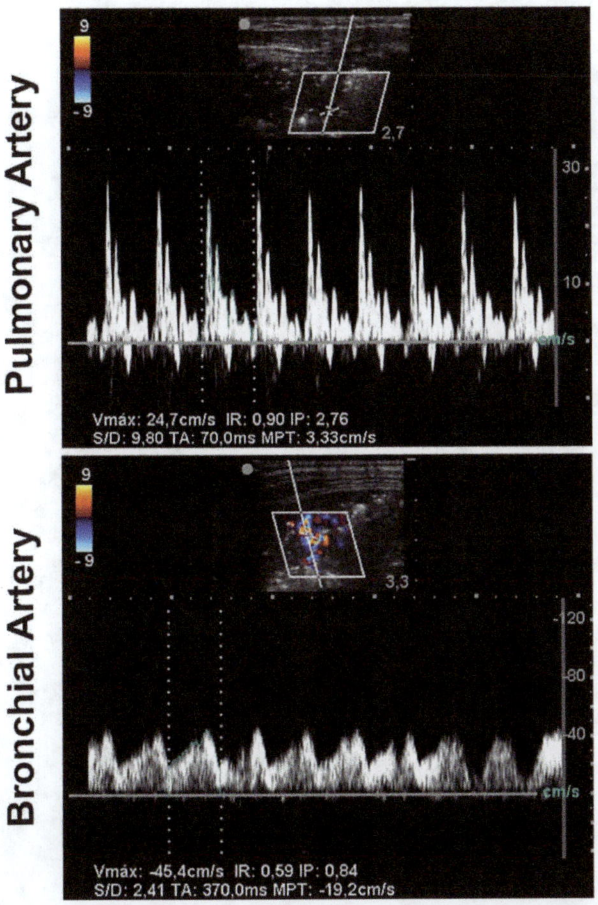

Fig. 3 Spectral Doppler analysis of the three types of vessels within the lung. Spectral Doppler analysis of a pulmonary artery (*upper*) and a bronchial artery (*lower*) within a representative anesthesia-induced atelectasis in 4-year-old patient. Spectral Doppler was performed during a brief expiratory pause. Pulmonary artery showed lower Doppler maximal velocity and higher resistance (IR) and pulsatile (IP) indexes than the bronchial artery presumably due to hypoxic pulmonary vasoconstriction

be conducted to answer these and many other related questions and to determine the potential clinical value of the presented Doppler-based shunt analysis.

Most published evidence was obtained in spontaneously breathing adults and is thus directly related neither to mechanically ventilated nor pediatric patients. Recently, Mongodi et al. [21] published color Doppler images of vessels within consolidated lung areas of mechanically ventilated critically ill adults and Yekeler et al. [22] presented similar images in spontaneously breathing children suffering from pneumonia. While our findings are in line with those of the latter publications, the demonstration of shunting blood within the atelectasis of mechanically ventilated children with previous healthy lungs is novel and unique.

Conclusions

Lung ultrasound can easily detect the presence of anesthesia-induced atelectasis and Doppler shunting within them in pediatric patients. Beyond the effects on gas exchange, the clinical impact of this shunting on pulmonary circulation must be analyzed in future studies.

Additional file

Additional file 1. The video belong to two mechanically ventilated anesthetized children. **1** 1 year old and **2** 2 months old. **A** Atelectasis are observed as subpleural consolidation with air bronchograms and coalescents B-lines. **B** Color Doppler revealed lung vessels within the atelectasis showing a radial distribution to the lung periphery. **C** Normal lung tissue after successful treatment of the atelectasis by a recruitment maneuver, the normal aeration prevents the pulmonary vessels from being seen by lung sonography.

Authors' contributions

CMA, MC, CE, and GT participated in the acquisition of data in the operating room. CMA, GT, SHB and FSS worked on the interpretation of the findings and in the final edition of the manuscript. All authors read and approved the final manuscript.

Author details

[1] Department of Anesthesia, Hospital Privado de Comunidad, Córdoba 4545, 7600 Mar Del Plata, Buenos Aires, Argentina. [2] Department of Radiology, Hospital Privado de Comunidad, Mar Del Plata, Buenos Aires, Argentina. [3] Department of Pediatric Surgery, Hospital Privado de Comunidad, Mar Del Plata, Buenos Aires, Argentina. [4] Section of Anesthesia and Critical Care Hedenstierna Laboratory, Department of Surgical Sciences, Uppsala University Hospital, Uppsala, Sweden. [5] CIBER de Enfermedades Respiratorias, Instituto de Salud Carlos III, Madrid, Spain. [6] Swisstom AG, Landquart, Switzerland.

References

1. Sargent MA, McEachen AM, Jamieson DH, Kahwaji R (1999) Atelectasis on pediatric chest CT: comparison of sedation techniques. Pediatr Radiol 29:509–513
2. Lutterbey G, Wattjes MP, Doerr D, Fischer NJ, Gieseke J, Schild HH (2007) Atelectasis in children undergoing either propofol infusion or positive pressure ventilation anesthesia for magnetic resonance imaging. Paediatr Anaesth 17:121–125
3. Serafini G, Cornara G, Cavalloro F, Mori A, Dore R, Marraro G, Braschi A (1999) Pulmonary atelectasis during paediatric anaesthesia: CT scan evaluation and effect of positive end expiratory pressure (PEEP). Paediatr Anaesth 9:225–228
4. Tusman G, Böhm SH, Tempra A, Melkun F, Garcia E, Turchetto E, Mulder PG, Lachmann B (2003) Effects of recruitment maneuver on atelectasis in anesthetized children. Anesthesiology 98:14–22
5. Rothen HU, Sporre B, Engberg G, Wegenius G, Hedenstierna G (1998) Airway closure, atelectasis and gas exchange during general anaesthesia. Br J Anaesth 81:681–686
6. Gunnarsson L, Tokics L, Gustavsson H, Hedenstierna G (1991) Influence of age on atelectasis formation and gas exchange impairment during general anesthesia. Br J Anaesth 66:423–432
7. Xue FS, Huang YG, Tong SY, Liu QH, Liao X, An G, Luo LK, Deng XM (1996) A comparative study of early postoperative hypoxemia in infants, children, and adults undergoing elective plastic surgery. Anesth Analg 83:709–715
8. Steinberg JM, Schiller HJ, Halter JM, Gatto LA, Lee HM, Pavone LA, Nieman GF (2004) Alveolar instability causes early ventilator-induced lung injury independent of neutrophils. Am J Respir Crit Care Med 169:57–63

9. Pavone LA, Albert S, Carney D, Gatto LA, Halter JM, Nieman GF (2007) Injurious mechanical ventilation in the normal lung causes a progressive pathologic change in dynamic alveolar mechanics. Crit Care 11:R64
10. Hauser GJ, Ben-Ari J, Covin MP, Dalton HJ, Hertzog JH, Bear M, Hopkins RA, Walker SM (1998) Interleukin-6 levels in serum and lung lavage fluid of children undergoing open heart surgery correlate with postoperative mortality. Intensive Care Med 24:481–486
11. Acosta CM, Maidana GA, Jacovitti D, Belaunzarán A, Cereceda S, Rae E, Ananda M, Gonorazky S, Bohm SH, Tusman G (2014) Accuracy of transthoracic lung ultrasound for diagnosing anesthesia-induced atelectasis in children. Anesthesiology 120:1370–1379
12. Yu X, Zhenping Z, Zhao Y, Zhu Z, Tong J, Yan J, Ouyang W (2016) Performance of lung ultrasound in detecting peri-operative atelectasis after general anesthesia. Ultrasound Med Biol. doi:10.1016/j.ultrasmedbio.2016.06.010
13. Tusman G, Acosta CM, Nicola M, Esperati M, Böhm SH, Suarez-Sipmann F (2015) Real-time images of tidal recruitment using lung ultrasound. Crit Ultrasound J 7:19
14. Yuan A, Chang DB, Yu CJ, Kuo SH, Luh KT, Yang PC (1994) Color Doppler sonography of benign and malignant pulmonary masses. AJR 163:5545–5549
15. Yang PC (1996) Color Doppler ultrasound of pulmonary consolidation. Eur J Ultrasound 3:169–178
16. Görg C, Seifart U, Görg K, Zugmaier G (2003) Color Doppler sonographic mapping of pulmonary lesions: evidence of dual arterial supply by spectral analysis. J Ultrasound Med 22(10):1033–1039
17. Volpicelli G, Elbarbary M, Blaivas M, Lichtenstein DA, Mathis G, Kirkpatric AW, Melniker L, Gargani L, Noble VE, Via G, Dean A, Tsung JW, Soldati G, Copetti R, Bouhemad B, Reissig A, Agricola E, Rouby JJ, Arbelot C, Liteplo A, Sargsyan A, Silva F, Hoppmann R, Breitkreutz R, Seibel A, Neri L, Storti E, Petrovic T (2012) Conference Reports and Expert Panel: international evidence-based recommendations for point-of-care lung ultrasound. Intensive Care Med 38:577–591
18. Cattarossi L (2013) Lung ultrasound: its role in neonatology and pediatrics. Early Hum Dev 89(Suppl 1):S17–S19
19. Yuan A, Yang PC, Lee L et al (2000) Reactive pulmonary artery vasoconstriction in pulmonary consolidation by color Doppler ultrasonography. Ultrasound Med Biol 26:49–56
20. Tusman G, Bohm SH (2010) Prevention and reversal of lung collapse during the intra-operative period. Best Pract Res Clin Anaesthesiol 24:183–197
21. Mongodi S, Bouhemad B, Iotti GA, Mojoli F (2015) An ultrasonographic sign of intrapulmonary shunt. Intensive Care Med. doi:10.1007/s00134-015-4169-3
22. Yekeler E, Ucar A, Yilmaz R, Cheikahmad I, Sharifov R, Somer A (2011) Predictive value of Doppler ultrasound in childhood pneumonia. J Inter Med Res 39:1536–1540

22

Social media to supplement point-of-care ultrasound courses: the "sandwich e-learning" approach

Dorothea Hempel[1*], Stephanie Haunhorst[2], Sivajini Sinnathurai[2], Armin Seibel[3,4], Florian Recker[5], Frank Heringer[6], Guido Michels[7] and Raoul Breitkreutz[4,8]

Abstract

Background: Point-of-care ultrasound (POC-US) is gaining importance in almost all specialties. E-learning has been used to teach theoretical knowledge and pattern recognition. As social media are universally available, they can be utilized for educational purposes. We wanted to evaluate the utility of the *sandwich e-learning* approach defined as a pre-course e-learning and a post-course learning activity using Facebook after a one-day point-of-care ultrasound (POC-US) course and its effect on the retention of knowledge.

Methods: A total of 62 medial students were recruited for this study and randomly assigned to one of four groups. All groups received an identical hands-on training and performed several tests during the study period. The hands-on training was performed in groups of five students per instructor with the students scanning each other. Group 1 had access to pre-course e-learning, but not to post-course e-learning. Instead of a pre-course e-learning, group 2 listened to presentations at the day of the course (classroom teaching) and had access to the post-course learning activity using Facebook. Group 3 had access to both pre- and post-course e-learning (*sandwich e-learning)* activities, while group 4 listened classroom presentations only (classroom teaching only). Therefore only groups 2 and 3 had access to post-course learning via Facebook by joining a secured group. Posts containing ultrasound pictures and videos were published to this group. The students were asked to "like" the posts to monitor attendance. Knowledge retention was assessed 6 weeks after the course.

Results: After 6 weeks, group 3 achieved comparable results when compared to group 2 (82.2 % + −8.2 vs. 84.3 + −8.02) ($p = 0.3$). Students who participated in the post-course activity were more satisfied with the overall course than students without post-course learning (5.5 vs. 5.3 on a range from 1 to 6).

Conclusions: In this study, the *sandwich e-learning* approach led to equal rates of knowledge retention compared to classroom lectures and post-course learning. Students appreciate new media for learning experiences and are more satisfied with their learning activity. The sandwich e-learning can be used to maximize hands-on training during courses.

Background

Social Media such as Facebook, Twitter, and YouTube are changing the way medical educators are teaching today. A significant percentage of students already use online resources and social media as means of self-directed learning [1–3]. The most popular and widely used network is Facebook with over 1.32 billion registered users, 945,000,000 of them using mobile devices [4]. Facebook allows users to communicate through chats or via private messages on an individual basis or in defined groups. Students already use Facebook for educational purposes on a daily basis [5, 6].

Ultrasound is an increasingly important diagnostic tool and is amenable to online learning. Facebook offers a broad variety of communication tools (messages, videos

*Correspondence: Doro.Hempel@gmail.com
[1] Department of Cardiology, Angiology and Intensive Care, University Medical Center Mainz, Mainz, Germany
Full list of author information is available at the end of the article

via walls, posts, etc.) that distinguish it from other media such as Twitter that are limited to 140 characters. A challenge in medical education has always been to teach not only for the moment but to achieve retention of knowledge over time. E-learning using social media and other forms such as password-secured platforms are increasingly being used by medical schools and in post-graduate education. The advantage of e-learning is that the learner can autonomously define time, pace, and location of the activity. As the use of social media is increasing, recommendations for the integration into educational programs have been published [7–9].

Hands-on training still is an integral part of every ultrasound course and is expected by the participants [10]. The time spent on this activity should be maximized.

In this study, we intended to assess the value of a pre-course e-learning combined with a post-course activity using Facebook, a concept we defined as *sandwich e-learning*. Our primary goal was to analyze the effect of this combined pre- and post-course e-learning (*sandwich e-learning*) activities on the retention of knowledge compared to standard lectures and post-course learning; the secondary aim was to evaluate the utility of post-course activity using social media.

Methods

We developed a one-day course based on emergency ultrasound courses offered by the DEGUM (German Society for Ultrasound in Medicine) and the German Society of Anesthesiology and Intensive care (Deutsche Gesellschaft für Anästhesie und Intensivmedizin; DGAI; curriculum of AFS module 5). The curriculae incorporate the E-FAST exam (extended focused assessment with sonography in trauma) and clinical applications of thoracic ultrasound such as pleural effusion, B-lines, and pulmonary edema, pneumothorax, and consolidations [11].

Participants

We recruited medical students without prior ultrasound experience (3rd year and higher) from two medical schools in Germany (University of Frankfurt and University of Bonn). Participation in the course was not required for completing the curriculum at university and had no influence on the progress or grading of their medical studies. For participating in the study, all students received an expense allowance of 50 Euros and a compensation for their traveling expenses. All were given ultrasound pocket-sized cards (www.SonoABCD.org) and a textbook summarizing the content of AFS Module 5 after the end of the study. The cards are pocket-sized cards summarizing scanning techniques, physiologic, and pathologic findings. We developed five different cards covering POC-US as an introduction, the FAST exam, thoracic ultrasound, the FEEL exam (focused echocardiographic evaluation in life support [12]), and deep vein thrombosis. Every student received the FAST and the thoracic ultrasound pocket cards. The textbook handed out to the students was published by two of the authors (RB and AS) as complementary material to the certified ultrasound courses. To motivate the students, the three top scorers were invited to participate in another ultrasound course free of cost. All participants gave written consent for their data being used for research purposes and publication; an approval by the ethics committee was waived.

Study design

The study was designed as a randomized, controlled, parallel group study. Students were randomized into four groups (G 1–4) (Fig. 1).

All students were required to take a multiple choice test (Test A) consisting of 20 questions including multiple choice questions (MC) and drag-and-drop tasks during the 4 weeks prior to the course.

The pre-course e-learning consisted of 14 case-based screencasts with a maximum duration of 5 min. The content of the screencasts is listed in Table 1. The screencasts, defined as digital recordings of a computer screen output enhanced with audio narration [13], were produced by seven experienced physicians using a standard template. All physicians were certified POCUS instructors and were taught how to use the free online program screencast-o-matic (www.screencast-o-matic.com) for production of the screencasts. Every presentation included a standard structure of the following slides: *title, presentation of the case/problem, ultrasound images or clips, interpretation/progress of the case, key messages, conclusion, questions*, and *title again* [14]. Screencasts were uploaded as an e-learning curriculum onto a password-secured platform.

G 1 and G 3 were given access to a case-based e-learning curriculum 4 weeks prior to the course and participated in a discussion (60 min) on the day of the course. The discussion was moderated by two tutors and intended to clarify all issues that arose during the e-learning.

G 2 and 4 (classroom groups) had no access to the pre-course e-learning and listened to standardized classroom-based presentations on the day of the course. The classroom teaching consisted of nine lectures lasting 15 min each, covering identical content as that for the pre-course e-learning (Table 1).

All groups participated in a hands-on training (HT) identical in structure and content (180 min in total). HT was performed in small groups of five students rotating

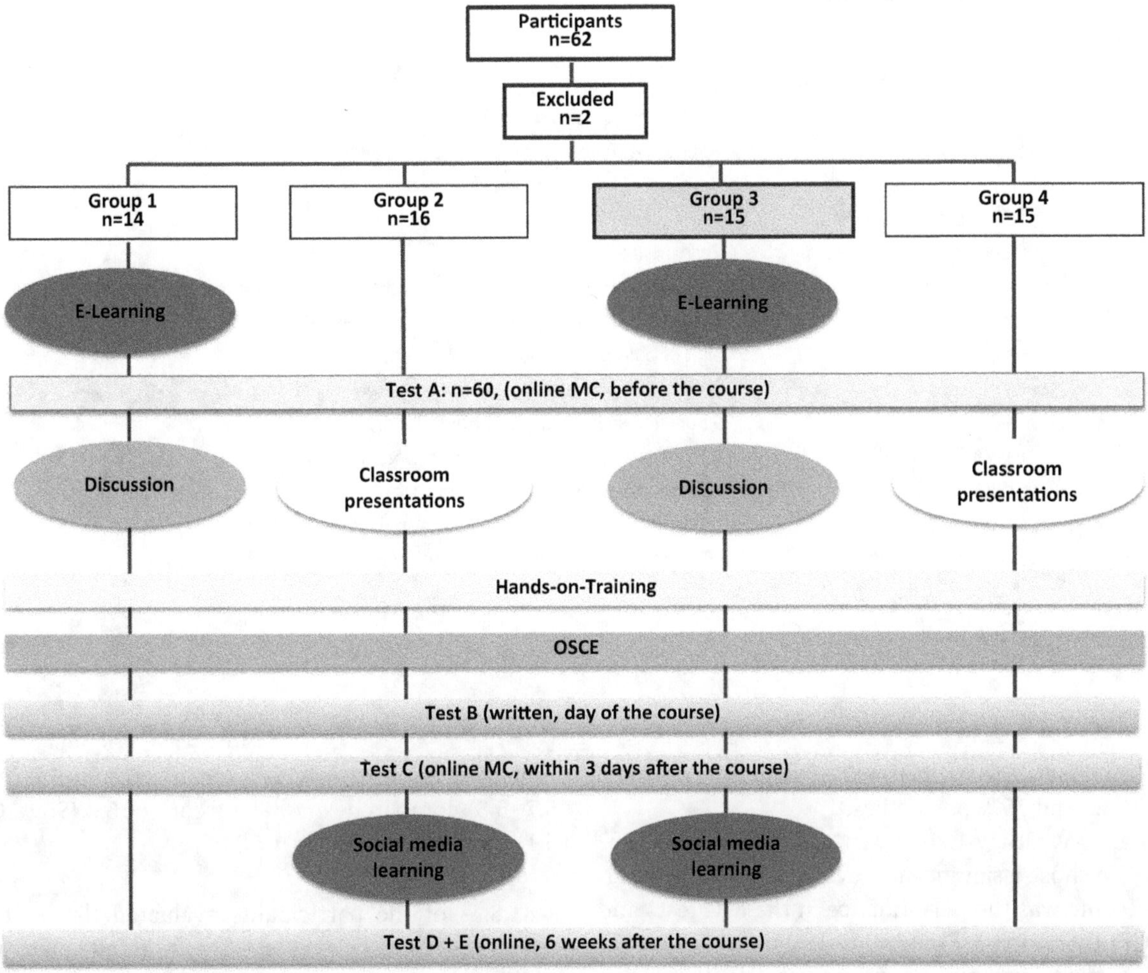

Fig. 1 Study design: Group 3 underwent the *sandwich e-learning* approach

through six stations with the students scanning each other under supervision of an experienced instructor who was not compensated for the activity (stations 1–3: thoracic ultrasound; stations 4–6: FAST).

After the HT, every participant performed a standardized objective clinical skills examination (OSCE) with the maximum score of 50. The test required the students to perform a defined exam, i.e., FAST, and name structures displayed. The instructors evaluated the tasks as right (1 point) or wrong (0 points). With a total of 50 tasks, the maximum score that could be achieved was 50.

After the course, G 2 and G 3 were invited to join a password-protected group in the social network Facebook. Every weekday, a Facebook post was posted to the group for a total of 6 weeks (30 tweets). Each post had a maximum word count of 140 characters; 17 out of 30 included an ultrasound video or image (Fig. 2). To monitor attendance, students were instructed to like each of the posts. The original posts can be found in the Additional file 1: Table S1.

All students performed a MC test (test B) on the day of the course; an online MC test within 3 days after the course (test C); and an online MC test 6 weeks after (test D). Another test (test E) consisted of 20 questions including pictures and videos showing physiologic or pathologic findings. These questions had to be answered in free text and were intended to assess the pattern/image-recognition ability of the students.

Students were also asked to answer a questionaire after the day of the course and after completion of the study protocol grading items from one (poor) to six (very good). The survey covered every phase of the study (pre-course, classroom lectures, HT, post-course, tests, etc.) and asked about their satisfaction with organization, layout, content, and applicability.

Statistical analysis

Statistical analysis was performed using GraphPad Prism version 6.0 (GraphPad software, Inc. La Jolla, CA 92037,

Table 1 Contents of the screencasts and the lectures

Screencast no.	Case vignette	Content	Corresponding lecture (no.)
1	Fall from 3 m height	FAST algorithm and probe positioning	7
2	Motorcycle accident	Positive FAST: free fluid in right upper quadrant	9
3	Bicycle accident	Positive FAST: free fluid in left upper quadrant	9
4	Syncope in a pregnant patient	Positive FAST: free fluid in pelvis	9
5	Resuscitation after thoracic surgery	Pericardial effusion	8
6	Dyspnea after central line placement	Physiologic artifacts in lung ultrasound: lung sliding, A-lines, lung pulse	1
7	Weaning failure and intubation	Pleural effusion, compression atelectasis, B-lines	4
8	Dyspnea I	Sign of pulmonary fluid: multiple B-lines	5
9	Dyspnea II	B-lines: Pathophysiology and scanning technique	2
10	Dyspnea III	Pleural effusion, ultrasound-guided thoracentesis	4
11	Dyspnea IV	Consolidations, aerobronchogram, pneumonia	5
12	Car crash	Rib fracture, exclusion of pneumothorax	6
13	Tracheostomy	Ultrasound of the trachea, tracheotomy under ultrasound-guidance	3
14	Respiratory distress after subclavian line placement	Lung ultrasound signs of pneumothorax	6

USA). Test results were analyzed and presented in % score with 25 and 75 % percentiles.

The Mann–Whitney-U test was used for group comparison. We chose a significance level of $\alpha = 5$ %. The primary outcome was the performance in the MC tests and the OSCE; therefore, a Bonferroni–Holm correction for multiple testing was applied, and power calculation was performed for $\alpha = 2.5$ %.

Results and discussion

A total of 62 students were recruited from the universities of Bonn and Frankfurt. Two students did not attend the course, while three students did not complete test C, leaving 57 students for this statistical analysis. When comparing group 3 (sandwich e-learning) with the other groups (post-course learning alone, pre-course learning only, and classroom-based), no significant differences were found both in test D and test E ($p = 0.3$; $p = 0.5$) (Fig. 3). Groups 1 and 3 performed significantly better in test A compared to groups 2 and 4 ($p < 0.05$). Results of tests B and C did not show any significant difference. The results and a detailed discussion of tests A, B, and C have previously been published elsewhere [14].

The evaluation by the participants showed that the post-course learning raised the satisfaction as G 2 and 3 evaluated the course with a mean score of 5.5 (95 % CI 5.7–5.3) compared to a mean score of 5.3 (95 % CI 5.5–5.1) given by G 1 and 4 ($p < 0.05$).

81.8 % of the participants evaluated the post-course activity as good or very good with an adequate amount of time spent on this activity. 60.6 % of students felt their increase in knowledge was good; this was only their subjective judgement.

In this study, we designed and applied the *sandwich e-learning* technique, a novel approach defined as a learning pathway including a pre-course e-learning curriculum, a hands-on training (HT) session, and a post-course activity using social media after the course.

Teaching POC-US ultrasound has to incorporate different aspects of learning. They are the sensor–motor component of moving the ultrasound probe, the skill of pattern recognition, and the skill of incorporation of the findings into the clinical setting. Pattern-recognition training can be imparted utilizing e-learning. The integration into the clinical context can be partially trained unsing e-learning by adding short case vignettes. Description, for example, of the history of present illness, vital signs, etc., in combination with an ultrasound picture or video, can instead be used in the training for the integration of the ultrasound findings into the clinical context. The motor skills of probe

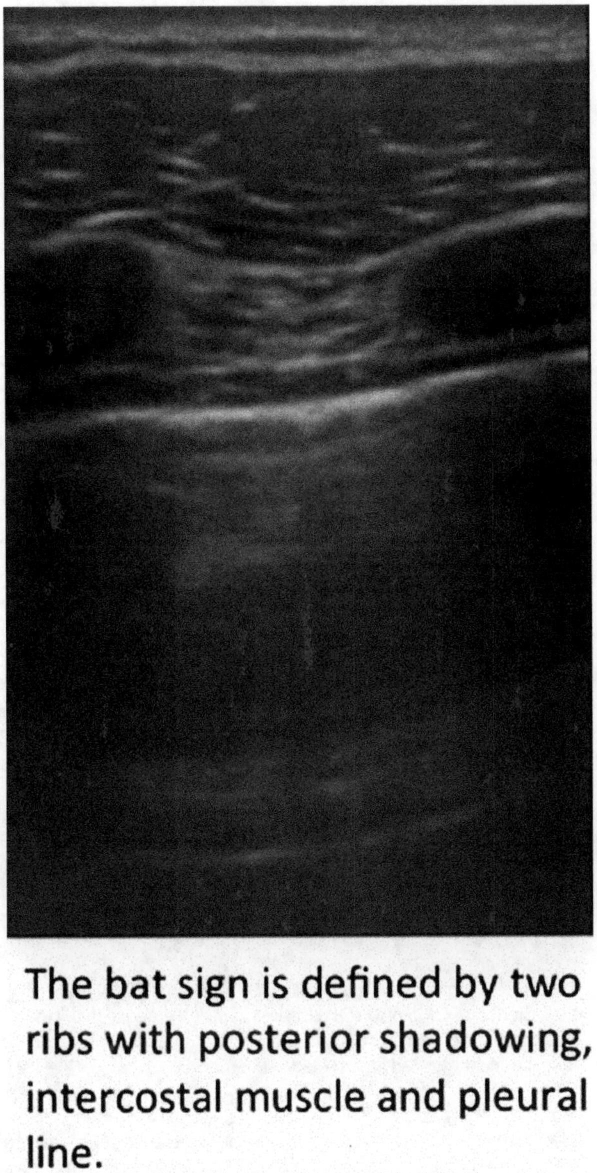

Fig. 2 Example of a post with a picture and a short text

placement on the patient can most effectively be learned via hands-on training [15]. Many studies have evaluated educational methods for teaching procedural skills [16, 17]. Hands-on training is very staff-intensive as the number of students trained by one teacher should be as small as possible to allow the individual student enough time. Many physicians and students learn the basics of POC-US in focused courses lasting only one to 2 days [18, 19]. Therefore, hands-on time during these courses should be maximized.

E-learning both traditional methods such as online curricula and new methods utilizing social media such as Facebook can be used to teach theoretical knowledge and pattern recognition [5, 6]. The advantages of e-learning are flexibility regarding space, time, and duration [20], and in contrast to generic courses, the form of a self-organized learning pathway over time which can enhance retention of knowledge. It is important to point out that every educational activity using social media needs to be rigorous regarding the appropriate use and privacy policies that apply [7].

Conclusions

In our study, students trained with the *sandwich e-learning* approach achieved similar test results after 6 weeks compared to the groups with traditional teaching methods such as classroom lectures. Therefore, we argue that e-learning might be an alternative to classroom lectures as it offers the possibility to maximize the time spent on hands-on training and seems to be a feasible method of learning in addition to hands-on training for POC-US.

Limitations

In this study, we only analyzed the effect of the sandwich e-learning approach on a limited number of medical students; further research is needed applying this approach to postgraduate training where the use of social media is not as common, especially regarding ultrasound education. We assume that all participating students had a high motivation, but we did not perform a motivational analysis. The results of the online tests are limited by the fact that students could have used other resources while completing the tests. As all groups would have this possibility, this does not contradict the results and conclusion of our study. Our study is further limited by the fact that we only assessed the retention of knowledge after 6 weeks. Further study comparing different models of sandwich e-learning, i.e., social media-based pre-course and post-course versus a structured curriculum-based pre-course and post-course, is needed to explore the efficacy of this technique. More detailed investigation is also needed to

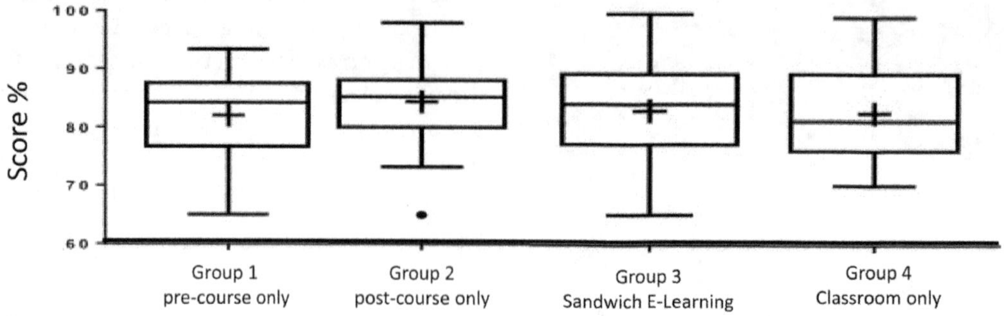

Fig. 3 Results of test D: no difference in performance between the groups

ascertain if knowledge is retained over longer periods of time and when it is applied in clinical practice.

Additional file

Additional file 1: Table S1. The posts that were sent to the Facebook group.

Authors' contributions

DH was involved in drafting the study, contributed to the screencasts used in this study and wrote the manuscript. SH and SS were involved in drafting and designing the study; both carried out the study and data collection. SH was involved in data analysis and approved the final manuscript after critical revision. AS contributed to the study conception and critically revised the manuscript. He has given approval of the final version. FR contributed significantly to recruitment of participants and data collection. He has given approval of the final version. FH contributed significantly to recruitment of participants and data collection. He was involved in designing the study. He has given approval of the final version. GM has been involved in data analysis and drafting of the manuscript. He has also given approval of the final version. RB has contributed to the study design and conception, supervised data analysis, and has critically revised data and manuscript. He has given approval of the final version. All authors read and approved the final manuscript.

Author details

[1] Department of Cardiology, Angiology and Intensive Care, University Medical Center Mainz, Mainz, Germany. [2] Department of Anesthesiology and Intensive Care Medicine, Kliniken Maria Hilf, Moenchengladbach, Germany. [3] Department of Anesthesiology, Intensive Care and Emergency Medicine, Diakonie Klinikum Jung Stilling, Siegen, Germany. [4] Ultrasound Network in Acute and Critical Care, SonoABCD, Frankfurt am Main, Germany. [5] Sono4Students, University Hospital Bonn, Bonn, Germany. [6] FINeST Frankfurt Institute of Interdisciplinary Emergency Medicine and und Simulation Training, Johann Wolfgang Goethe University, Frankfurt am Main, Germany. [7] Department III of Internal Medicine, Heartcenter, University Hospital of Cologne, Cologne, Germany. [8] Emergency Department, Hospital of the City of Frankfurt (Höchst), Gotenstr. 6-8, 65929 Frankfurt am Main, Germany.

Acknowledgements

The authors thank tutors (S. Schellhaas, T. ElAnsari, K. Kunz, Y. Trusau, C. Schrader, and T. Schröder) for their help during this study. The authors also want to thank Sono4students and FINEST Frankfurt for the cooperation. Regional network of ultrasound in acute and critical care www.SonoABCD.org designed and supported this study. The authors are also indebted to J. Geib for her organizational help. Studying the effects of Tweets to enhance student's performance was inspired by David P. Bahner, Ohio State University, USA and is gratefully acknowledged.
Parts of the data was presented at the World Congress of Ultrasound in Medical Education meeting, Portland, USA October 2014.

References

1. Hollinderbäumer A, Hartz T, Rückert F (2013) Education 2.0—How has social media and Web 2.0 been integrated into medical education? A systematical literature review. GMS Z Med Ausbild 30(1):1–12
2. Barry DS, Marzouk F, Chulak-Oglu K, Bennett D, Tierney P, O'Keeffe GW (2015) Anatomy education for the YouTube generation. Anat Sci Educ 9(1):90–96
3. Choi-Lundberg DL, Low TF, Patman P, Turner P, Sinha SN (2015) Medical student preferences for self-directed study resources in gross anatomy. Anat Sci Educ. doi:10.1002/ase.1549
4. Wikipedia. https://de.wikipedia.org/wiki/Facebook. Accessed 17 Oct 2014
5. Pander T, Pinilla S, Dimitriadis K, Fischer MR (2014) The use of Facebook in medical education—a literature review. GMS Z Med Ausbild 31(3):Doc33. doi:10.3205/zma000925
6. Gray K, Anabell L, Kennedy G (2010) Medical students' use of Facebook to support learning: Insights from four case studies. Med Teach 32(12):971–976
7. Pearson D, Cooney R, Bond MC (2015) Recommendations from the Council of Residency Directors (CORD) Social Media Committee on the Role of Social Media in Residency Education and Strategies on Implementation. West J Emerg Med 16(4):510–515
8. Chang TP, Pham PK, Sobolewski B, Doughty CB, Jamal N, Kwan KY, Little K, Brenkert TE, Mathison DJ (2014) Pediatric emergency medicine asynchronous e-learning: a multicenter randomized controlled Solomon four-group study. Acad Emerg Med 21(8):912–919
9. Chu LF, Ngai LK, Young CA, Pearl RG, Macario A, Harrison TK (2013) Preparing interns for anesthesiology residency training: development and assessment of the successful transition to anesthesia residency training (START) e-learning curriculum. J Grad Med Educ 5(1):125–159
10. Röhrig S, Hempel D, Stenger T, Armbruster W, Seibel A, Wlcher F, Breitkreutz R (2014) Which learning methods are expected for ultrasound training? Blended learning on trail. Anaesth 63(10):745–752
11. Röhrig S, Seibel A, Zechner PM, Steigerwald M, Kummer T, Groesdonk HV, Armbruster W, Breitkreutz R (2011) Thoracoabdominal sonography (E-FAST plus)- AI training module 5 in anaesthesiologist-performed focussed sonography. Anasthesiol Intensivmed Notfallmed Schmerzther. 46(11–12):772–781
12. Breitkreutz R, Price S, Steiger HV, Seeger FH, Ilper H, Ackermann H, Rudolph M, Uddin S, Weigand MA, Müller E, Walcher F (2010) Emergency Ultrasound Working Group of the Johann Wolfgang Goethe-University Hospital, Frankfurt am Main (2010) Focused echocardiographic evaluation in life support and peri-resuscitation of emergency patients: a prospective trial. Resuscitation. 81(11):1527–1533
13. http://en.wikipedia.org/wiki/Screencast. Accessed 22 Aug 2015
14. Hempel D, Sinnathurai S, Haunhorst S, Seibel A, Michels G, Heringer F, Recker F, Breitkreutz R (2015) Influence of case based E-learning on students' performance in point-of-care ultrasound courses: a randomized trail. Eur J Emerg Med. doi:10.1097/MEJ.0000000000000270
15. Cartier RA, Skinner C, Laselle BJ (2014) Perceived effectiveness of teaching methods for point of care ultrasound. Emerg Med. 47(1):86–91

16. Jayaraman V, Feeney JM, Brautigam RT, Burns KJ, Jacobs LM (2014) The use of simulation procedural training to improve self-efficacy, knowledge, and skill to perform cricothyroidotomy. Am Surg 80(4):377–381
17. Andreatta P, Chen Y, Marsh M, Cho K (2011) Simulation-based training improves applied clinical placement of ultrasound-guided PICCs. Support Care Cancer 19(4):539–543
18. Mozzini C, Garbin U, Fratta Pasini AM, Cominacini L (2015) Short training in focused cardiac ultrasound in an Internal Medicine department: what realistic skill targets could be achieved? Intern Emerg Med 10(1):73–80
19. Gaspar HA, Morhy SS, Lianza AC, de Carvalho WB, Andrade JL, do Prado RR, Schvartsman C, Delgado AF (2014) Focused cardiac ultrasound: a training course for pediatric intensivists and emergency physicians. BMC Med Educ 14:25
20. Platz E, Goldflam K, Mennicke M, Parisini E, Christ M, Hohenstein C (2010) Comparison of Web-versus classroom-based basic ultrasonographic and EFAST training in 2 European hospitals. Ann Emerg Med 56(6):660–667
21. Walcher F, Weinlich M, Conrad G et al (2006) Prehospital ultrasound imaging improves management of abdominal trauma. Br J Surg 93(2):238–242

23

Estimating the accuracy of optic nerve sheath diameter measurement using a pocket-sized, handheld ultrasound on a simulation model

Garrett G. R. J. Johnson[1], Frederick A. Zeiler[2,3], Bertram Unger[4], Gregory Hansen[5], Dimitrios Karakitsos[6] and Lawrence M. Gillman[2*]

Abstract

Background: Ultrasound measurement of optic nerve sheath diameter (ONSD) appears to be a promising, rapid, non-invasive bedside tool for identification of elevated intra-cranial pressure. With improvements in ultrasound technology, machines are becoming smaller; however, it is unclear if these ultra-portable handheld units have the resolution to make these measurements precisely. In this study, we estimate the accuracy of ONSD measurement in a pocket-sized ultrasound unit.

Methods: Utilizing a locally developed, previously validated model of the eye, ONSD was measured by two expert observers, three times with two machines and on five models with different optic nerve sheath sizes. A pocket ultrasound (Vscan, GE Healthcare) and a standard portable ultrasound (M-Turbo, SonoSite) were used to measure the models. Data was analyzed by Bland–Altman plot and intra-class correlation coefficient (ICC).

Results: The ICC between raters for the SonoSite was 0.878, and for the Vscan was 0.826. The between-machine agreement ICC was 0.752. Bland–Altman agreement analysis between the two ultrasound methods showed an even spread across the range of sheath sizes, and that the Vscan tended to read on average 0.33 mm higher than the SonoSite for each measurement, with a standard deviation of 0.65 mm.

Conclusions: Accurate ONSD measurement may be possible utilizing pocket-sized, handheld ultrasound devices despite their small screen size, lower resolution, and lower probe frequencies. Further study in human subjects is warranted for all newer handheld ultrasound models as they become available on the market.

Keywords: Point-of-care ultrasound, Optic nerve sheath diameter, Ultrasound, Intra-cranial pressure, Handheld ultrasound

Background

Elevated intra-cranial pressure (ICP) is a frequent and grave complication of neurological injury secondary to conditions, such as traumatic brain injury, hydrocephalus, hepatic encephalopathy, and central nervous system infection. Close ICP monitoring is fundamental to the early detection and appropriate management [1]. Direct ventricular or intra-parenchymal monitoring is considered the gold standard for measuring ICP; however, the procedure is invasive, carries the risk of infection and bleeding, and is resource intensive [2, 3]. Other modalities for estimating ICP, such as lumbar puncture, computed tomography, or magnetic resonance imaging, have their own limitations, and can be impractical or dangerous in a variety of patient care settings [4]. A variety of non-invasive techniques utilizing ultrasound have been

*Correspondence: gillmanlm@yahoo.ca
[2] Departments of Surgery, University of Manitoba, GF439, 820 Sherbrook Street, Winnipeg, MB R3A 1R9, Canada
Full list of author information is available at the end of the article

investigated including transcranial Doppler (TCD) ultrasonography and the pulsatility index calculated from its flow velocity waveform, and transorbital ultrasound measurement of optic nerve sheath diameter (ONSD). Both show promise in the emergency medicine and critical care literature for a variety of adult and pediatric patient populations [5–14]. Ultrasound is readily available, rapid, and non-invasive, making it a potentially excellent tool for monitoring the neurocritically ill.

With improvements in ultrasound technology, machines are becoming ultra-portable allowing for flexible point-of-care examinations, including at the scene of injury, in austere environments and during transport. Recent literature suggests that ONSD measurements by ultrasound show low inter- and intra-observer variability [6, 8, 9, 15, 16]. However, to diagnose increased ICP, ONSD measurements require precise measurement of a 3–6 mm structure to the nearest 0.1 mm accuracy [8, 17] and it is unclear if these ultra-portable handheld units have the resolution to make these precise measurements.

In this study, we estimate the accuracy of ONSD measurement in a pocket-sized ultrasound unit (Vscan, GE Healthcare) utilizing a locally developed model of the eye and optic nerve sheath, and compare it to previously validated portable unit (M-Turbo, SonoSite) as a reference standard.

Methods

Model

All measurements were made using our previously developed and validated optic nerve sheath models [16, 18] with varying sheath diameters of known size (simulated from 3-D printed discs), and conducted by expert point-of-care ultrasonographers (LG and GH).

Ultrasound technique

We used the standard ultrasound technique for measuring ONSD on our models as previously described [16, 18]. Both a handheld unit (Vscan with Dual Probe utilizing the linear transducer, GE healthcare, Little Chalfont, United Kingdom) and a conventional transducer using a 13–6 MHz linear array (L25x transducer with a SonoSite M-Turbo Ultrasound Machine, SonoSite Inc, Bothell, WA) were used. Sonographers measured each model with both machines (Fig. 1). The models were presented randomly, and the operators were blinded to the color and actual size of each disc. Trials were blocked by machine, where each operator made all of their SonoSite measurements consecutively, before making their Vscan readings.

Sample size

To compare the level of agreement between the two technologies, we powered our study by assuming a minimum Pearson correlation of 0.6, since less would likely preclude a useful conversion algorithm. Using the Fisher Z transformation with a significance level of 0.05 and a two-sided alternate hypothesis, we calculated that we required 24 measurements to be done with each ultrasound to achieve a 90% power. Therefore, we constructed five different models to be measured in triplicate by two expert operators with both machines for a total of 30 measurements per machine. The disc sizes measured 5.6 (light blue), 5.5 (pink), 6.9 (dark blue), 4.9 (black), and 3.8 (dark green) mm. Disc sizes were chosen to approximate the range of ONSD in patients with normal or elevated ICP found in vivo [6, 8].

Statistical analysis

Inter-rater reliabilities between operators and between machines were analyzed by intra-class correlation coefficient. Inter-rater reliability between machines ("inter-machine reliability") was also examined by the Bland–Altman agreement analysis [19]. Finally, both a simple Pearson correlation and quadratic regression were used to compare measurements between machines.

Results

The ICC between raters for the SonoSite was 0.878, and that for the Vscan was 0.826. The between-machine agreement ICC was 0.752.

The Bland–Altman agreement analysis between the SonoSite and the Vscan is shown in Figs. 2 and 3. The Vscan measurements tended to be 0.33 mm higher than the SonoSite on average, with a standard deviation of their difference of 0.64 mm.

Simple Pearson correlation between machines demonstrated a correlation coefficient of 0.803. Using a quadratic regression, the correlation can be improved and a quadratic equation generated to predict the SonoSite measurement from the Vscan one (Fig. 4). The equation is:

$$y = 8.54 - 2.86x + 0.405x^2$$

where x is the Vscan measurement and y represented the predicted measurement if using the SonoSite machine. After adjusting the Vscan data with this formula, the new mean difference is 0 ± 0.53 mm.

Discussion

It is currently unknown if pocket ultrasound devices have the resolution to make ONSD measurements as accurately as their larger counterparts. We attempted to assess the accuracy of ONSD measurement in an ultra-portable ultrasound (Vscan) and compare it to a conventional sized portable unit (SonoSite). This was achieved by utilizing our previously validated model,

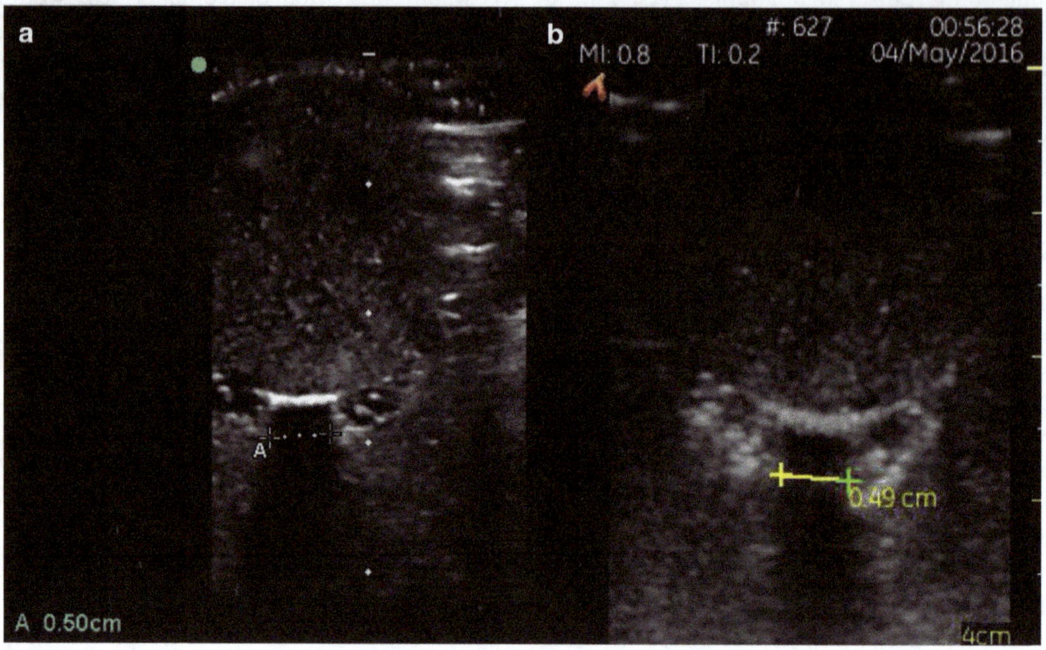

Fig. 1 Ultrasound images of ONSD measurements utilizing the SonoSite (**a**) and Vscan (**b**) ultrasound units

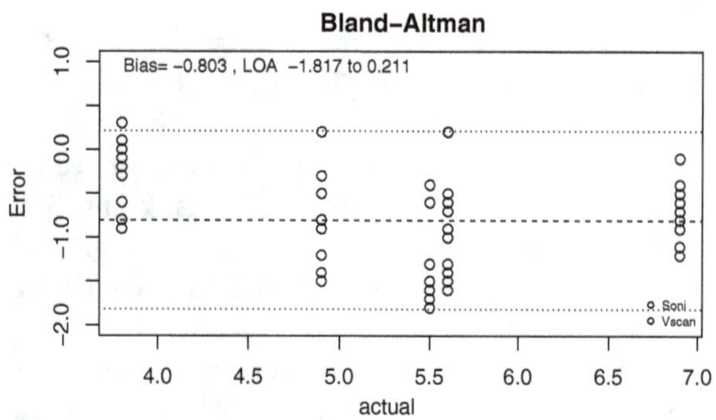

Fig. 2 Bland–Altman plot demonstrating the variability of SonoSite (*black*) and Vscan (*red*) measurements over the range of ONSD sizes

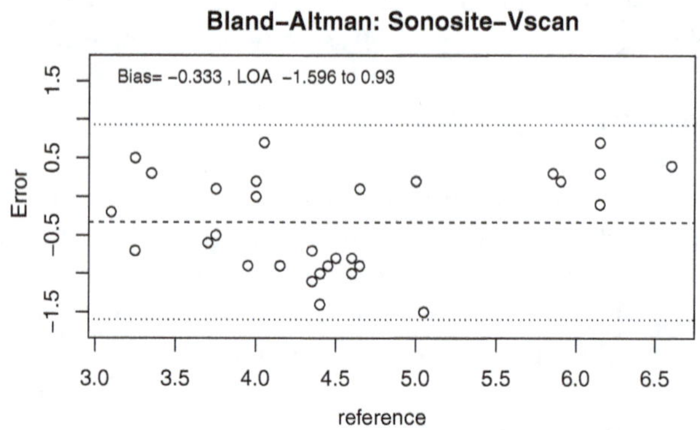

Fig. 3 Bland–Altman plot demonstrating the variability of SonoSite–Vscan measurements over the range of ONSD sizes

which evaluated intra- and inter-observer variability [16, 18]. We report that the ICC between raters was 0.826 for the Vscan and 0.878 for the SonoSite and the between-machine agreement ICC was 0.752.

Our high inter-rater agreement for both ultrasound devices is equivalent and larger than we have previously reported (ICC = 0.643) using our ONSD model with the same SonoSite device [16]. These improvements are likely due to our exclusive reliance on expert operators for our data this time, as our results are comparable to those found in the previous studies examining inter-rater reliability of experts in small populations in vivo [7, 15, 20, 21]. Although achieving competency in ONSD ultrasonography is not very arduous [22], errors in probe positioning and caliper placement can lead to incorrect measurement with novice operators.

The inter-machine agreement ICC between the SonoSite and the Vscan was 0.752. This is only slightly lower than the ICC between different observers for either machine implying an "excellent" agreement, and that the variation in measurements between the machines was only slightly greater than the variation in measurements between two observers using an identical machine. This suggests that a skilled operator may be able to use either machine to make ONSD measurements with a similar degree of accuracy as two operators using the same machine.

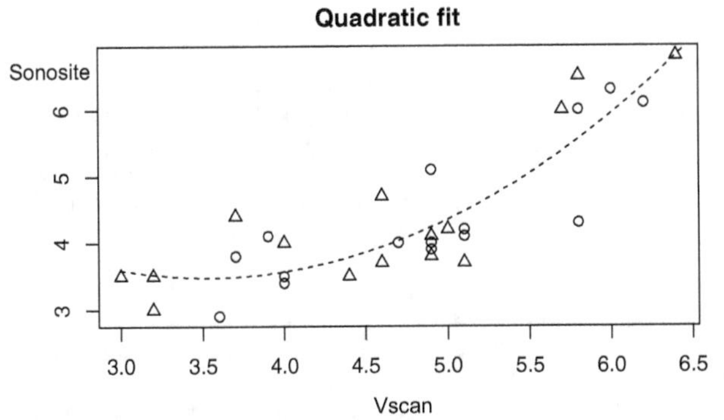

Fig. 4 Quadratic regression model comparing VScan to SonoSite measurements

In the Bland–Altman analysis comparing level of agreement between Vscan and SonoSite measurements, there was an even spread across the range of disc sizes suggesting no systematic bias. It did find that the Vscan tended to over-estimate ONSD by a small amount (0.33 ± 0.65 mm). We hypothesize that this may be due to the screen size and resolution of the Vscan as compared to the SonoSite. Since the screen on the Vscan device was smaller than that of the SonoSite, attempts to position, the calipers on the edge of the optic nerve sheath may have lead to an overestimation. Importantly, this strong agreement between ONSD measurements by both devices allows us to create a quadratic conversion formula between the two measures. After adjusting the Vscan results using this formula, the mean difference shrinks to 0 ± 0.53 mm. A conversion formula could potentially be used to translate previously established normal reference ranges from the SonoSite into those more useful for the Vscan. This conversion formula requires further validation in a prospective study.

The advantage of our ONSD model is: it creates a controlled environment where the known disc size was consistent across different measurements and readers. This allows for an isolated comparison of measurement accuracy inherent to each technique and observer. On the surface, comparing the resolution of two ultrasound units to measure a fixed structure may seem like a simple task. The Vscan linear probe has a frequency range of 8–3.4 MHz which is significantly lower than the SonoSite's 13–6 MHz probe. However, one must consider more than just sheer resolution of the unit, as ultrasound imaging is an operator dependent task that involves optic nerve sheath interpretation, caliper measurement, and ease of software and probe usage. Hence, the primary outcome of agreement between the two measurements is not only important, but also the secondary outcomes of inter-rater and within-subject reliability.

Pocket ultrasound units are not currently approved in Canada or the United States for the measurement of ONSD in human subjects as the existing units do not have the required presets to make these measurements safely. For this reason, we elected to perform this initial pilot study utilizing our ONSD model. The recommended settings for ONSD ultrasound in human subjects requires a thermal index (TI) ≤1 and mechanical index (MI) ≤0.23 [23] which are not achievable with the current Vscan firmware. We, therefore, do not encourage the "off-label" usage of these machines in live human subjects until the appropriate presets are made available.

Despite the importance of our findings, there are limitations to our study. First, all of the data comparing the relative accuracies of the ultrasound devices were obtained in a controlled setting on a simulation model. This was done to limit external variables and limit random error to more precisely study machine and observer effects between devices. However, it is difficult to extrapolate our findings to in vivo as the model does not necessarily account for effects, such as patient variation in anatomy or movement, fluctuations in ICP, and time constraints. Our model may itself introduce some random error of its own, such as imaging the 3D printed disc on an angle causing the disc to produce a larger shadow than usual, or that the shadow generated by the disc is not the same size as the disc itself. We also used a relatively small group of "experts", as ultrasound evaluation of ONSD is still largely considered experimental in our centre, and there are relatively few experts to recruit. In addition, by having the sonographers both measure using the SonoSite first followed by the Vscan, we may have unintentionally introduced some bias into the measurements, however, looking at the Bland–Altman plot (Fig. 2), the similar variability around the mean for both machines would suggest if present this was likely inconsequential. Finally, our model simulates what is known as the "black stripe method" of ONSD measurement—meaning that the operator measures the edges of the internal diameter of the ONS. However, new quality criteria recently introduced [24] suggest that instead the external hypo-echogenic layers surrounding the optic nerve should be measured. To date, we have been unable to simulate this appearance in our model. This does not invalidate the comparison between ultrasound units are we are still measuring the same structure, but the authors wish to caution the reader that in vivo images may appear different and the ability of the units to clearly differentiate the borders of the ONS may be different in vivo as well.

Conclusions

This represents the first ONSD study utilizing a pocket-sized, handheld ultrasound device. Despite its small size, lower screen resolution, and significantly lower probe frequency, the ONSD measurements appear accurate and consistent when compared with the conventional portable units. Further study is needed to determine if pocket ultrasound can be accurately used in vivo to measure ONSD.

Abbreviations
ONSD: Optic nerve sheath diameter; ICP: Intra-cranial pressure; TI: Thermal index; MI: Mechanical index; ICC: Intra-class correlation coefficient.

Authors' contributions
All authors were involved in study design, data analysis, and manuscript composition. LG, GJ, BU, and GH were involved in data collection. All authors read and approved the final manuscript.

Author details
[1] Undergraduate Medical Education, University of Manitoba, Winnipeg, MB, Canada. [2] Departments of Surgery, University of Manitoba, GF439, 820 Sherbrook Street, Winnipeg, MB R3A 1R9, Canada. [3] Clinician Investigator Program, University of Manitoba, Winnipeg, MB, Canada. [4] Department of Internal Medicine, Section of Critical Care, University of Manitoba, Winnipeg, MB, Canada. [5] Pediatrics and Child Health, University of Manitoba, Winnipeg, MB, Canada. [6] Department of Critical Care, Keck Medical School, USC, Los Angeles, CA, USA.

Acknowledgements
This research was supported by a General Operating Grant from the Health Science Centre Foundation and a GFT Research Grant from the Department of Surgery, University of Manitoba, both in Winnipeg, Manitoba, Canada.

References

1. Pickard JD, Czosnyka M (1993) Management of raised intracranial pressure. J Neurol Neurosurg Psychiatry 56:845–858
2. Bernuau J, Durand F (2006) Intracranial pressure monitoring in patients with acute liver failure: a questionable invasive surveillance. Hepatology 44:502–504. doi:10.1002/hep.21243
3. Brain Trauma Foundation, American Association of Neurological Surgeons, Congress of Neurological Surgeons (2007) Guidelines for the management of severe traumatic brain injury. J Neurotrauma 24(Suppl 1):S1–S106
4. Chmrc CFRN (2016) Optic nerve sheath diameter ultrasound and the diagnosis of increased intracranial pressure. Crit Care Nurs Clin N Am 28:95–99. doi:10.1016/j.cnc.2015.10.005
5. Dubourg J, Javouhey E, Geeraerts T et al (2011) Ultrasonography of optic nerve sheath diameter for detection of raised intracranial pressure: a systematic review and meta-analysis. Intensiv Care Med 37:1059–1068. doi:10.1007/s00134-011-2224-2
6. Bäuerle J, Lochner P, Kaps M, Nedelmann M (2010) Intra- and interobsever reliability of sonographic assessment of the optic nerve sheath diameter in healthy adults. J Neuroimaging 22:42–45. doi:10.1111/j.1552-6569.2010.00546.x
7. Moretti R, Pizzi B, Cassini F, Vivaldi N (2009) Reliability of optic nerve ultrasound for the evaluation of patients with spontaneous intracranial hemorrhage. Neurocrit Care 11:406–410. doi:10.1007/s12028-009-9250-8
8. Goeres P, Zeiler FA, Unger B et al (2015) Ultrasound assessment of optic nerve sheath diameter in healthy volunteers. J Crit Care 31:168–171. doi:10.1016/j.jcrc.2015.10.009
9. Ballantyne SA, O'Neill G, Hamilton R, Hollman AS (2002) Observer variation in the sonographic measurement of optic nerve sheath diameter in normal adults. Eur J Ultrasound 15:145–149
10. Bellner J, Romner B, Reinstrup P, Kristiansson KA, Ryding E, Brandt L (2004) Transcranial Doppler sonography pulsatility index (PI) reflects intracranial pressure (ICP). Surg Neurol 62:45–51 **(discussion 51)**
11. Brandi G, Béchir M, Sailer S, Haberthür C, Stocker R, Stover JF (2010) Transcranial color-coded duplex sonography allows to assess cerebral perfusion pressure noninvasively following severe traumatic brain injury. Acta Neurochir 152:965–972
12. Homburg AM, Jakobsen M, Enevoldsen E (1993) Transcranial Doppler recordings in raised intracranial pressure. Acta Neurol Scand 87:488–493
13. Bouzat P, Francony G, Declety P et al (2011) Transcranial Doppler to screen on admission patients with mild to moderate traumatic brain injury. Neurosurgery 68:1603–1609
14. Gura M, Elmaci I, Sari R, Coskun N (2011) Correlation of pulsatility index with intracranial pressure in traumatic brain injury. Turk Neurosurg 21:210–215
15. Bäuerle J, Schuchardt F, Schroeder L et al (2013) Reproducibility and accuracy of optic nerve sheath diameter assessment using ultrasound compared to magnetic resonance imaging. BMC Neurol 13:187. doi:10.1186/1471-2377-13-187
16. Zeiler FA, Unger B, Zhu Q et al (2014) A unique model for ONSD part II: inter/intra-operator variability. Can J Neurol Sci 41:430–435
17. Asghar A, Hashmi M, Hussain A (2015) Optic nerve sheath diameter evaluated by transorbital sonography in healthy volunteers from Pakistan. Anaesth Pain Intensiv Care 19:282–286
18. Zeiler FA, Unger B, Kramer AH et al (2013) A unique model for ultrasound assessment of optic nerve sheath diameter. Can J Neurol Sci 40:225–229
19. Bland JM, Altman DG (1986) Statistical methods for assessing agreement between two methods of clinical measurement. Lancet 1:307–310
20. Bäuerle J, Lochner P, Kaps M, Nedelmann M (2012) Intra- and interobserver reliability of sonographic assessment of the optic nerve sheath diameter in healthy adults. J Neuroimaging 22:42–45. doi:10.1111/j.1552-6569.2010.00546.x
21. Steinborn M, Fiegler J, Ruedisser K et al (2011) Measurement of the optic nerve sheath diameter in children: comparison between transbulbar sonography and magnetic resonance imaging. Ultraschall Med. doi:10.1055/s-0031-1273491
22. Potgieter DW, Kippin A, Ngu F, McKean C (2011) Can accurate ultrasonographic measurement of the optic nerve sheath diameter (a non-invasive measure of intracranial pressure) be taught to novice operators in a single training session? Anaesth Intensiv Care 39:95–100
23. US Food and Drug Administration center for devices and Radiological Health (2008) Guidance for industry and FDA staff-information for manufacturers seeking marketing clearance of diagnostic ultrasound systems and transducers. US Department of Health and Human Services. Available at http://www.fda.gov/MedicalDevices/DeviceRegulationandGuidance/GuidanceDocuments/ucm070856.htm. Accessed 7 Nov 2016
24. Sargsyan AE, Blaivas M, Geeraerts T, Karakitsos D (2014) "Ocular ultrasound in the intensive care unit" in critical care ultrasound. In: Lumb P, Karakitsos D (ed). Elsevier, Amsterdam

24

Right heart thrombus in transit: a series of two cases

Eva Otoupalova[1*], Bhavinkumar Dalal[2] and Brian Renard[3]

Abstract

Right heart thrombus in transit is an increasingly recognized medical emergency with very high mortality rate. Echocardiography helps to establish the diagnosis and can differentiate between right heart thrombi that result from atrial fibrillation and those originating from deep venous thrombosis. We present two cases of right heart thrombus in transit diagnosed with echocardiography that were managed with different approaches.

Background

Increased use of echocardiography has led to greater detection of atrial thrombi in recent years. In absence of atrial fibrillation, right heart thrombi mostly represent an embolus in transit originating from a deep venous thrombosis. Right heart thrombi occur in about 4% [1] of cases of acute PE and have very high mortality rate. Treatment options include surgery, thrombolysis, and catheter-based interventions. We present two cases of right heart thrombus in transit diagnosed by echocardiography.

Case 1

79-year-old female with history of hypertension presented with acute abdominal pain for 1 h. She was hypotensive in the emergency room. Initial ECG showed inferior Q-waves and ST depressions in the lateral leads. Right-sided ECG revealed 1.5 mm ST elevation in right-sided lead V4 (RV4). Laboratory workup was significant for troponin elevation 0.14 ng/mL. Emergent heart catheterization was done and revealed non-obstructive moderate coronary artery disease.

An urgent bedside transthoracic echocardiography (TTE) was performed and revealed large, free-floating thrombus in right atrium, septal flattening, and severely decreased right ventricular systolic function (Figs. 1, 2; Additional files 1, 2). Right ventricular systolic pressure (RVSP) elevated at 56 mmHg.

Patient was taken to surgery and underwent atriotomy and pulmonary arteriotomy on cardiopulmonary bypass. Despite successful surgery, patient developed infectious complications and passed 5 days later.

Case 2

89-year-old female presented with dyspnea for 1 day. In the emergency room, she was normotensive but tachycardic and tachypneic. Initial ECG revealed normal sinus rhythm, right bundle brunch block, and T wave inversion in V1–V3. Initial laboratory workup showed elevated troponin 2.60 ng/mL. TTE was performed and showed mobile thrombus in the right atrium and severely enlarged right ventricle with RVSP 45–50 mmHg (Figs. 3, 4; Additional files 3, 4). Akinesis of mid-free wall of the right ventricle and normal motion of apex consistent with Mc Connell's sign was present.

Patient was taken to cardiac catheterization laboratory to undergo catheter directed AngioVac thrombus extraction. However, upon obtaining access, patient became hypotensive and bradycardic. A transesophageal echocardiography demonstrated markedly worsened dilation of the right ventricle with a very small left ventricle indicative of severe right heart strain. The right atrial thrombus was still visible and appeared unchanged. Resuscitative measures were undertaken; unfortunately, the patient did not respond and passed.

*Correspondence: eva.otoupalova@beaumont.edu
[1] Department of Internal Medicine, Oakland University William Beaumont School of Medicine, 3601 W 13 Mile Rd., Royal Oak, MI 48073, USA
Full list of author information is available at the end of the article

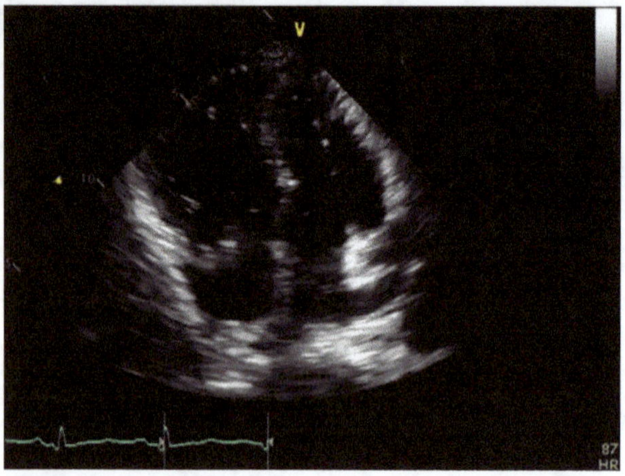

Fig. 1 Apical 4-chamber view with a large mobile thrombus in the right atrium crossing into the right ventricle. The right ventricle is severely enlarged

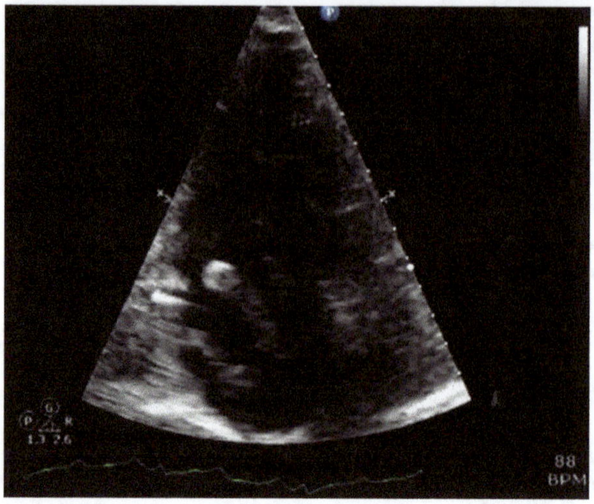

Fig. 3 Apical 4-chamber view with a large mobile thrombus in the right atrium crossing into the right ventricle. There is flattening of the interventricular septum consistent with right ventricular pressure overload. Mc Connell's sign is present

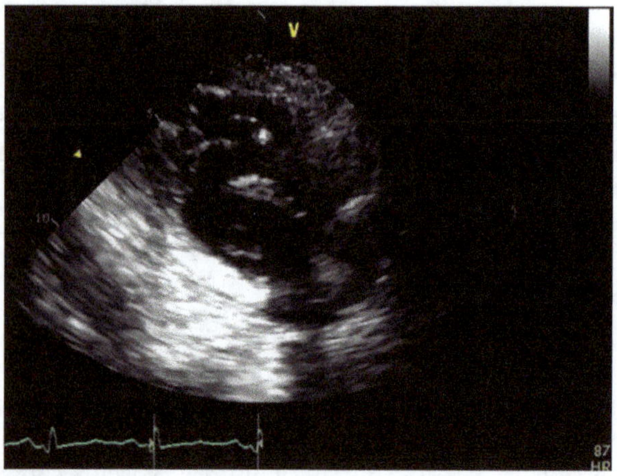

Fig. 2 Right ventricular inflow view with large mobile thrombus crossing into the right ventricle

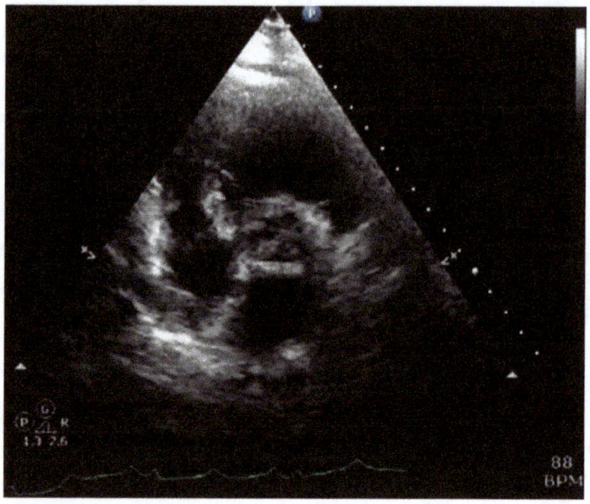

Fig. 4 Parasternal short axis view of large mobile thrombus in the right atrium

Discussion and literature review

Both of our patients died; however, our first patient died due to infectious complications and not due to obstructive shock itself. As appropriately described in literature, our first patient had surgical embolectomy and survived from acute problem of right heart thrombus (RHT), while in the second case, there was not enough time before patient deteriorated and died. This feature describes the importance of early diagnosis and aggressive treatment of RHT. In current era, many bedside echocardiographs are performed not only by cardiology team but also by emergency and internal medicine house staff; recognition of RHT and its aggressive treatment is crucial.

Right heart thrombi occur in about 4% of pulmonary embolism (PE) [1]. They result either from dislodging clot from deep venous thrombosis, or form in situ mostly due to atrial fibrillation. They can also be associated with intracardiac foreign bodies such as pacemakers and prosthetic valves.

Mortality rate in patients with RHT is about 28%, with mortality rates in untreated patients of 80–100%. In contrast, the in-hospital mortality rate for acute pulmonary embolism (PE) is about 2.5% [1]. Patients with RHT have shorter duration of symptoms, lower systolic blood pressure, more frequent right ventricular hypokinesis and congestive heart failure [2].

Three major types of right heart thrombus can be distinguished on echocardiography [2]: type A is most common, is usually the result of deep venous thrombosis and has the highest risk of embolization. It is elongated, with a worm-like appearance and is freely mobile within the heart chambers. Type B thrombus is thought to originate within the atrium or ventricle, and is firmly attached to the chamber wall and ovoid shape. Type C thrombi are rare, highly mobile and resembling cardiac myxomas. Transesophageal echocardiography (TEE) provides better visualization of the thrombus and should be considered when TTE is suboptimal or non-diagnostic [3]; it can localize thrombus in pulmonary artery or lodged in patent foramen ovale.

Both of our patients had type A thrombus. In addition, both of our patients had signs of severe right ventricular pressure overload. Akinesis of mid-free wall of the right ventricle and normal motion of apex such as in our second patient (McConnell's sign) is particularly suggestive of PE [4].

Treatment modalities for RHT include anticoagulation therapy, systemic thrombolysis and surgical embolectomy. Optimal therapeutic approach is still subject of discussion as no randomized controlled trials have directly compared the treatment methods. In a meta-analysis of 119 patients by Kinney from 1989, there was a small survival benefit with anticoagulation (70%) when compared to surgical embolectomy or thrombolysis (62%) [5]. However, not all patients had a pulmonary embolism in the study. A multicenter observational European study from the same year reported a markedly lower mortality with surgical embolectomy (27%) as compared to anticoagulation (>60%) [2]. A meta-analysis by Rose from 2002 of 177 patients with RHT demonstrated a superiority of thrombolytic therapy over surgical embolectomy (OR for mortality: 2.83, 95% CI 1.04–7.69) and anticoagulation (OR for mortality: 3.03, 95% CI 1.02–3.125) [6]. These results were confirmed by the largest meta-analysis to date by Ganesh et al. from 2015 that evaluated total 328 patients. In this meta-analysis, 70 patients received anticoagulation, 122 patients received thrombolysis and 120 patients had surgical embolectomy. Mortality rates were 37.1, 18.3 and 13.9%, respectively. After adjusting for age and hemodynamic status, the OR for survival was 4.83 (95% CI 1.51–15.36) with thrombolysis and 2.61 (95% CI 0.90–7.58) with surgical embolectomy [7]. Data on catheter-based interventions are scarce.

Conclusion

As our two cases illustrate, right heart clot in transit is a medical emergency with high mortality that requires immediate evaluation and treatment. TTE is preferred diagnostic method and helps distinguish between clot formed in situ and clot in transit. Thrombolysis and surgical embolectomy are superior to anticoagulation, with thrombolysis possibly offering a modest survival benefit.

Additional files

Additional file 1. Apical 4-chamber view with a large mobile thrombus in the right atrium crossing into the right ventricle. The right ventricle is severely enlarged.

Additional file 2. Right ventricular inflow view with large mobile thrombus crossing into the right ventricle.

Additional file 3. Apical 4-chamber view with a large mobile thrombus in the right atrium crossing into the right ventricle. There is flattening of the interventricular septum consistent with right ventricular pressure overload. Mc Connell's sign is present.

Additional file 4. Parasternal short axis view of large mobile thrombus in the right atrium.

Abbreviations

ECG: electrocardiogram; TTE: transthoracic echocardiography; TEE: transesophageal echocardiography; RHT: right heart thrombus; RVSP: right ventricular systolic pressure; PE: pulmonary embolism.

Authors' contributions

EO has written main portion of the manuscript. BD has reviewed and edited the manuscript. BR has been responsible for the discussion of the echo findings in each case and reviewing the imaging portion of the manuscript. All authors read and approved the final manuscript.

Author details

[1] Department of Internal Medicine, Oakland University William Beaumont School of Medicine, 3601 W 13 Mile Rd., Royal Oak, MI 48073, USA. [2] Department of Pulmonary and Critical Care, Oakland University William Beaumont School of Medicine, 3601 W 13 Mile Rd., Royal Oak, MI 48073, USA. [3] Department of Cardiology, Oakland University William Beaumont School of Medicine, 3601 W 13 Mile Rd., Royal Oak, MI 48073, USA.

Acknowledgements

None.

References

1. Carson JL, Kelley MA, Duff A et al (1992) The clinical course of pulmonary embolism. N Engl J Med 326:1240–1245
2. European Working Group on Echocardiography (1989) The European cooperative study on the clinical significance of right heart thrombi. Eur Heart J 10(12):1046–1059
3. Ragland MM, Tak T (2006) The role of echocardiography in diagnosing space-occupying lesions of the heart. Clin Med Res. 4:22–32
4. Sosland RP, Gupta K (2008) McConnell's Sign. Circulation 118:e517–e518
5. Kinney EL, Wright RJ (1989) Efficacy of treatment of patients with echocardiographically detected right-sided heart thrombi: a meta-analysis. Am Heart J 118:569–573
6. Rose PS, Punjabi NM, Pearse DB (2002) Treatment of right heart thromboemboli. Chest 121:806–814
7. Athappan G, Sengodan P, Chacko P, Gandhi S (2015) Comparative efficacy of different modalities for treatment of right heart thrombi in transit: a pooled analysis. Vasc Med 20(2):131–138

Permissions

All chapters in this book were first published by Springer; hereby published with permission under the Creative Commons Attribution License or equivalent. Every chapter published in this book has been scrutinized by our experts. Their significance has been extensively debated. The topics covered herein carry significant findings which will fuel the growth of the discipline. They may even be implemented as practical applications or may be referred to as a beginning point for another development.

The contributors of this book come from diverse backgrounds, making this book a truly international effort. This book will bring forth new frontiers with its revolutionizing research information and detailed analysis of the nascent developments around the world.

We would like to thank all the contributing authors for lending their expertise to make the book truly unique. They have played a crucial role in the development of this book. Without their invaluable contributions this book wouldn't have been possible. They have made vital efforts to compile up to date information on the varied aspects of this subject to make this book a valuable addition to the collection of many professionals and students.

This book was conceptualized with the vision of imparting up-to-date information and advanced data in this field. To ensure the same, a matchless editorial board was set up. Every individual on the board went through rigorous rounds of assessment to prove their worth. After which they invested a large part of their time researching and compiling the most relevant data for our readers.

The editorial board has been involved in producing this book since its inception. They have spent rigorous hours researching and exploring the diverse topics which have resulted in the successful publishing of this book. They have passed on their knowledge of decades through this book. To expedite this challenging task, the publisher supported the team at every step. A small team of assistant editors was also appointed to further simplify the editing procedure and attain best results for the readers.

Apart from the editorial board, the designing team has also invested a significant amount of their time in understanding the subject and creating the most relevant covers. They scrutinized every image to scout for the most suitable representation of the subject and create an appropriate cover for the book.

The publishing team has been an ardent support to the editorial, designing and production team. Their endless efforts to recruit the best for this project, has resulted in the accomplishment of this book. They are a veteran in the field of academics and their pool of knowledge is as vast as their experience in printing. Their expertise and guidance has proved useful at every step. Their uncompromising quality standards have made this book an exceptional effort. Their encouragement from time to time has been an inspiration for everyone.

The publisher and the editorial board hope that this book will prove to be a valuable piece of knowledge for researchers, students, practitioners and scholars across the globe.

List of Contributors

Joseph Dahine
Department of Intensive Care, Université de Montréal, Montreal, QC, Canada

Annie Giard
Department of Emergency Medicine, Hôpital Sacré-Coeur de Montréal, Montreal, QC, Canada

David-Olivier Chagnon
Department of Radiology, Centre Hospitalier de l'Université de Montréal, Montreal, QC, Canada

André Denault
Department of Anesthesiology and Division of Critical Care, Montreal Heart Institute, Université de Montréal, 5000 Belanger Street, Montreal, QC H1T 1C8, Canada
Division of Critical Care, Centre Hospitalier de l'Université de Montréal, Montreal, QC, Canada

Jennifer R. Marin
Children's Hospital of Pittsburgh, 4401 Penn Ave, AOB Suite 2400, Pittsburgh, PA 15224, USA

Alyssa M. Abo
Children's National Medical Center, Washington DC, USA

Alexander C. Arroyo
Maimonides Medical Center, Brooklyn, NY, USA

Stephanie J. Doniger
New York Methodist Hospital, Brooklyn, NY, USA

Jason W. Fischer
Hospital for Sick Children, Toronto, Ontario, Canada

Rachel Rempell, Jason A. Levy and Rebecca L. Vieira
Boston Children's Hospital, Boston, MA, USA

Brandi Gary
Queens Medical Center, Honolulu, HI, USA

James F. Holmes
University of California-Davis, Sacramento, CA, USA

David O. Kessler, Lorraine Ng and Lindsey Chaudoin
Morgan Stanley Children's Hospital, New York, NY, USA

Samuel H. F. Lam
University of California-San Diego, San Diego, CA, USA

Marla C. Levine
Dell Children's Medical Center, Austin, USA

Alice Murray
Boston Medical Center, Boston, MA, USA

Vicki E. Noble
Massachusetts General Hospital, Boston, MA, USA

Daniela Ramirez-Schrempp
Boston University Medical Center, Boston, NY, USA

David C. Riley
Columbia University Medical Center, New York, NY, USA

Vaishali Shah
Montefiore Medical Center, Bronx, NY, USA

Adam B. Sivitz
Newark Beth Israel Medical Center, Newark, NJ, USA

Ee Tein Tay and James W. Tsung
Mount Sinai Hospital, New York, NY, USA

David Teng
Cohen Children's Medical Center, New Hyde Park, USA

Yaffa M. Vitberg
Weill Cornell Medical Center, New York, NY, USA

Sachita P. Shah
Division of Emergency Medicine, Harborview Medical Center, University of Washington School of Medicine, 325 9th Ave, Seattle, WA 98104, USA

Sachin P. Shah and David M. Venesy
Division of Cardiology, Lahey Hospital and Medical Center, Burlington, MA, USA

Reginald Fils-Aime, Walkens Desir and Joanel Joasil
Hopital Bon Sauveur, Zanmi Lasante/Partners In Health, Central Plateau, Cange, Haiti

Krithika Meera Muruganandan
Department of Emergency Medicine, Boston Medical Center, Boston, MA, USA

Vigil James, Aswin Warier, Khai Pin Lee and Gene Yong-Kwang Ong
Children's Emergency, KK Women's and Children's Hospital, 100 Bukit Timah Road, Singapore 229899, Singapore

Resa E. Lewiss
Department of emergency medicine, Department of Radiology, University of Colorado Hospital, Aurora, CO, USA

Jessica Cook
Department of emergency medicine, Yale-New Haven Hospital, New Haven, CT, USA

Jeffrey Rabrich, Sebastian D. Siadecki and Allison Sauler
Department of emergency medicine, Mount Sinai St. Luke's Mount Sinai West, New York, NY, USA

Turandot Saul
St. Lukes-Roosevelt Hospital, New York, NY, USA
Department of emergency medicine, Mount Sinai St. Luke's Mount Sinai West, New York, NY, USA

Nicholas Avitabile
Department of emergency medicine, St. Barnabas Hospital, Bronx, NY, USA

Nicole L. Kaban
Department of emergency medicine, Mount Sinai Beth Israel Hospital, New York, NY, USA

Dan Wiener
Bronx-Lebanon Hospital Center, Bronx, NY, USA

Rachel Spevack
Internal Medicine Training Program, Department of Medicine, Jewish General Hospital, McGill University, 3755 Chemin de la Cote St Catherine, Montreal H3T 1E2, Canada

Mohamed Al Shukairi
Critical Care Fellowship Training Program, McGill University, Montreal, Canada

Dev Jayaraman
Division of General Internal Medicine, Department of Medicine, MUHC, McGill University & Adult Critical Care, Jewish General Hospital, McGill University, Montreal, Canada

Jerrald Dankoff
Department of Emergency Medicine, Jewish General Hospital, McGill University, Montreal, Canada

Lawrence Rudski
Division of Cardiology, Department of Medicine, Jewish General Hospital, McGill University, Montreal, Canada
Department of Adult Critical Care, Jewish General Hospital, McGill University, Montreal, Canada

Jed Lipes
Division of General Internal Medicine, Department of Adult Critical Care, Jewish General Hospital, McGill University, Montreal, Canada

Jesper Weile
Emergency Department, Regional Hospital Herning, Herning, Denmark
Research Center for Emergency Medicine, Aarhus University Hospital, Nørrebrogade 44, Building 1B, 8000 Aarhus C, Denmark

Klaus Nielsen
Department of Medicine, Section of Respiratory Medicine, University Hospital Hvidovre, Hvidovre, Denmark

Stine C. Primdahl
Aarhus University, Aarhus, Denmark

Christian A. Frederiksen
Department of Cardiology, Aarhus University Hospital, Aarhus, Denmark

Christian B. Laursen
Department of Respiratory Medicine, Odense University Hospital, Odense, Denmark

Erik Sloth
Department of Anesthesiology and Intensive Care, Aarhus University Hospital, Aarhus, Denmark

Hans Kirkegaard
Research Center for Emergency Medicine, Aarhus University Hospital, Aarhus, Denmark

Philippe Le Conte, David Trewick, Philippe Pes and Eric Batard
Service des Urgences, CHU de Nantes, 44093 Nantes, France

Eric Frampas
Radiologie centrale, CHU de Nantes, Nantes, France

Christian Tingström and Jon Karlsson
Department of Orthopedics, Sahlgrenska University Hospital, Instititute of Clinical Sciences, Sahlgrenska Academy, University of Gothenburg, Gothenburg, Sweden

Hanna Hebelka
Department of Radiology, Institute of Clinical Sciences, Sahlgrenska Academy, University of Gothenburg, Gothenburg, Sweden

Henrik Hedelin
Department of Orthopedics, Sahlgrenska University Hospital, Instititute of Clinical Sciences, Sahlgrenska Academy, University of Gothenburg, Gothenburg, Sweden
Barnortopeden Östra sjukhuset, Sahlgrenska Universitetssjukhuset, Smörslottsgatan 1, 416 78 Gothenburg, Sweden

Elizabeth C. Lee and Marc F. Kurtzman
Department of Medicine, Oregon Health & Science University, Portland, USA

Renee K. Dversdal
Division of Hospital Medicine, Department of Medicine, Oregon Health & Science University, 3181 SW Sam Jackson Park Road, OP-30, Portland, OR 97239, USA

Ryan D. Clay
Department of Medicine, Oregon Health & Science University, Portland, USA Mayo Clinic Minnesota, 200 First Street SW, Rochester, MN, USA

Stephan H. Böhm
Hepa Wash GmbH, Munich, Germany
Swisstom AG, Landquart, Switzerland

Andreas D. Waldmann
Swisstom AG, Landquart, Switzerland

Carlos Ferrando
Department of Anesthesiology, University Hospital Valencia, Valencia, Spain

Manuel Perez Marquez
Department of Intensive Care Medicine, Instituto de Investigación Sanitaria Fundación Jiménez Díaz, IIS-FJD, Madrid, Spain

Fernando Suarez Sipmann
Hedenstierna Laboratory, Department of Surgical Sciences, Section of Anesthesia and Critical Care, Uppsala University Hospital, Uppsala, Sweden
CIBERES, Madrid, Spain
Department of Critical Care, Hospital La Fe, Valencia, Spain

Maria Teresa Giordani
Infectious and Tropical Diseases Unit, San Bortolo Hospital, Via Rodolfi 37, 36100 Vicenza, Italy

Francesca Tamarozzi
Center for Tropical Diseases, Sacro Cuore-Don Calabria Hospital, Negrar, Verona, Italy

Daniel Kaminstein
Department of Emergency Medicine and Hospitalist Service, Medical College of Georgia at Augusta University, Augusta, GA, USA

Enrico Brunetti
Division of Infectious and Tropical Diseases, University of Pavia, IRCCS S. Matteo Hospital Foundation, Pavia, Italy

Tom Heller
Lighthouse Clinic, Lilongwe, Malawi

Scott J. Millington, Robert T. Arntfield, Robert Jie Guo, Seth Koenig, Pierre Kory, Vicki Noble, Haney Mallemat and Jordan R. Schoenherr
Division of Critical Care, University of Ottawa, 501 Smyth Road, Ottawa, ON K1H 8L6, Canada

Cameron Green
Department of the Intensive Care Unit, Frankton Hospital, Frankston, VIC 3199, Australia

Kavi Haji
Department of the Intensive Care Unit, Frankton Hospital, Frankston, VIC 3199, Australia
Faculty of Medicine, Nursing and Health Sciences, Monash University, Melbourne, Australia

Darsim Haji
Frankston Hospital, Frankston, VIC, Australia
Department of Surgery, University of Melbourne, Melbourne, Australia

David J. Canty
Department of Surgery, University of Melbourne, Melbourne, Australia
Department of Medicine, Health Sciences and Nursing, Monash University, Melbourne, Australia
Royal Melbourne Hospital, Melbourne, Australia

Alistair G. Royse
Ultrasound Education Group, Department of Surgery, The University of Melbourne, Melbourne, Australia
Department of Cardiothoracic Surgery, The Royal Melbourne Hospital, Melbourne, Australia

Colin F. Royse
Ultrasound Education Group, Department of Surgery, The University of Melbourne, Melbourne, Australia
Department of Anaesthesia and Pain Management, The Royal Melbourne Hospital, Melbourne, VIC, Australia

Stephanie J. Doniger
Department of Pediatric Emergency Medicine, St. Christopher's Hospital for Children, Philadelphia, PA, USA
Department of Emergency Medicine, NYU Winthrop Hospital, Mineola, NY, USA

Alexander Wang
Department of Emergency Medicine, New York-Presbyterian, Brooklyn Methodist Hospital, Brooklyn, NY, USA

Lindsay A. Taylor, Michael J. Vitto, Michael Joyce, Jordan Tozer and David P. Evans
Virginia Commonwealth University Emergency Medicine, 1250 E Marshall Street, 2nd Floor, Suite 500, Richmond, VA 23298, USA

Annie Heffernan Rominger
Department of Pediatrics, Division of Emergency Medicine, University of Louisville, 571 South Floyd Street, Suite 412, Louisville, KY 40202, USA

Gerardo Antonio Aguilar Gomez and Patrick Elliott
Compañeros En Salud, Calle Primera Poniente Sur #25, 30370 Angel Albino Corzo (Jaltenango), Chiapas, Mexico

Joe Betcher
Department of Emergency Medicine, Lake Michigan Emergency Specialists, Mercy Health Muskegon, Muskegon, USA

Al Majkrzak
Department of Emergency Medicine, Emergency Physicians Medical Group, St. Joseph Mercy Ann Arbor, Ann Arbor, USA

Jim Cranford
Department of Psychiatry, University of Michigan, Ann Arbor, MI, USA

Ross Kessler, Nik Theyyunni and Rob Huang
Department of Emergency Medicine, University of Michigan, Ann Arbor, MI, USA

Cecilia M. Acosta, Nadia Rudzik, Nicolás Venturin, Sebastián Gerez and Gerardo Tusman
Department of Anesthesiology, Hospital Privado de Comunidad, Córdoba 4545, 7600 Mar del Plata, Buenos Aires, Argentina

Giovanni Volpicelli
Department of Emergency Medicine, San Luigi Gonzaga University Hospital, Orbassano, Torino, Italy

Lila Ricci and Marcela Natal
Department of Mathematics, Facultad de Ciencias Exactas, Universidad Nacional de Mar del Plata, Mar del Plata, Argentina

Pavitra Kotini-Shah, Felix Huang and Joseph S. Colla
Department of Emergency Medicine, University of Illinois at Chicago, 808 S. Wood Street (MC 724), Chicago, IL 60612, USA

Susana Cuadros
University of Illinois at Chicago, College of Medicine, Chicago, USA

James Griffiths
School of Clinical Medicine, University of Cambridge, Cambridge, UK

Richard Kendall and Rajeev Madan
Emergency Department, Cambridge University Hospitals NHS Foundation Trust, Cambridge, UK

Amadeus Carnegie
School of Clinical Medicine, University of Cambridge, Cambridge, UK
Robinson College, Grange Road, Cambridge CB3 9AN, UK

Mauro Costantini
Department of Anesthesia, Hospital Privado de Comunidad, Córdoba 4545, 7600 Mar Del Plata, Buenos Aires, Argentina

Camila Echevarría
Department of Radiology, Hospital Privado de Comunidad, Mar Del Plata, Buenos Aires, Argentina

Sergio Pollioto and Diego Abrego
Department of Pediatric Surgery, Hospital Privado de Comunidad, Mar Del Plata, Buenos Aires, Argentina

Fernando Suarez-Sipmann
Section of Anesthesia and Critical Care Hedenstierna Laboratory, Department of Surgical Sciences, Uppsala University Hospital, Uppsala, Sweden
CIBER de Enfermedades Respiratorias, Instituto de Salud Carlos III, Madrid, Spain

Dorothea Hempel
Department of Cardiology, Angiology and Intensive Care, University Medical Center Mainz, Mainz, Germany

Stephanie Haunhorst and Sivajini Sinnathurai
Department of Anesthesiology and Intensive Care Medicine, Kliniken Maria Hilf, Moenchengladbach, Germany

Armin Seibel
Department of Anesthesiology, Intensive Care and Emergency Medicine, Diakonie Klinikum Jung Stilling, Siegen, Germany
Ultrasound Network in Acute and Critical Care, SonoABCD, Frankfurt am Main, Germany

Florian Recker
Sono4Students, University Hospital Bonn, Bonn, Germany

Frank Heringer
FINeST Frankfurt Institute of Interdisciplinary Emergency Medicine and und Simulation Training, Johann Wolfgang Goethe University, Frankfurt am Main, Germany

Guido Michels
Department III of Internal Medicine, Heartcenter, University Hospital of Cologne, Cologne, Germany

Raoul Breitkreutz
Ultrasound Network in Acute and Critical Care, SonoABCD, Frankfurt am Main, Germany
Emergency Department, Hospital of the City of Frankfurt (Höchst), Gotenstr. 6-8, 65929 Frankfurt am Main, Germany

Garrett G. R. J. Johnson
Undergraduate Medical Education, University of Manitoba, Winnipeg, MB, Canada

Lawrence M. Gillman
Departments of Surgery, University of Manitoba, GF439, 820 Sherbrook Street, Winnipeg, MB R3A 1R9, Canada

Frederick A. Zeiler
Departments of Surgery, University of Manitoba, GF439, 820 Sherbrook Street, Winnipeg, MB R3A 1R9, Canada
Clinician Investigator Program, University of Manitoba, Winnipeg, MB, Canada

Bertram Unger
Department of Internal Medicine, Section of Critical Care, University of Manitoba, Winnipeg, MB, Canada

Gregory Hansen
Pediatrics and Child Health, University of Manitoba, Winnipeg, MB, Canada

Dimitrios Karakitsos
Department of Critical Care, Keck Medical School, USC, Los Angeles, CA, USA

Eva Otoupalova
Department of Internal Medicine, Oakland University William Beaumont School of Medicine, 3601 W 13 Mile Rd., Royal Oak, MI 48073, USA

Bhavinkumar Dalal
Department of Pulmonary and Critical Care, Oakland University William Beaumont School of Medicine, 3601 W 13 Mile Rd., Royal Oak, MI 48073, USA

Brian Renard
Department of Cardiology, Oakland University William Beaumont School of Medicine, 3601 W 13 Mile Rd., Royal Oak, MI 48073, USA

Index